HOW CAN
I GET
BETTER?

Also by Richard I. Horowitz

Why Can't I Get Better?
Solving the Mystery of Lyme and Chronic Disease

HOW CAN
I GET
BETTER?

{ An Action Plan for Treating
Resistant Lyme and Chronic Disease }

Richard I. Horowitz, MD

ST. MARTIN'S GRIFFIN
NEW YORK

To my wife, Lee,
and the millions of people suffering from Lyme
and associated tick-borne disorders

Contents

Acknowledgments

This book couldn't have been written without the help of many people. Jennifer Weis at St. Martin's Press has been an invaluable supporter for many years, and I'm thrilled that I was able to work with her. Pam Liflander has been helpful in getting my thoughts onto these pages clearly and coherently.

A huge thanks goes out to my wife, Lee, for her understanding and support, as long hours (including on vacation) were needed to get this book into its present form. Her love has graced my life.

My office staff also deserves a special thank-you for their dedication, hard work, skill, knowledge, and compassion, which has allowed me to help so many stricken with chronic illness. These people include John Fallon, FNP-C (Batman); Janet M. Cosh, AAS; Lisa Haynes; Danielle Passineau; Angela Jacobs; Diamond Elting; Renee Nelson; Kalah Matthews, BSN; Sonja Siderias, AAS, LPN; Etheldria Walker, MA; and Barbara Semanick, BSN, RN. A special thanks and large debt of gratitude goes to Phyllis R. Freeman, PhD, senior researcher at our center, whose skill, compassion, and hard work has allowed us to publish new groundbreaking research on Lyme and co-infections.

I would also like to acknowledge Dr. Mark Hyman and the speakers from the Institute for Functional Medicine (IFM) conference in San Diego, California, as well as Dr. Leo Galland and Dr. Chris Melitis, from the Integrative Health Symposium conference in New York City, who contributed material. Dr. Eva Sapi, from the University of New Haven, shared her original research on biofilms. A debt of gratitude also goes out to Dr. Alan McDonald for his groundbreaking work on Borrelia and permission to reprint his slides on its cystic form and biofilms, as well as Dr. Judith Miklossy, who provided photos of the atypical and cystic forms of Borrelia in neurological Lyme disease. Dr. Claire Riendeau provided her insight on biotoxin illness. I also wish to thank Dr. Garth Nicolson for reviewing the initial manuscript and for his assistance in providing extensive scientific literature on mycoplasmal infections and mitochondrial dysfunction. I would also like to recognize the heroes of Lyme disease, who have consistently put their patients before themselves, sometimes at the risk of their own careers. This includes Dr. Joseph Burrascano (who also provided a short history of Lyme disease for this book, and information on Advanced Labs and the new Lyme culture); Dr. Sam Donta; Dr. Charles Ray Jones; Dr. Kenneth Leigner; and many others.

I am also grateful for the assistance of several colleagues who lent their expertise and reviewed individual chapters: Allan Warshowsky, MD, for his work on the endocrinology chapter; David H. Haase, MD, for reviewing the GI autonomic nervous system dysfunction and allergy chapters; Andrea Gaito, MD, for her help with the immunity and inflammation chapters; Sunil Khurana, MD, for helping with the GI and liver function chapters; Fred Harvey, MD, for his assistance in reviewing the chapter on environmental medicine; and David Perlmutter, MD, FACN, who reviewed the brain and pain chapters. Dr. Elizabeth Maloney and Dr. Bea Szantyr also provided their feedback on the manuscript, and I am grateful for their help.

A huge debt of gratitude goes to my spiritual teachers who have guided and supported me perfectly through this life.

Finally, thanks to all of the Lyme-MSIDS sufferers, who have been some of the greatest teachers to me in this lifetime. Your courage and perseverance to regain health has inspired me to constantly look for answers, and has been the inspiration for this book.

Introduction

Lyme and associated tick-borne diseases are rapidly spreading worldwide, mimicking a host of common illnesses such as chronic fatigue syndrome (CFS, now renamed as systemic exertional intolerance disease—SEID), fibromyalgia (FM), and autoimmune diseases like rheumatoid arthritis (RA), lupus, and multiple sclerosis (MS). These tick-borne diseases can even imitate psychiatric conditions such as depression, anxiety, obsessive-compulsive disorder (OCD), and psychosis. Lyme is known as "the great imitator," and I have witnessed tremendous suffering among the twelve-thousand-plus patients I have treated during the past twenty-nine years.

Lyme disease may also be one of the driving forces underlying multiple chronic diseases. People from all over the United States and abroad come to my office complaining of chronic fatigue and varying pain syndromes, as well as cognitive and neuropsychiatric problems. These symptoms often are severe and can result in long-term disability. Many of my patients have the same story. They have gone from doctor to doctor looking for answers and only ended up getting help once their Lyme, associated co-infections, and multiple overlapping medical illnesses were all simultaneously addressed.

In 2013 I published my first book, *Why Can't I Get Better? Solving the Mystery of Lyme and Chronic Disease*. It has been tremendously satisfying that this book is often referred to as the "Lyme Bible" and that it has changed the way doctors both understand and treat this debilitating disease. This new book is an updated and simpler version, and it includes some of the most important scientific discoveries to emerge since the original publication. For instance, we now know that there are bacterial "persisters"— bacteria that can survive short courses of antibiotics—and how pulsing medication, treating biofilms that protect bacteria, and using established "persister drugs" for other chronic bacterial diseases may lead to better outcomes. I have done studies in my office on these newer protocols, taking the research from the laboratory into the clinical setting, and I am seeing successful outcomes in patients who have failed prior therapies. This is very exciting, as our team at the Hudson Valley Healing Arts Center has searched for close to thirty years to find answers for people who are suffering with persistent/resistant symptoms. Details of these new and effective protocols are in this book to help you get better.

LYME IS SPREADING

While you may know of the health epidemics of obesity, diabetes, cardiovascular disease, strokes, heart attack, and cancer, unless you or a family member has faced Lyme disease, you might not know that we are also witnessing epidemics of bacterial, viral, and parasitic illnesses. Lyme disease is the number one "vector borne" spreading infectious disease in the United States and in Europe (while rapidly expanding to other countries like Canada, Australia, and China).

Several months after my first book was published, the Centers for Disease Control and Prevention (CDC) reported that 1.3 percent of respondents of a survey in the United States in 2009, and 0.9 percent in 2012, had been diagnosed with Lyme disease. Of the respondents in 2012, 0.3 percent had been diagnosed in the last year. This forced the CDC to revise their figures and increase the rate of annual infection by a factor of ten, from thirty thousand to over three hundred thousand individuals a year. These numbers have more recently been revised and found to be even higher. A 2015 CDC study, published in the journal *Emerging Infectious Diseases*, discussed the geographic distribution and expansion of Lyme disease in the United States over the past twenty years. They found a 320 percent increase in the northeastern states, and in the north-central states where the number of counties having a high incidence of Lyme disease increased by greater than 250 percent for the same period. According to the CDC, "The center of the high-incidence focus in the northeastern United States generally moved westward and northward, away from the coast of northern New Jersey and into east-central Pennsylvania. In the north-central high-incidence focus, the geographic center remained relatively stable in northwestern Wisconsin, moving northward and southward between adjacent counties over time." Their conclusion was that "relatively constant rates of geographic expansion (were happening) in all accessible directions."

A population-based, cross-sectional study was also conducted several years ago by Professor Holly Ahearn, which was published in the *Journal of Microbiology Research*. She concluded that we were underestimating the risk of *Borrelia burgdorferi*, the etiologic agent of Lyme disease, and the spread of borreliosis, diseases caused by borrelia, a genus of spirochetal (corkscrew-shaped) bacteria. In her study, 2 percent of respondents reported being diagnosed with Lyme according to the CDC criteria for "probable" Lyme disease, which is significantly higher than the number of reported cases by the CDC. Another 16 percent of undiagnosed survey respondents also reported subjective signs and symptoms consistent with "late stage" Lyme disease, which is consistent with the CDC study, in which 10.5 percent of respondents in 2011 reported personally knowing someone described as having "Chronic Lyme disease." These figures imply that millions of people have been bitten by ticks and infected with Lyme disease and associated co-infections, and yet the numbers are probably significantly underestimating the risk and true incidence.

Other studies reveal that 3.5 percent of the U.S. population was diagnosed with Chronic Fatigue Syndrome (CFS/SEID), and up to 1.5 percent was diagnosed with Fibromyalgia (FM). That means over 17 million people have a chronic fatiguing, musculoskeletal disorder of "unknown etiology" or cause. There are no reliable tests for either of these syndromes, as the diagnosis is primarily made by relying on clinical criteria—like Lyme disease. Chronic fatigue, sleep disturbances, musculoskeletal pain, and neurocognitive difficulties are exactly the same symptoms that are seen in Lyme, and I have helped many suffering with CFS/SEID, FM, autoimmune diseases, and even patients with major psychiatric manifestations who failed classical treatments for their diseases, simply by treating Lyme disease, associated co-infections, and the overlapping causes that can lead to what I now call Multiple Systemic Infectious Disease Syndrome (MSIDS).

THE SEVEN RULES OF LYME DISEASE:
AN ACTION PLAN

This book is a compilation of everything I've discovered about Lyme disease and, subsequently, about chronic disease in general. By reading it and learning from my patient anecdotes, my hope is that you will be able to identify your own symptoms and work with your doctor for the best possible treatment outcome.

Many people are confused when they first get a diagnosis of Lyme disease. You might be suffering from a myriad of seemingly unconnected symptoms, or have received conflicting diagnoses and/or treatments from your healthcare providers, some of which may work and others may not. The reason for this confusion is not just that Lyme disease is complex, but more to the point, that you are unique. Your genetic makeup, and even the bacterial populations within the microbiome of your gut, is specific to you. These factors affect how you react to infections as well as how you absorb nutrients, detoxify chemicals, create hormones, and handle inflammation. Each of us also carries different infectious burdens, including bacteria, parasites, viruses and/or fungi, varying levels of inflammation and immune dysfunction, possible food and environmental allergies, different toxic loads, detoxification abilities, hormone levels, and sleep and exercise habits, as well as different levels of cellular and organ damage from previous or underlying infections. In short, your prior and current medical status determine exactly how Lyme disease will affect your health.

Consequently, there is no single "right way" to treat this illness, and this is why general guidelines to diagnose and treat Lyme and associated co-infections will never be adequate. Each regimen must be customized to your unique patterns of illness. However, there are some basic rules to help you heal from Lyme and chronic illness that I have found after effectively treating thousands of patients. In this book, you will learn how to apply these rules to your individual situation so that you can get better.

Rule One: Symptoms Drive Diagnosis and Treatment

The focus on symptoms driving a diagnosis and treatment for Lyme and co-infections is the hallmark of what I call the Horowitz Method. You will learn why the blood tests for Lyme and associated co-infections are not 100 percent accurate, and how to begin to parse through your symptoms to arrive at what I call a comprehensive differential diagnosis. I will teach you how to become a medical detective by understanding your clinical history, identifying symptoms, and ruling out other diseases. You will also learn how to listen to the messages your body is sending. For instance, when you take a medication or an herb, or eat a certain food, how do you feel? The body has wisdom, and by following your symptoms and the response to treatment we can determine your underlying problems and the best course of action for you to take.

The majority of people who come to see me have multiple overlapping etiologies, or causes of their symptoms, that are keeping them sick. That is why I refer to this illness as Lyme-MSIDS, or Multiple Systemic Infectious Disease Syndrome. My sixteen-point MSIDS map described in this book is a road map to healing this disease and many other chronic "unexplained" illnesses.

I often use the analogy of a patient going into a doctor with sixteen nails in his or her foot. If the doctor only pulls out one nail, the patient is not going to feel better. The medical paradigm that many healthcare providers subscribe to for chronic diseases, that there is one cause for one illness, is also an outdated medical model. There are often multiple overlapping causes for chronic illness, and each person is different. Medicine is moving toward personalized/precision care, and the MSIDS model incorporates the most up-to-date science to help you create an individualized plan to help you regain your health.

Rule Two: Lower Inflammation

The one common denominator underlying most chronic illness is inflammation. We now know that heart attacks, strokes, Parkinson's disease, Alzheimer's disease, dermatitis, cataracts, cancer, and the symptoms of chronic Lyme disease—including ongoing fatigue, joint and muscle pain, nerve pain, headaches, memory and concentration problems, sleep and mood disorders—are all influenced by inflammation. This inflammation may be due to different infections, autoimmune processes, toxins, unhealthy bacteria in our colons (dysbiosis), an improper diet and/or nutritional deficiencies, lack of sleep, and a variety of other environmental factors. You will learn how to identify all of the underlying causes of inflammation so that you can achieve optimal health.

Rule Three: Detoxify, Detoxify, Detoxify

Our bodies are designed to naturally remove toxins, but often these detoxification systems are overburdened and no longer work optimally. In order to get better, you will learn how to both decrease your load of infections, including Lyme and associated co-infections (our infectious burden, i.e., IB), and to assist your body in detoxifying chemicals, such as heavy metals and mold, as well as the inflammatory chemical messengers produced during illness.

Many infections and toxins produce inflammatory chemicals called cytokines. These molecules, such as tumor necrosis factor alpha (TNF-alpha), interleukin-1 (IL-1), interleukin-6 (IL-6), interferon gamma (IFN-gamma), and others cause a "fire" to be produced in the body, which leads to symptoms. Infections, toxins, and inflammatory cytokines can damage our cell membranes, DNA, joints, and sensitive nervous system, leading to many of the common symptoms seen in chronic Lyme disease with MSIDS.

Rule Four: Repair the Damage

We must also repair the damage to the body that has resulted from chronic infections and toxins if we are to feel well. Infections and toxins create free radicals. Free radicals are not hippies who recently graduated from California universities, but rather unpaired electrons that bounce around in the body, causing oxidative stress and damaging our cells and mitochondria. These mitochondria play an important role in our health. They are the organelles inside our cells that make energy and are necessary for proper functioning of the heart, liver, kidneys, GI tract, brain, and nervous system. Without healthy, functioning mitochondria, we can't expect to function at full capacity. This damage also occurs at the level of our autonomic nervous system, which is the part of the body that controls our blood pressure, heart rate, stomach/intestines, and bladder. This frequently leads to resistant symptoms of fatigue, dizziness, palpitations, anxiety, and cognitive difficulties. You will learn how to repair this damage through proper medication and effective nutrient supplementation.

Rule Five: Provide Internal Balance

Homeostasis is a term that means to have balance in the body. When we are out of balance with regards to cytokines, chemokines (specialized signaling molecules that modulate inflammation), hormones, and infections (bacterial, viral, parasitic, and fungal), our cells and organs do not work properly. Some chemical messengers help to lower inflammation, and others increase inflammation. TNF-alpha, IL-1, and IL-6 are molecules produced during infection with Lyme and associated co-infections, and these increase inflammation. These molecules cause the symptom flares experienced by the majority of people suffering from Lyme and other chronic illness. It is therefore necessary to decrease these molecules if we are to feel better. This can be done by properly treating the infections with medication and natural supplements to decrease the infectious burden (IB) and associated autoimmune reactions, while detoxing the body, using antioxidants (food, supplements), replacing essential minerals, avoiding allergic/sensitive foods, getting enough exercise and sleep, and making sure that we have the right bacterial growth in our GI tract. And if we do not achieve a proper balance of cytokines in the body, our hormones may not work properly, leading to symptoms including resistant fatigue, pain, weight gain, sluggishness, poor memory and concentration, and low libido.

Rule Six: Master the Big Three: Sleep, Food, and Exercise

An unhealthy lifestyle that is high in stress and low in rest can also make your internal health unbalanced. Lack of sleep increases inflammation and adversely affects hormone levels. Even if you properly treated the infections, decreased autoimmune reactions, detoxified chemicals and toxins, repaired the damage to the mitochondria, and tried to balance the cytokines, hormones, and microbiome, it is impossible to get back to full health without getting regenerative sleep. Improper sleep patterns and poor exercise habits have been linked to cardiovascular disease, strokes, and cancer, and they interfere with healing from Lyme disease.

The foods you eat also strongly influence your health. You are what you eat. Your ability to heal from infections, detoxify chemicals, lower inflammation in the body, produce hormones, make neurotransmitters in the brain, and have your internal organs function properly depends on the nutrition you provide your body. An imbalance in proteins, carbohydrates, fats, minerals, and vitamins will interfere with the healing process and prevent a fully successful outcome. You will learn which foods to avoid and which ones to enjoy, to ensure that you are on the path to better health.

Rule Seven: Heal Your Emotional Wounds

Many people who come to see me have had very difficult life experiences, which influence their ability to get better. I affectionately call these patients the "walking wounded." Some suffer from post-traumatic stress disorder (PTSD) either caused by abuse, whether physical, emotional, or sexual, or from insensitive healthcare providers who do not believe that a patient's illness is due to Lyme and treat them as if they were simply psychiatric patients "making it all up." No matter what the cause of the emotional wounding, the body and mind work as one, and oftentimes the immune system will not work correctly if underlying emotional trauma is not properly addressed and healed. You will learn why healing involves forgiveness, self-compassion, and loving ourselves. Love and compassion are some of the greatest healing forces in the universe, and if accessed they can be a powerful force in helping us to recover from illness and find peace.

Part of loving ourselves is allowing us the proper time and space to heal. Some of that healing may be with gifted healthcare professionals, and some of the healing is learning to be alone with ourselves, and at peace, at the deepest level of our being. This state can be accessed with meditation. When we meditate, we give ourselves the ultimate gift of time, which we can use to connect with our inner peace and deepest wisdom and go beyond relative suffering to experience our wholeness. Meditation has also been shown to have numerous health benefits, including helping mood, balancing the sympathetic nervous system, lowering cortisol levels (our stress hormone), and decreasing inflammation.

LET'S GET STARTED

This Action Plan will help you get started on the road to recovery and health. The first step is to fill out the Horowitz Lyme-MSIDS Questionnaire (HMQ), which you'll find on page 23. Then, read through the book so that you can create a comprehensive plan with your doctor that will allow you to get better. Have your physician read the book and review the extensive scientific references on these newer diagnostic and treatment regimens so that you can work together in a healing partnership. You may find that doctors trained in integrative medicine are more familiar with some concepts, and can be part of your medical team, in order to implement the functional medicine testing and treatment protocols that I've described.

If you bring the results of this questionnaire to your healthcare provider and find that he or she is not responsive to the philosophy or the diagnostic and treatment plans outlined in this book, it may be due to the fact that this person is not fully informed. Science and medicine are ever-changing, and some treatment regimens using the MSIDS model reported in this book have only recently been published in the medical literature. Bringing this information to your doctor may put you in a position of being perceived as "pushy" or "misguided," but this is a risk you might want to take if you want to get better.

In treating over twelve thousand patients over the last twenty-nine years, I have seen 90 percent to 95 percent of my chronically ill patients improve by applying the MSIDS model as a map to get to the multifactorial causes of their illness. Some get slightly better, some moderately better, and some significantly better, while some become symptom-free. Let's find out, together, how much better you can feel by uncovering the source of your health issues.

PART I

Testing and Treating Lyme Disease

ONE

Identifying Lyme Disease and Other Tick-Borne Illnesses

To understand Lyme disease, we need to go back to the mid-1970s, when portrait painter Polly Murray first noticed an outbreak of what had been called "juvenile rheumatoid arthritis" in the town of Lyme, Connecticut, which had affected her and her children from decades earlier. Dr. Alan Steere, a rheumatologist at Yale University, was called in to investigate the epidemic, as were researchers from the National Institutes of Health (NIH) and Rocky Mountain Labs. Dr. Willy Burgdorfer, a researcher at Rocky Mountain Labs, identified a microscopic spirochete, a spiral-shaped bacterium that resembles the bacteria that causes syphilis. This was eventually identified as the causative agent of the newly identified disease, and the spirochete was named *Borrelia burgdorferi* (Bb) after Dr. Burgdorfer's discovery, and the related disease was called Lyme after its initial outbreak in the town of Lyme, Connecticut.

Although patients may have had other manifestations of the disease, Dr. Steere primarily investigated those with rashes and rheumatologic manifestations, including hot, swollen joints, for the Connecticut Department of Public Health. He was instrumental in determining that many became ill in summer or early fall and lived in geographic clusters in mostly rural areas. He recognized that these patients were very ill and not just psychologically disturbed. But what caused this enigmatic new illness?

This mysterious illness was actually not a new discovery at all. Lyme disease had already been reported in Europe in the late 1800s as a rash of the hands. Dr. Alfred Buchwald described a skin lesion; others in Europe and the United States reported the same lesion to be part of a condition called Bannwarth syndrome, a triad of radiculitis (a pain radiating along a nerve), Bell's palsy (the sudden onset of facial paralysis), and meningitis (an inflammation occurring in the membranes covering the brain and spinal cord). In 1909, Dr. Arvid Afzelius described an expanding ring-like skin rash, later named erythema chronicum migrans or ECM. (In 1990, dermatologist Dr. Bernard Berger recognized that the rash was not chronic in all cases and renamed it erythema migrans or, simply, EM.) Ten years later, Dr. Afzelius connected the disease with joint problems and speculated that they are somehow related to the bite of a tick.

In 1922 the disease was found to be associated with neurological problems, and in 1930 the diagnosis further included psychiatric disturbances. A few years later, arthritic problems were added. In 1965 Dr. Sidney Robbin, a semiretired internist living in Montauk, New York, described expanding circular rashes that responded to penicillin treatment, which appeared in conjunction with a peculiar type of arthritis that he named Montauk knee. Five years later, Dr. Rudolph Scrimenti, a Wisconsin dermatologist, published the first report of an ECM rash in the United States. As Dr. Robbin had observed, Dr. Scrimenti also reported that the rash responded to penicillin.

No one, however, had put all the pieces together, or connected these symptoms to the patients who were so ill in rural Connecticut. Was this a new illness, and if so, where did it come from, and how should we treat it? By 1977, Dr. Steere, the Yale rheumatologist who first investigated the Connecticut outbreak, was reporting a whole host of specific and often bizarre signs of this new disease, including fever, fatigue, headache, and migratory joint pains as well as multiple cardiovascular and neurological abnormalities. As the result of treating patients with antibiotics for (only) seven to ten days, many patients went on to develop other symptoms. It appeared that antibiotics just wouldn't help Lyme patients. Perhaps Lyme was caused by a virus, or it was an autoimmune disorder.

When you have been trained in a particular medical specialty, you see the world through certain lenses and diagnostic paradigms. A gastroenterologist, for example, sees the world through the lens of the gastrointestinal (GI) tract and tries to link up a patient's symptoms to diseases known in that person's specialty. The same approach is true for neurology or infectious disease or, in the case of Dr. Steere, a rheumatologist, for diseases of the joints, which include autoimmune diseases. It is not that the thinking of these doctors and subspecialists is necessarily wrong, as Lyme can cause an autoimmune response and affect different organ systems of the body, but it may be that their worldview only includes part of the whole picture. There is relative truth, and then there is absolute truth. When the three blind men are feeling the elephant, they each describe a different part. One describes the elephant as having a long, movable nose, another tough skin with thick legs and big nails, and the third might just describe a thin, coarse tail. Each has described a certain relative truth, and none is incorrect, but none of them have seen the big picture: It's an elephant!

So it is with Lyme disease. The initial paradigm created for diagnosis and treatment was through a rheumatologist's narrowly focused eyes. Soon the infectious disease doctors claimed Lyme disease as part of their turf.

I was trained as an internist to be a medical detective, with a wide diagnostic perspective: We have to know something about all of the medical subspecialties. The vision of an internist must be broad and inclusive of all possibilities, since his or her job is to diagnose and effectively determine who needs to be referred to subspecialists. An internist, therefore, will not necessarily have some of the inherent biases or diagnostic schema associated with subspecialists. As Lyme diagnosis and treatment fell into the domains of the rheumatologists and infectious disease doctors early on, a paradigm was forming based on the way these subspecialists viewed the world. In addition, traditional medical education has always taught doctors to find one cause for all of the patient's symptoms. This is deeply ingrained in every physician's education. We generally are not taught to look for multifactorial causes of an illness. Therefore, if a Lyme disease patient presents with thirty-five different symptoms, the established paradigm would be to try and explain these complaints according to the accepted medical model of one primary diagnosis. If the doctor could not find a single etiology, or cause, for your symptoms, it must be because it is psychological in nature, and you are crazy. Or the answer might be elusive because the symptoms can't be understood in the HMO-dictated fifteen-minute time frame. Or perhaps the physician hasn't looked hard enough, or just sees the world through one narrow diagnostic lens.

IS IT POSSIBLE THAT I HAVE LYME DISEASE?

There has been a 320 percent increase in the number of counties identified as having a high incidence of Lyme disease over the past twenty years, according to the CDC. This means that it is becoming increasingly likely that you have been or will be exposed, especially if you live in or have traveled to certain highly endemic areas of the United States (the Northeast, Pacific Coast, and certain parts of the Midwest). Many people also have gotten Lyme disease from visiting supposedly "non-endemic" areas, including parts of Texas, Florida, and the Carolinas. We now know that there are other species of borrelia, apart from Lyme disease, that have been found in ticks, including *Borrelia sensu lato* and the recently diagnosed species *Borrelia miyamotoi, Borrelia bisettii,* and *Borrelia mayonii.* These other species can cause Lyme-like syndromes and may not be identified by standard blood tests used to diagnose Lyme, like the enzyme-linked immuno-sorbent assay (ELISA) test and the Western blot.

No matter where you live, you may have been exposed to ticks. Regular enjoyment of gardening, hiking, biking, boating, the beach, or any activity that puts you in contact with high grass or woody areas makes it likely that you have crossed paths with ticks. But how can we know for certain if we have been exposed?

Lyme disease is known as the great imitator, and it can mimic a broad range of other diseases. If you or a loved one suffer from ongoing fatigue, muscle and joint pain, tingling, numbness, burning sensations, headaches, memory and concentration problems, and/or mood and sleep disorders, and the doctors have told you that they can't find anything wrong with you—that it is in your head—they may be right. You may have Lyme spirochetes, co-infections, and neurotoxins inside your brain that are making you sick.

Unfortunately, the blood tests for diagnosing Lyme and certain associated tick-borne disorders like Babesia (a malaria type parasite) and Bartonella (a species of bacteria, one of which is "cat scratch fever"), which you will learn about later, are not 100 percent reliable, and most physicians do not do testing for multiple neurotoxins (like mold, heavy metals, pesticides, and volatile organic solvents). Therefore, you may have tick-borne infections and associated toxins, and your healthcare providers either may not have looked for these problems or were not able to find them, and given you a label of another illness.

You may also have Lyme disease that is either influencing or occurring along with other chronic illnesses. The CDC recognizes that chronic illness may be a complex interplay of genetics, environmental factors, infections, and trauma. But in day-to-day practice, doctors often do not use this broad framework to understand and treat chronic illness. Usually, the HMO model encourages limited time for visits and referring patients to specialists who, if they get approval, will perform long lists of expensive tests. Yet these same insurance companies often place limits on medically necessary treatment options for economic reasons. Few physicians have the time to uncover the multifactorial causes of chronic illness. In order to discover if you have Lyme disease, I believe that a paradigm shift must begin with primary care physicians. These first-line physicians must use a broader and more inclusive framework to break down chronic illness into layers by examining the mental, emotional, and physical aspects of each illness.

Then we must go even further and break physical symptoms down into the anatomy of an illness, the biology, biochemistry, and immunology of an illness, and the genetics behind the illness. Functional medicine and abnormalities in the biochemical pathways that drive chronic illness are a start. These often need to be examined to discover clues as to why the chronically ill patient has persistent symptoms.

In medical school, doctors are not adequately taught about environmental medicine or chronic infections and how they interact with each other. How toxins cause damage to the body is not emphasized, nor is how detoxification pathways work, or how toxins and chronic infections increase inflammatory cytokines (the protein molecules that are secreted by cells that can communicate with each other), causing sickness syndrome in a broad range of chronic diseases. Physicians are trained to recognize and treat some chronic infections, but many believe that the list of chronic diseases is limited to those like tuberculosis, leprosy, syphilis, chronic Q fever, or chronic viral infections such as hepatitis B, hepatitis C, or HIV. In truth, we now know that Lyme disease and many co-infections have been shown to persist, and adversely interact with environmental toxins, causing chronic illness.

If we wish to get to the source(s) of a disease process, I believe that each person's symptoms need to be considered individually, then collected and put into likely disease categories to try and find the common denominator.

This is a process doctors call "the differential diagnosis." Each chronic illness is complex, and its causes are likely interrelated.

For example, a woman comes to my office complaining of night sweats. She is forty years old and not in menopause. After obtaining a history and performing a physical, I begin my investigation to identify the most common causes of night sweats. Is it tuberculosis or non-Hodgkin's lymphoma? Is there a cough, hemoptysis (blood in the sputum), or weight loss, or has there been exposure to someone who contracted tuberculosis? A simple chest X-ray and tuberculosis test (PPD) could help rule out these two differential diagnoses while I check the patient for hard, enlarged, non-mobile lymph nodes, which can be seen with a lymphoma. Has she been traveling to countries where she could have been exposed to malaria? Did she get a febrile illness while she was there? Examining a blood smear under the microscope (Giemsa stain) to rule out malaria could be helpful. Does she live in a tick-endemic area, or has she traveled to one where she could have contracted babesiosis, which is a malaria-like illness? Performing Babesia titers (antibody testing), a Giemsa stain, a polymerase chain reaction (PCR) DNA test, or a fluorescent in situ hybridization (FISH) test of ribonucleic acid (RNA), looking for Babesia, would be helpful in this circumstance. Is the patient having hormonal issues even though she is young? Checking follicle-stimulating hormone (FSH), luteinizing hormone (LH), estradiol, progesterone, testosterone, and free-testosterone levels, as well as sex-hormone-binding globulin (SHBG), would help rule out this possibility. Is she hyperthyroid? Is she suffering from weight loss, palpitations, tremors, anxiety, diarrhea, and sweats? Checking a full thyroid panel would be helpful. Has she undergone any recent trauma that might be triggering an anxiety disorder? By simply listing these six to seven most common differential diagnoses for night sweats and ruling out each one with a proper history, physical, and laboratory testing, answers can be found.

We need to get to the source of the problems in medicine because the world, now more than ever, is out of balance. The ancient adage "as above, so below" could now be applied to medicine in terms of "as without, so within." When does the illness of the world become our own personal illness? When does our own personal illness impact the balance of the world? If we identify the source of illness within us, it also informs us about what is out of balance in the world, and perhaps can teach us how to remedy it.

For example, is it normal to be losing your memory as you get older, and that every sixty-seven seconds someone is diagnosed with Alzheimer's in the United States? Or is it possible that there are multiple etiologies at the root of this condition? We find that the majority of our Lyme disease patients with co-infections have severe memory and concentration problems. An early hint of the connection between infection and dementia can be found in a report from pathologist Dr. Alan B. MacDonald, who examined brain biopsies from the McLean Hospital (an affiliate of Harvard University) data bank from patients with confirmed Alzheimer's disease (AD). His PCR analysis showed that seven out of ten of these patients had the DNA of *Borrelia burgdorferi* in their brain, the etiologic agent of Lyme disease. Dr. MacDonald has discovered biofilms as well as other borrelia species, like *Borrelia miyamotoi,* in patients with neurological problems, and Dr. Judith Miklossy has published extensively on the role of spirochetal infections in Alzheimer's disease. Their research was corroborated by scientists at Drexel University in 2016, who found borrelia in biofilms during brain autopsies of Alzheimer's patients, and other researchers have found similar results, implicating Lyme as well as other infections. It turns out that the higher your infectious burden (IB), the greater your risk for Alzheimer's, yet other factors are being implicated.

We also find that the majority of our chronically ill patients with Lyme disease and co-infections have been exposed to high levels of heavy metals, such as mercury and lead, and occasionally to aluminum. Heavy metal exposure can cause memory and concentration problems as well as the production of elevated levels of free radicals, which can increase inflammation. Similarly, we are exposed to hundreds of environmental chemicals every day that are fat-soluble and find their way to the brain. These can and do affect cognitive processing. Medical researchers published in the *Journal of the American Medical Association (JAMA)* in 2014 that pesticides have been found in the brains of Alzheimer's patients; we know that environmental toxins, with or without infections, drive inflammation, and an inflammatory process is at work in Alzheimer's disease that causes the production of amyloid (an insoluble fibrous protein that in excess can lead to neurodegenerative diseases). Apart from a rising infectious burden of bacteria and viruses being linked to AD, ultrafine particle pollution containing toxic combinations of hydrocarbons, sulfates, nitrates, and heavy metals are now suspected agents in neurodegenerative brain disease, according to a 2015 article in *the Journal of Alzheimer's Disease*. Are Lyme disease, co-infections, environmental toxins, and heavy metals some of the agents causing the severe memory and concentration problems associated with Alzheimer's disease? People who are inactive, and/or have diabetes/glucose intolerance and sleep disorders, are also at risk. If we then include patients who have undiagnosed B_{12} deficiency, which we would identify through blood tests for B_{12}, methylmalonic acid, and homocysteine levels, and/or patients who suffer from undiagnosed hypothyroidism, we have enough causes for an epidemic of dementia in the general population.

I have seen elderly individuals with a diagnosis of dementia, with cognitive deficits, given drugs prescribed for Alzheimer's such as Aricept and Namenda that slow down (but do not reverse) their cognitive decline. But I have also seen improvements in cognitive functioning after treating chronic tick-borne infections; by removing fat-soluble toxins with glutathione; by using oral chelating agents to remove mercury, lead, and aluminum; by getting their blood sugar under control; by getting them a good night's sleep; and by identifying and treating B_{12} deficiencies and/or hypothyroidism. This is why I believe that identifying the multifactorial causes of chronic illness is now the most important paradigm shift in medicine, and it may be the key to keeping down rising healthcare costs, decreasing suffering, and unlocking the mystery of Lyme disease and other chronic illnesses.

How Do I Know If I Have Lyme and Tick-Borne Disease?

There are hundreds of species of borrelia worldwide, so when we talk about "Lyme disease" we are really talking about a disease complex caused by a large family of spirochetal bacteria. For example, if you get an erythema migrans (EM) rash, the classic expanding ringlike skin rash that is seen with Lyme disease, it could have been caused by more than one species of borrelia. Although Lyme disease and Lyme-like illnesses were not supposed to exist in certain parts of the southern United States, Dr. Kerry Clark found the DNA of *Borrelia burgdorferi sensu lato* as well as other species, including *B. americana* and *B. andersoni*, in patients from southern states.

Although many EM rashes are due to *Borrelia burgdorferi*, the agent of Lyme disease, other borrelia species like *Borrelia sensu lato* can cause an EM type rash in the Midwest, like Southern tick-associated rash illness (STARI), and occasionally the relapsing fever borrelia, *Borrelia miyamotoi*, can also cause an EM rash. Standard blood tests for Lyme disease may not pick up these other species.

Other types of rashes due to tick-borne infections are also possible. The newly discovered borrelia species *Borrelia mayonii* can cause a widespread, spotted rash that is not classic for Lyme disease. There is a violaceous (purplish) skin rash of the extremities called acrodermatitis chronica atrophicans (ACA) caused by a borrelia species commonly found in Europe called *Borrelia afzelii*, as well as skin rashes that appear from tick-borne diseases like Bartonella, which cause stretch marks to appear on different parts of the body. Other tick-borne infections like ehrlichiosis can cause a macular (flat) or maculopapular (raised) rash, and rarely can cause small red spots (petechiae) to appear, like Rocky Mountain spotted fever or other rickettsia of the spotted fever group. Any of these rashes tell you that you have been exposed to a bacterial infection from ticks (although Bartonella species can also be transmitted from a cat scratch as well as from lice, black flies, sand flies, and fleas, but more on that in Chapter 5).

Many people, however, never see a rash following a tick bite. Less than half of the people exposed to Lyme disease get a rash, and if they do, it doesn't necessarily look like a bullseye. It can also have the appearance of a solid red rash that resembles a bacterial infection of the skin (cellulitis), or a spider bite, and therefore can be misdiagnosed and improperly treated.

Because Lyme disease so often goes undiagnosed, I have developed the Horowitz Lyme-MSIDS Questionnaire (HMQ), a screening symptom questionnaire to determine if people have Lyme disease or other tick-borne illnesses, and if this is one of the contributing factors to their chronic illness. Without this tool I know that many important clues would be missing, as these are often the symptoms that are essential for making an accurate diagnosis. This questionnaire was initially validated in my medical office several years ago, and it was validated statistically again in 2016 by researchers at SUNY New Paltz. Over 1,500 patients participated, and we found that the HMQ reliably differentiates Lyme disease patients from non–Lyme disease participants. This questionnaire determines a probability of suffering from Lyme and associated tick-borne illness and can help differentiate between those who are suffering with Lyme and those with a non-Lyme-like illness (although it can't differentiate between

Lyme and other chronic diseases). This strategy can help improve your diagnosis and can lead to earlier treatment, making long-term suffering and disability less likely.

Most people with chronic complex illnesses come into my office with a stack of medical records and a long list of complaints. By meticulously reviewing their records and using the questionnaire to further delineate the full extent of their symptoms, I am ensuring that I am complete in obtaining a proper history. This questionnaire also provides me an opportunity to formulate the most probable differential diagnoses while interviewing the patient. Taking a proper history that will uncover these highly complex conditions, with patients who may have been to ten to twenty doctors in the past several years, usually takes at least one hour. Then I spend another two or three hours to complete a social history, family history and environmental exposure history, and then review their symptoms, conduct a complete physical examination and assessment, and devise a treatment plan.

When I arrive at the final assessment and plan, I try to make sure that every symptom on the questionnaire that was circled has one or several potential differential diagnoses. This ensures that each symptom receives the appropriate testing and has an appropriate plan.

Why Use the Questionnaire Instead of Simply Relying on Blood Tests?

The blood tests for diagnosing Lyme and associated co-infections are inadequate and, at best, problematic. They cannot easily detect all of the new emerging species of bacteria, parasites, and viruses found in ticks, and they cannot pick up all of the different species of borrelia. For example, there are over a hundred strains of borrelia in the United States, and three hundred strains worldwide. Although not all of these strains are pathogenic, the sensitivity and specificity of the present two-tiered testing for Lyme disease, using an ELISA followed by a Western blot, misses the majority of these strains. A perfect example is *Borrelia miyamotoi*, the relapsing fever borrelia causing a Lyme-like illness. It is missed on standard Lyme testing and was found in up to 4 percent of individuals living in New England. The same situation exists for intracellular infections like Bartonella and Mycoplasma. Parasites like Babesia also have over one hundred different species, which can be missed on standard testing.

Researchers are looking at developing better diagnostics for Lyme disease, including more sensitive PCRs (polymerase chain reactions, a DNA test to identify the bacteria) and utilizing specific inflammatory markers (CXCL-19, an inflammatory molecule associated with Lyme, identified by Johns Hopkins researchers), which can be found early on in the illness before antibodies are produced.

Until we develop more sensitive PCR testing (direct detection tests), as well as better indirect testing (antibody tests), we must rely on taking a good clinical history, looking for common clinical manifestations of these diseases. That's why I suggest you use the HMQ as a first-line screening tool to determine your probability of having Lyme and associated tick-borne infections.

THE HOROWITZ LYME-MSIDS QUESTIONNAIRE (HMQ)

The HMQ is necessary for following the first rule of the Action Plan: Discover how your symptoms will drive your diagnosis and treatment. You will begin to determine the probability of a Lyme-MSIDS diagnosis for yourself. I also highly recommend that new and experienced physicians use this as a screening tool to determine if their patients might have Lyme disease. This process ensures that no symptoms are left out and gives the provider an initial opportunity to develop a broad range of differential diagnoses while reviewing the symptom list early on in the patient visit. It provides the healthcare provider with clues that point to whether the patient has a high probability of having Lyme disease, a possible case of Lyme disease, or is unlikely to have Lyme disease. It also reassures patients that the provider will pay close attention to all of their complaints.

All of the points on the list in Section 1 of the questionnaire are symptoms that can be seen with Lyme disease. They are not specific to Lyme disease in and of themselves, and can be found in many other illnesses. However, the gestalt that can be perceived by looking at all of the symptoms simultaneously helps the clinician reach a probability as to whether the patient may suffer from Lyme disease and associated tick-borne disorders. At the same time this list can also be used to identify simultaneous overlapping disease states, so that multiple sources of the patient's suffering can be discovered. These multifactorial causes of illness are often at the heart of most chronic disease states, and this led me to create the MSIDS model. It can be immensely helpful in ruling out other disease processes on the MSIDS map while looking for specific symptom complexes that are frequently seen in Lyme disease (such as symptoms coming and going with good and bad days, migratory joint and muscle pain, neuralgia that comes and goes and migrates, headaches, and sleep disorders with associated cognitive deficits).

Sections 2 and 3 of the questionnaire represent those signs and symptom complexes most associated with Lyme and MSIDS, which I have compiled after examining hundreds of patient charts over the last decade. Section 4 is based on two of the four questions in the Healthy Days Core Module used by the CDC to track population trends nationally and identify healthcare disparities, and it helps us identify the frequency of physical and mental health problems in the preceding month.

Answer the following questions as honestly as possible. Think about how you have been feeling over the previous month and how often you have been bothered by any of the following problems. Score the occurrence and frequency of each symptom on the following scale: never, sometimes, most of the time, all the time.

SECTION 1: SYMPTOM FREQUENCY SCORE

0 Never/Not applicable   **1** Sometimes   **2** Most of the time   **3** All the time

1. Unexplained fevers, sweats, chills, or flushing
2. Unexplained weight change; loss or gain
3. Fatigue, tiredness
4. Unexplained hair loss
5. Swollen glands
6. Sore throat
7. Testicular or pelvic pain
8. Unexplained menstrual irregularity
9. Unexplained breast milk production; breast pain
10. Irritable bladder or bladder dysfunction
11. Sexual dysfunction or loss of libido
12. Upset stomach
13. Change in bowel function (constipation or diarrhea)
14. Chest pain or rib soreness

15. Shortness of breath or cough
16. Heart palpitations, pulse skips, heart block
17. History of a heart murmur or valve prolapse
18. Joint pain or swelling
19. Stiffness of the neck or back
20. Muscle pain or cramps
21. Twitching of the face or other muscles
22. Headaches
23. Neck cracks or neck stiffness
24. Tingling, numbness, burning, or stabbing sensations
25. Facial paralysis (Bell's palsy)
26. Eyes/vision: double, blurry
27. Ears/hearing: buzzing, ringing, ear pain
28. Increased motion sickness, vertigo
29. Lightheadedness, poor balance, difficulty walking
30. Tremors
31. Confusion, difficulty thinking
32. Difficulty with concentration or reading
33. Forgetfulness, poor short-term memory
34. Disorientation: getting lost; going to wrong places
35. Difficulty with speech or writing
36. Mood swings, irritability, depression
37. Disturbed sleep: too much, too little, early awakening
38. Exaggerated symptoms or worse hangover from alcohol

Tally your answers and record your score.

Score: _____

SECTION 2: MOST COMMON LYME SYMPTOMS SCORE

If you rated a 3 for all the following symptoms in section 1, give yourself five additional points:

- Fatigue
- Forgetfulness, poor short-term memory
- Joint pain or swelling
- Tingling, numbness, burning, or stabbing sensations
- Disturbed sleep: too much, too little, early awakening

Score: _____

SECTION 3: LYME INCIDENCE SCORE

Now please circle the points for each of the following statements you can agree with:

1. You have had a tick bite with no rash or flulike symptoms. *3 points*
2. You have had a tick bite, an erythema migrans, or an undefined rash, followed by flulike symptoms. *5 points*
3. You live in what is considered a Lyme-endemic area. *2 points*
4. You have a family member who has been diagnosed with Lyme and/or other tick-borne infections. *1 point*
5. You experience migratory muscle pain. *4 points*
6. You experience migratory joint pain. *4 points*
7. You experience tingling/burning/numbness that migrates and/or comes and goes. *4 points*
8. You have received a prior diagnosis of chronic fatigue syndrome or fibromyalgia. *3 points*
9. You have received a prior diagnosis of a specific autoimmune disorder (lupus, MS, or rheumatoid arthritis), or of a nonspecific autoimmune disorder. *3 points*
10. You have had a positive Lyme test, such as an immunofluorescent assay (IFA), ELISA, Western blot, PCR, lymphocyte transformation tests (LTT and/or ELISPOT), and/or borrelia culture. *5 points*

Score: _____

SECTION 4: OVERALL HEALTH SCORE

1. Thinking about your overall physical health, for how many of the past thirty days was your physical health not good? _____ days
Award yourself the following points based on the total number of days:
0–5 days=1 point
6–12 days=2 points
13–20 days=3 points
21–30 days=4 points

2. Thinking about your overall mental health, for how many days during the past thirty days was your mental health not good? _____ days
Award yourself the following points based on the total number of days:
0–5 days=1 point
6–12 days=2 points

13–20 days=3 points
21–30 days=4 points
Score: _____

SCORING:

Record your total scores for each section below and add them together to achieve your final score: _____

A score of 63 or greater indicates a high probability of a tick-borne disorder; scores between 45 and 62 indicate a "probable" tick-borne disorder; scores between 25 and 44 indicate a "possible" tick-borne disorder, and scores under 25 indicate that you are not likely to have a tick-borne disorder. My updated study involves over 1,500 patients from both an online survey and several physicians' offices treating Lyme disease (paper submitted for publication). Verified Lyme patients at different stages of treatment scored an average of 59. Those who self-reported "suffering Lyme now" from an online survey (with no way of identifying their current treatment protocols) scored, on average, 89, and self-identified "healthy" participants had an average score of 25.

Certainly, if you scored 63 or more on this questionnaire, you have a high probability of a tick-borne disorder and should see a healthcare provider for further evaluation. If you scored between 45 and 62, you probably have a tick-borne disorder based on our recent study and should see a healthcare provider for further evaluation. If you scored between 25 and 44 you have a possible tick-borne disorder and should see a healthcare provider for further evaluation. If you scored under 25, you are not likely to have Lyme with associated tick-borne infections.

The results of our study demonstrated that the HMQ does reliably differentiate Lyme disease patients from non–Lyme disease participants ("healthy"), and that it is a valid measure of the probability of having Lyme disease. It is an inexpensive, easy, and accurate screening tool to determine your initial probability of having a tick-borne disorder.

Interpreting the Results

We see a high frequency of Section 1 symptoms, including fatigue, joint and muscle pain that often migrates, sleep disorders, as well as memory and concentration problems, and a high frequency of Section 3 symptoms, especially neuropathic pain that comes and goes and migrates (tingling, numbness, burning, and stabbing sensations). These form a cluster of presenting symptoms that are characteristic of individuals with a high probability of having Lyme-MSIDS.

In one prior study conducted in our office of one hundred consecutive patients, we found that more than 25 percent reported that the following symptoms were present most or all of the time in the month preceding their office visit. Many reported that these symptoms affected their quality of life: 71 percent reported that their physical health was not good and 47 percent reported that their mental health was not good on at least fifteen days in the previous month. The most common symptoms related to Lyme and MSIDS are:

- Fatigue
- Headaches
- Stiffness of the neck or back
- Joint pain or swelling
- Tingling, numbness, and/or burning of the extremities
- Confusion, difficulty thinking
- Difficulty with concentration or reading
- Forgetfulness, poor short-term memory
- Disturbed sleep: too much, too little, early awakening
- Difficulty with speech or writing

In the statistical survey done through SUNY New Paltz in 2015–2016, the common hallmarks of late-stage Lyme disease were migratory muscle pain, migratory joint pain, and tingling/burning/numbness (neuropathy) that migrates and/or comes and goes. In fact, 78 percent of patients experienced all three migratory symptoms. These symptoms were more likely reported in the patient and self-identified groups suffering from Lyme disease than in the "self-identified healthy group." So, if you are currently suffering from several of these presenting symptoms, and your healthcare provider can't find a reason for your illness, or has told you that you suffer from CFS/SEID, fibromyalgia, a nonspecific autoimmune disorder, MS, an early dementia, or a pure psychiatric condition, then get tested for tick-borne disorders. The list of most common symptoms we found also corresponds to the symptom cluster identified in Nancy Shadick's work on Lyme disease, which was published in the medical literature years ago. She examined 186 patients, each with a history of Lyme disease, and used CDC case status and 167 controls (no history of Lyme disease) in a population-based, retrospective cohort design. We have therefore identified a symptom complex that healthcare providers can refer to when patients come to their offices, and if that symptom cluster is positive, they can be tested and considered for a diagnosis of Lyme disease. Using the questionnaire in this manner will help to identify chronically ill patients with undiagnosed tick-borne diseases, improving their diagnosis and treatment.

CONFIRM YOUR RESULTS WITH THE BEST TESTING AVAILABLE

Talk to your doctor about the results of this questionnaire. Depending on your score, you may want to follow up with blood tests for Lyme disease, including indirect and direct testing. Indirect testing measures antibodies, indicating prior exposure, and includes an IFA (immunofluorescent assay), ELISA (enzyme-linked immuno-sorbent assay), C6 ELISA, IgM and IgG antibodies on Western blots, as well as lymphocyte transformation tests (LTT or ELISPOT). The newer Spirotest, which is under development, is also an indirect test, which measures important inflammatory molecules called chemokines, seen in early and late Lyme (like CCL19). This may help to identify an early infection before antibodies are produced, and prove chronic infection. Direct testing may also be performed, and includes PCR studies, antigen testing (Lyme Dot Blot, Nanotrap test), and culture testing. The Nanotrap test is a specific urine antigen test for Lyme, and the Lyme Dot Blot can be done both on urine and cerebral spinal fluid (CSF). Although culture tests are available through Advanced Laboratories, their accuracy has been questioned by the CDC, and validation studies are still pending for the FDA. The test has however passed other federal regulatory standards including the Clinical Laboratory Improvement Amendments (CLIA).

No one test has sufficient sensitivity to be 100 percent reliable and pick up the disease, so a broad screening approach using indirect and direct testing is usually necessary to determine exposure to borreliosis. Do not just rely on the CDC criteria of using an ELISA followed by a Western blot in a two-tiered testing protocol, as this is only meant as a tool for health departments to screen large populations for Lyme disease, and never meant to be used for an individual diagnosis (as per the CDC). Remember, Lyme disease is a clinical diagnosis, and blood tests only help to confirm your clinical suspicion.

These tests should be performed with testing for other tick-borne diseases as well, since ticks may transmit multiple infections simultaneously. A positive test for relapsing fever species like *Borrelia hermsii* and *Borrelia miyamotoi*, Ehrlichia, Neo-Ehrlichia species, Anaplasma, Babesia species, Bartonella species, rickettsial species (Rocky Mountain spotted fever, Q fever, typhus), and/or tularemia also implies that you may have been bitten by a tick (although some of these infections can be transmitted by other routes), increasing the probability of having been exposed to Lyme disease.

With so many different strains of borrelia, when using standard labs like Quest or LabCorp, which only check for one strain, we can't expect to always pick up Lyme disease or other borrelia species. We therefore use speciality laboratories like IGeneX in California, which uses several strains of borrelia for their Lyme testing, resulting in more borrelia-specific bands showing up on the Western blot (23, 31, 34, 39, 83/93). Even one of these borrelia-specific bands in the right clinical setting can indicate exposure to Lyme or a related borrelia species and help establish the diagnosis. IGeneX also does a Babesia FISH test and a Bartonella FISH test, which is an RNA test not run by standard labs, helping to discover the presence of Babesia and Bartonella species when antibody or DNA tests are negative. Galaxy Diagnostics in North Carolina also check for multiple strains of Bartonella, helping to establish the diagnosis.

Testing should be based on exposure risk and symptoms. My experience has taught me that sending out a broad tick-borne screen on the initial visit may help to better define the illness, as there may have been exposure to less frequently seen infections, such as Q fever, tularemia, or Brucella, requiring specific treatment regimens early on in the course of therapy.

The following list of tests can be ordered by a healthcare provider, which can be an MD, DO, ND, PA, NP, chiropractor, or any other licensed health professional in your state. However, not every test is available in all states. After performing a complete history and physical, depending on your chief complaints, clinical history, social, family, and environmental history, as well as examination findings, your doctor should choose the appropriate tests from the list below to help establish a differential diagnosis. Most standard U.S. laboratories will perform the tests listed, except for some specialty testing for tick-borne disorders. Functional medicine testing that evaluates levels of toxins, mold, heavy metals, oxidative stress and detoxification pathways, hormone levels, as well as specific markers of GI health, are usually done through speciality laboratories, which are identified below:

ROUTINE BLOOD WORK: A CBC (complete blood count) and CMP (comprehensive metabolic profile, including electrolytes, liver and kidney function) is needed on the first visit and on follow-up visits, especially if taking antibiotics for tick-borne diseases. An EKG at the first visit is advisable, as Lyme (and co-infections) can affect the heart. Check for any evidence of arrhythmias, heart block, and/or other electrical abnormalities, such as prolongation of the QT interval on the electrocardiogram. A lengthened QT interval is a marker for potential ventricular arrhythmias, which could be impacted by certain medications used for treating MSIDS, like macrolides or quinolones, as well as other common medications like SSRIs, and PPIs.

LYME DISEASE/BORRELIOSIS: If you are doing testing for the first time, testing with a Lyme ELISA, or C6 ELISA, and IgM/IgG Western blot is generally a good idea, along with IgM and IgG Anaplasma/ Ehrlichia and Babesia testing, since these are the most commonly transmitted tick-borne infections (with *Borrelia miyamotoi*). If the ELISA is negative, perform a C6 ELISA, which is more sensitive. For the IgM and IgG Western blots, consider IGeneX laboratory in the United States, as it uses two strains of borrelia, the B-31 and 297 strains, which improves recognition of borrelia-specific bands versus using only the B-31 strain used by most commercial labs. Use other indirect tests such as the IFA and LTT (ELISPOT) if the above tests are indeterminate or negative, and consider antibody testing through Imugen for *Borrelia miyamotoi*, if it is available in your state. Direct testing using PCR for *B. burgdorferi* and *B. miyamotoi*, as well as the Lyme Dot Blot Assay (LDA), the Nanotrap test, and culture tests (Advanced Laboratory) can also be used. The LDA can be useful when initial Lyme panel tests on blood samples are negative (including PCR) and symptoms for Lyme disease are present, however cross reactions may occur with other non-Lyme antigens, so use caution.

The Nanotrap test was published in 2015, as a new urine antigen test for detecting early stage Lyme and can also evaluate treatment. PCRs can be performed on whole blood, serum, urine, breast milk, skin, and CSF, but due to the low numbers of bacteria usually present in specimens, samples can be negative and multiple tests may be necessary. TGen in Arizona is presently working on a newer generation PCR test to improve sensitivity.

EHRLICHIA/ANAPLASMA: human monocytic ehrlichiosis (HME) and human granulocytic anaplasmosis (HGA) titers with IgM/IgG antibodies.

BABESIOSIS/PARASITES: Babesia IFA (*microti, duncani*/WA-1), Babesia PCR/FISH assay (IGeneX), and Giemsa stains are available. A Babesia panel approach, using multiple tests, may be necessary to prove infection. Babesia suppresses the ability of the immune system to clear other parasites, so other parasitic testing should be considered, including FL-1953 (*Protomyxoa rheumatica*, Fry Labs), Toxoplasma IgM/IgG antibodies, and intestinal parasites if GI symptoms are present (amoeba, giardia, cryptosporidium, hookworm, pinworm, roundworm, including filariasis, and strongyloides). Filarial worms are also in black flies and mosquitos, and have recently been found in ticks and human specimens. Direct pathological examination and finding circulating antigens in the blood may help establish the diagnosis.

BARTONELLA: Bartonella IFA (multiple species, i.e., *B. henselae, B. Quintana, B. bacilliformis*)/PCR/FISH (IGeneX), and Bartonella panel through Galaxy labs in North Carolina (specialty laboratory). The vascular endothelial growth factor (VEGF) is an indirect marker of Bartonella activity, and can be positive when antibody testing is negative.

Talk with your doctor about further testing listed below, based on the results from the questionnaire. The HMQ can help you formulate, with your doctor, differential diagnoses that will explain your current health status. Using the HMQ, in combination with the Horowitz sixteen-point differential diagnostic MSIDS map on page 49 as well as Table 2.1 on pages 51–64, will help you create an effective healthcare plan.

OTHER BACTERIA: *Chlamydia pneumonia* IFA, Mycoplasma IFA + PCR (i.e., *M. fermentans*, Clongen Laboratories), RMSF, Q fever (phase I and phase II antibodies), typhus, Brucella IgM/IgG antibodies with an ag-glutination test (confirmatory), tularemia titers (IgM/IgG) if indicated, and *Yersinia enterocolitica* if reactive arthritis.

VIRAL INFECTIONS: IFAs/PCRs for Epstein Barr virus (EBV), human herpes virus-6 (HHV6), cytomegalovirus (CMV), West Nile, Coxsackie, Parvovirus. Consider a viral encephalitis panel if severe neurological symptoms: Testing is usually sent to state health departments for Powassan encephalitis, Eastern equine encephalitis, Western equine encephalomyelitis, Heartland, Bourbon, and Tacaribe viruses.

CANDIDA/FUNGI/MOLD BIOTOXINS: Stachybotrys titers can be done through most local laboratories as an initial screen for black mold. Consider Real Time Labs urine mycotoxin assay if there is a strong exposure history or resistant symptoms with a nasal swab/culture for mold and MARCoNS (Multiple Antibiotic Resistant Coagulase Negative Staphylococci); Histoplasmosis, Aspergillosis, Coccidiomycosis titers can also be done if clinically indicated.

RHEUMATOLOGY PANEL: antinuclear antibody (ANA), rheumatoid factor (RF), erythrocyte sedimentation rate (ESR), high sensitivity C-reactive protein (HS-CRP), complement studies (C3, C4, CH50, C1Q), HLA DR-2,4. If there is a suspicion of other autoimmune diseases, consider a single-stranded DNA (SS DNA), double-stranded DNA (dsDNA), especially if suspecting true lupus, Smith antigen (Sm Ag), seen in lupus, anti-cyclic citrullinated peptide antibody (CCP) if suspecting true rheumatoid arthritis, and Sjögren's SSA and SSB (Sjögren's syndrome). Antimitochondrial antibodies (AMA) can be checked if suspecting primary biliary cirrhosis (PBC). C3a, C4a, Transforming growth factor beta 1 (TGF-β1) and Matrix metalloproteinase 9 (MMP9) can be used to monitor inflammation, especially if there is mold exposure and joint involvement. A uric acid level should be done if there is a history of metabolic syndrome or gout.

FOOD ALLERGY PANEL: IgE, IgG antibodies with subclasses, antigliadin antibodies (an expanded panel can be obtained through Cyrex Laboratories) and Tissue Transglutaminase (TTG) to rule out gluten sensitivity and celiac disease. Consider a Comprehensive Digestive Stool Analysis (CDSA) to look for dysbiosis/evidence of leaky gut. A serum and urine histamine level can be obtained for indirect evidence of allergies (environmental/food), as well as skin allergy tests. Check tryptase levels if suspecting mast cell disorders.

ENDOCRINOLOGY/HORMONE TESTING: thyroid function tests (TFTs) including T3, Free T3, T4, reverse T3, thyroid stimulating hormone (TSH), anti-thyroid antibodies including anti-thyroid peroxidase antibodies (Anti-TPO ABs), anti-thyroglobulin antibodies (Anti-Tg ABs); an adrenal hormone panel (salivary DHEA/cortisol levels) through speciality labs (i.e., Labrix, ZRT, Genova, Diagnostek labs), and consider additional blood (8 am serum cortisol), and 24-hour urine cortisol testing; sex hormones, including follicle-stimulating hormone (FSH), luteinizing hormone (LH), estradiol, progesterone, testosterone, free testosterone, dihydrotestosterone (DHT), DHEA-sulfate (DHEA-S), pregnenolone, sex hormone binding globulin (SHBG), insulin-like growth factor 1 (IgF1) for growth hormone deficiency, intact parathyroid hormone (PTH) and calcium with Vitamin D levels if there is hypo/hypercalcemia without another etiology (i.e., cancer/metastases). Melanocyte Stimulating Hormome (MSH) and Vasointestinal Peptide (VIP) can be checked if mold exposure. Antidiuretic hormone (ADH) if frequent unexplained urination. Insulin, leptin and adiponectin levels if problems with weight.

VITAMIN TESTING: B_{12}, folate, methylmalonic acid (MMA) for occult B_{12} deficiency, homocysteine levels (HC) as a marker of oxidative stress and B vitamin/folate deficiency/cardiovascular risk, methylenetetrahydrofolate reductase (MTHFR) to evaluate methylation status, and Vitamin D 25-hydroxy (OH) levels and 1/25 OH-Vitamin D levels. A ratio of 1–25/25 OH Vitamin D greater than 2 is indicative of inflammation, as per a meta-analysis in the *Lancet Diabetes & Endocrinology* (2013), where overall Vitamin D levels were indicative of inflammation and overall death. Other: Vitamin A, other B vitamins (B_1, B_2, B_3, B_6, B_7), and Vitamin E levels when indicated (i.e., malabsorption, severe nutritional deficiency, alcohol use).

NUTRITIONAL TESTING: amino acids (AA), fatty acids (FAs, Omega 3/6/9 levels), mineral levels: iron, total iron binding capacity (TIBC), ferritin, serum magnesium, red blood cell (RBC) magnesium, zinc (serum, RBC), iodine, copper (serum, RBC), and ceruloplasmin levels if suspecting copper overload.

DETOXIFICATION AND OXIDATIVE STRESS TESTING/MITOCHONDRIAL EVALUATION: glutathione levels (serum), CoQ10, carnitine levels; specialty labs: Organix/ION test (Genova); consider lipid peroxides, 8-oxo-dG (8-hydroxy-2'-deoxyguanosine), and protein carbonyls as markers of oxidative stress.

IMMUNOLOGY PANEL: SPEP (serum protein electrophoresis) with IgA, IgM, and IgG levels with subclasses: Secretory IgA (sIgA) deficiency is associated with food allergies; IgM deficiency is seen in Lyme, and elevated levels are seen in acute infections and Waldenstrom's macroglobulinemia; IgG deficiencies and subclass deficiencies can be seen with Lyme, common variable immune deficiency (CVID), and cases of resistant neuropathy; elevated IgG levels with monoclonal kappa and lambda chains are seen with monoclonal gammopathy of unknown significance (MGUS) and multiple myeloma; therefore do an immunoelectrophoresis (IEP) if there are elevated IgM/IgG levels. Some physicians follow CD-57 natural killer (NK) cells as a marker of the immune response to Lyme, but they are not specific, and also found in HIV, autoimmune disease, and mercury exposure.

OTHER IMMUNE MARKERS: Antiganglioside ABs (GM1, Mag, ASI) IgM/IgG and antimyelin ABs should be checked for neuropathy, to rule out an autoimmune component. Do a Cunningham panel which measures immunoglobulin G (IgG) levels against receptors in the brain if considering an autoimmune encephalitis for unexplained neuropsychiatric or motor disorders.

FUNCTIONAL MEDICINE TESTING: includes heavy metal testing through Doctor's Data (six-hour urine DMSA challenge to evaluate levels of mercury, lead, arsenic, cadmium, aluminum), ION/Organix test (includes urine organic acids, fatty acids, vitamins, minerals, and antioxidants) through Genova, evaluating nutritional imbalances and detoxification pathways, and consider genetic testing such as the DetoxiGenomic profile (Genova) for single nucleotide polymorphisms (SNPs) if there are difficulties detoxifying chemicals. PacTox laboratory and Great Plains laboratories (GPL) do further environmental toxin testing. The Toxic Organic Chemical Exposure Profile (GPL-Tox) measures 168 different toxic chemicals and Tiglyglycine (TG), a marker for mitochondrial disorders resulting from mutations of mitochondrial DNA.

GASTROINTESTINAL: based on symptomatology, includes an antigliadin/TTG (a Cyrex Laboratories panel for expanded markers of gluten sensitivity is available in some states); consider an *H. pylori* antibody (and breath test if suspecting active infection); a breath test for Small Intestinal Bacterial Overgrowth (SIBO), fructose malabsorption, leaky gut; a CDSA with Ova and Parasite testing, and antibodies/culture for Entamoeba, Giardia, Schistosoma, Strongyloides, Cryptosporidium, and worms if there is a history of chronic diarrhea and/or foreign travel exposure; bacterial stool testing for *Clostridium difficile*, Salmonella, Shigella, Yersinia, Campylobacter, E. coli 0:157 can be performed if there is acute/chronic diarrhea.

ELEVATED LIVER FUNCTIONS: includes a hepatitis panel (A, B, C), iron (Fe)/total iron binding capacity (TIBC), and ferritin levels for hemochromatosis (iron overload), serum/RBC copper, and ceruloplasmin levels (to rule out copper overload/Wilson's disease), antinuclear antibodies (ANA)/anti-mitochondrial antibodies (AMA) for autoimmune hepatitis/primary biliary cirrhosis, and alpha-1-antitrypsin levels.

The Six Biggest Signs That You Suffer from Lyme Disease and Co-infections

1. You have more than one symptom: Lyme disease is a multisystemic illness. Many of my patients present with a constellation of symptoms, which oftentimes include fatigue, pain, stiffness, tingling/numbness/burning/stabbing sensations, memory and concentration problems, and mood and sleep disorders. A score greater than 63 on the HMQ infers a high probability of exposure and a score of 45–62 indicates probable exposure.
2. Your symptoms come and go with good and bad days (without an obvious reason).

3. Your pain migrates around your body. Joint, muscle, and nerve pains that come and go and migrate around the body are classic for Lyme disease and are not seen in other diseases like CFS/SEID, fibromyalgia, or most autoimmune illnesses. One exception is inflammatory bowel disorders, where transient migratory arthritis can be part of the clinical picture; however, we would expect a predominance of gastrointestinal manifestations.

4. Women's symptoms tend to worsen right before, during, and after the menstrual cycle (hormonal changes and low estrogen levels often affect symptoms).

5. Symptoms often worsen or improve after antibiotic therapy (for Lyme or an unrelated infection like a urinary tract infection or upper respiratory infection). If you have been diagnosed with a nonspecific fatiguing, musculoskeletal illness and get better with antibiotics, it implies a bacterial origin to your illness. Worsening of symptoms can occur with antibiotic treatment due to a Herxheimer reaction (JH reaction), which is an inflammatory process secondary to the killing off of spirochetes (see Chapter 3). This usually resolves shortly after the antibiotic course is stopped, but symptoms may continue if you have angered the bacteria and "woke them up."

6. You have positive blood tests for Lyme and associated tick-borne diseases. As we discussed, the tests are not reliable (such as the ELISA and Western blot), and this is due in part to the different strains of borrelia that exist in the United States and Europe, which cannot all be picked up on standard testing. One way we can determine if you have been exposed to one of these borrelia species is that there are five bands (proteins) on the Western blot that are specific for borreliosis. These are the 23 (Osp C), 31 (Osp A), 34 (Osp B), 39, and 83–93 kdA (kilodalton) proteins. If you have many of the six signs and symptoms of Lyme disease, with a high score on the HMQ, and even one borrelia-specific band on a sensitive Western blot, this implies that you have been bitten by a tick and that your symptoms may be due to Lyme disease or other borrelia species, especially if you have ruled out overlapping medical conditions.

TWO

A Comprehensive Diagnosis: The Horowitz Sixteen-Point Differential Diagnostic Map

One of the most important axioms in medicine is "Do no harm." The second most important axiom is "An open mind doesn't mean that your brain will fall out." The information in this chapter may nudge some readers out of their diagnostic comfort zones. However, if you have a strong motivation to feel better, or to help sick and suffering patients, leaving your comfort zone can be rewarding.

Let's start with the basics. Naming an illness and prescribing a drug for it does not necessarily mean that you have properly understood the illness or adequately treated it. The medical system continues to struggle with the causes of many illnesses, like cancer and Alzheimer's disease. Is it possible that there are common denominators underlying these illnesses that can help us improve our prevention and treatment? As we continue to investigate, medicine has even come up with a term for diseases that we do not understand: We call them "idiopathic." One of my patients once translated this for me as the "pathetic idiocy" of chronic disease medicine today.

In the last chapter, we began the process of understanding and diagnosing Lyme disease and Multiple Systemic Infectious Disease Syndrome (MSIDS) by using the HMQ to identify the many different symptoms you may be experiencing. The next step is to divide these symptoms into component parts to discover their source. In some instances, we'll find that they stem from one disease process. However, it is much more likely that if you or your patient is suffering from a chronic disease, there may be both interconnected and overlapping medical problems responsible for the symptoms.

One of the essential problems with the traditional medical model is that doctors are taught that there is generally only one cause for each illness. Yet I believe that instead of looking for one answer, we should be looking for many. In fact, I have identified sixteen likely causes of illnesses that can occur simultaneously with Lyme disease (Lyme-MSIDS) or exacerbate the symptoms of other diseases that occur without Lyme disease (non–Lyme-MSIDS) by increasing inflammation.

The difficulty in establishing a diagnosis for Lyme disease is that it is considered to be "the great imitator." Like its cousin, syphilis, Lyme disease can mimic many illnesses and exacerbate previously existing medical problems, and it can cause symptoms that are seen with each of the sixteen separate medical conditions I've outlined below. For example, if you were always prone to headaches, you may begin to have migraines with Lyme or Lyme-MSIDS. The medical literature provides abundant evidence on this subject, even though it is not entirely clear why the disease manifests in different ways for each particular individual. It may be influenced by your genetic code and unique bioindividuality, as well as by the number of tick bites you received, other co-infections, your present immune status, the presence of other overlapping diseases and inflammatory conditions, your environmental toxin load and detoxification ability, your underlying psychological status, and the particular strain or species of borrelia with which you were infected.

Because of all of these disparate factors, each person can present with Lyme disease in a unique way. For example, although many of my patients were diagnosed with a primary psychiatric disorder before they first came to see me, Lyme disease has been known to cause a host of neuropsychiatric abnormalities. In fact, virtually every psychiatric diagnosis listed in the *Diagnostic and Statistical Manual (DSM),* the bible of mental health diagnoses, can be caused by Lyme disease and associated co-infections.

Similarly, Lyme disease can mimic a whole host of neurological syndromes: It can cause neurocognitive deficits in both children and adults, and it has even been associated with Tourette's and neurological syndromes such as Alzheimer's disease. The same problem exists with chronic fatigue syndrome (which has been renamed as systemic exertional intolerance disease, or SEID) and fibromyalgia. Lyme disease can also mimic autoimmune disorders such as rheumatoid arthritis, lupus, and multiple sclerosis. Therefore, resistant symptoms may possibly be the result of failing to diagnose and treat the underlying infections correctly, and of not having addressed enough of the abnormalities present on the MSIDS map.

I believe that the persistent symptoms of Lyme disease are more than simply one infection that will not go away. Of the more than twelve thousand patients seen in our medical center, almost none of them had "only" Lyme disease. In fact, most have a clinically recognizable syndrome, an association of several symptoms occurring together. Some typical Lyme symptoms are worsened by co-infections like Babesia and Bartonella, as well as by the presence of other multiple overlapping factors on the MSIDS map. Some of these abnormalities are caused by Lyme and co-infections, and some are unrelated but nevertheless affecting the clinical course.

I call this condition Multiple Systemic Infectious Disease Syndrome (MSIDS) because it better defines those patients for whom initial treatments for Lyme disease have not worked. MSIDS is a symptom complex of Lyme disease and multiple associated tick-borne co-infections that encompasses not only infections with *Borrelia burgdorferi* but also other bacterial, viral, parasitic, and fungal infections. Patients with MSIDS can also have evidence of associated immune dysfunction, inflammation, environmental toxins and heavy metal burdens, detoxification problems, nutritional deficiencies, hormonal abnormalities, sleep disorders, mitochondrial dysfunction, food allergies and sensitivities, and deconditioning and imbalances in their autonomic nervous system (ANS), the part of the body that controls the heart rate, blood pressure, and digestive system. All of these factors can keep you chronically ill.

By using this definition, I can treat my patients more effectively, because most patients are unable to recover their health unless the majority of these factors are properly addressed. This may be the reason why so many people don't improve with the standard Lyme treatments, such as one month of doxycycline or Rocephin. The design of many of the double-blind, placebo-controlled studies evaluating treatments for Lyme disease do not take into account these potential multifactorial causes, so giving only one or two antibiotics for a short period of time only addresses a small piece of the complex puzzle. The answers lie in a more holistic diagnostic and treatment approach.

WHY IS THERE CONFUSION OVER THE DIAGNOSIS AND TREATMENT OF LYME DISEASE?

As of 2016, there is only one current standard of care for the diagnosis and treatment of Lyme disease in the United States: the International Lyme and Associated Diseases Society (ILADS) guidelines. The Infectious Disease Society of America (IDSA) guidelines were recently removed from the National Guidelines Clearinghouse (NGC) because they contained outdated science. The NGC is part of the U.S. Department of Health and Human Services (HHS), and they recently accepted the ILADS standard of care, which used Institute of Medicine (IOM) criteria for developing trustworthy guidelines. The ILADS recommendations for the diagnosis and treatment of Lyme disease is the first set of guidelines to comply with these high IOM standards.

ILADS also integrated a specific methodology to develop their guidelines, known as the Grading of Recommendations Assessment, Development, and Evaluation (GRADE) process, which is used by top medical organizations across the globe, including the American College of Physicians (ACP), the World Health Organization (WHO), and the National Institute for Health and Clinical Excellence (NICE) in the United Kingdom. This means that the ILADS guidelines represent the best available medical evidence available at the time of their publication. These guidelines stress the importance of a doctor's clinical judgment in making the diagnosis, because the scientific literature has found that the existing testing is unreliable. The previously available IDSA guidelines narrowly restricted the diagnosis to just the CDC criteria. Accordingly, the Lyme blood tests were held to be reliable, and patients with persistent Lyme symptoms after standard treatment were felt to have post-treatment Lyme disease syndrome (PTLDS) with autoimmune phenomenon and/ or damage to tissue accounting for their ongoing symptoms. The problem with this approach is that the CDC uses a strict surveillance definition, which was developed for the national reporting of Lyme disease, and it is primarily used by health departments for epidemiological purposes. The CDC Surveillance Case Definition is narrow, meaning a minority of actual cases will meet its strict criteria. The definition can only be satisfied in the following two ways:

A. a case with an erythema migrans (EM) rash 5 centimeters or larger
B. a case with at least one late, objective manifestation, such as meningitis (inflammation occurring in the membranes covering the brain and spinal cord), cranial neuropathy (cranial nerve damage), brief attacks of arthritis, or AV block (an electrical conduction defect in the heart) that is laboratory confirmed.

According to this CDC Surveillance Case Definition, late manifestations require laboratory confirmation. This may involve obtaining a positive culture for *Borrelia burgdorferi* from blood, skin, a joint, or cerebral spinal fluid (CSF), or by identifying antibodies to the bacterium in the cerebrospinal fluid; the most common method, however, known as the two-tier testing algorithm, uses a specific sequence of blood tests. The first is an ELISA, the second is a Western blot. These are indirect tests of infection, because instead of identifying the organism itself, they look for antibodies to *Borrelia burgdorferi* that were made by the immune system. The ELISA tests measure the total amount of anti-*Borrelia burgdorferi* antibodies present, while Western blots identify individual antibodies and look for specific protein patterns that are unique to borrelia. If enough of these borrelia proteins are present, the test is considered to be positive. Although the surveillance case definition does firmly establish a Lyme disease diagnosis, many patients unfortunately do not meet these criteria because these tests are often inaccurate. That is why the CDC has publicly stated on their Web site: "This surveillance case definition was developed for national reporting of Lyme disease; it is not intended to be used in clinical diagnosis."

No one test or combinations of tests is perfect in establishing a laboratory diagnosis, and there are extensive scientific references in the medical literature documenting false-negative blood tests. The CDC points out that there are problems with testing, and that a patient with Lyme disease may not be diagnosed using these criteria. This has been confirmed in many studies. The first was a New York State Department of Health study conducted in 1996, which was reported to the CDC. Among the 1,535 patients studied, 81 percent of non-EM cases were not confirmed with the present two-tiered testing algorithm. In other words, the presently used two-tiered testing missed 81 percent of the Lyme cases, especially when they did not have a bull's-eye rash.

One of the most comprehensive reviews of the standard Lyme tests comes from a 2005 study at Johns Hopkins University, confirming the poor sensitivity of the ELISA. Working with early diagnosed Lyme disease patients from Pennsylvania and Maryland, the Hopkins scientists studied state-of-the-art blood and DNA tests (PCR testing) for Lyme and found serious flaws. Most tellingly, when the standard two-step method recommended by the CDC was used on patients with other laboratory evidence of Lyme disease, it was positive between 45 percent and 77 percent of the time. As for the DNA tests, the Hopkins researchers reported that these tests rarely pick up otherwise confirmed Lyme disease at all. In another study, published in the *Journal of Medical Microbiology* in 2005, Dr. Antonella Marangoni reported that three different commercial ELISA tests showed discrepant results. The sensitivity for the same blood tested varied between 36.8 percent and 70.5 percent. A study by Ang in 2011 confirmed that not only was the ELISA an insensitive test, but that various Western blot kits often gave discordant results on the same specimen. He concluded that the likelihood of a patient being diagnosed with Lyme disease was highly influenced by which ELISA–Western blot combination was used. This confirmed the results of a prior study done by Lori L. Bakken, published in the *Journal of the Clinical Microbiology* years before. Another study, published in 2007 in the *British Medical Journal* by Ray Stricker, MD, and Lorraine Johnson, found that the overall sensitivity of the combined ELISA–Western blot was only 56 percent. These findings mirror what I have found in my own practice: Many of my patients do have Lyme disease, but standard testing protocols are not sensitive enough to pick it up, and those who fail the ELISA may never go on to be tested with a confirmatory Western blot by doctors using IDSA guidelines.

The ILADS guidelines state that Lyme disease is a clinical diagnosis. Cases meeting the CDC criteria qualify under the ILADS definition, as do patients who have symptoms consistent with Lyme disease and a history of potential exposure to the ticks that transmit the illness, particularly if symptoms cannot be rightfully attributed to other diseases. Positive two-tier testing is not required, because they hold the view that the present available testing is unreliable. So you may have some Lyme-specific bands on the Western blot (e.g., 23 kDa, 31 kDa, 34 kDa, 39 kDa, 83–93 kDa) but do not have the exact pattern required to be considered positive by the CDC—and yet have a clinical presentation and treatment response consistent with the illness when other disease processes have been ruled out. The CDC criterion also demands looking for Lyme disease without testing for multiple strains: They recommend trying to find five out of ten positive bands on an IgG Western blot for *Borrelia burgdorferi*, or two out of three specific bands on an IgM Western blot (23 kDa, 39 kDa, 41 kDa) to confirm the diagnosis, and only if the ELISA is positive. Yet in clinical practice, patients with persistent Lyme disease symptoms rarely meet CDC criteria for a positive IgG Western blot, and more often, they have a positive IgM Western blot, seen in both early and late Lyme. The magnitude of real Lyme patients eluding the standard tests could be vast, as suggested by screening conducted to confirm the diagnosis in a study for the National Institutes of Health. When Dr. Brian Fallon, an internationally recognized expert in the neuropsychiatric aspects of Lyme disease, screened patients known to have been exposed to Lyme in an NIH double-blind study, approximately one out of one hundred patients actually met the CDC criteria for a positive IgG Western blot, although they clearly had been exposed to borrelia and remained ill.

Based on the review of prior randomized controlled trials, where patients did not have an optimal long-term response to the therapies used, the new ILADS guidelines take a patient-centered response, where there is no fixed duration or combination of antibiotics. Instead, the guidelines suggest tailoring the therapy to the patient's response, and adjusting therapy accordingly to reduce the risk of chronic complications due to inadequate treatment. This approach has been effective in the thousands of patients that I have treated over the past twenty-nine years.

The opposing guidelines have confused many healthcare providers as to the best way to diagnose and treat Lyme disease. The MSIDS model explains in part the differences between the IDSA and ILADS approach to identifying and treating Lyme disease. My model allows Lyme to be redefined as MSIDS: a clinical syndrome that encompasses multiple overlapping factors that keep you chronically ill. Many doctors have adopted the model, based on my having presented the MSIDS map as part of a large body of published scientific research with positive clinical outcomes. The value of this multifactorial model has also been published in the peer reviewed medical literature by myself and others.

Nine Clinical Diagnostic Standards for Lyme Disease

1. Lyme disease is a clinical diagnosis, and lab results support the clinical diagnosis.

2. An erythema migrans (EM) rash is definitive evidence of an infection with borrelia (like Lyme disease), and does not require laboratory confirmation to make a diagnosis. Although many EM rashes do resemble "bull's-eye rashes," there are also other Lyme-related rashes. One is a solid red, expanding rash that may look like a cellulitis (bacterial infection of the skin) or spider bite. Multiple EM rashes are indicative of a disseminated borrelia infection, as are EM rashes with central nervous system (CNS) manifestations (stiff neck, headache, light and sound sensitivity, dizziness, cognitive difficulties, tingling/numbness/burning of the scalp or face) or peripheral nervous system (PNS) manifestations (tingling, numbness, burning, and/or stabbing sensations of the extremities).

3. Patients often have negative blood tests if tested too early, or if antibiotics have been used early in the course of the disease, since this may prevent antibodies from being produced.

4. The two-tiered protocol of using a Lyme ELISA followed by a Western blot will miss approximately half of those affected, due to the insensitivity of the tests.

5. The Western blot may provide us with useful information, but it also has its limitations. The utility of the Western blot is based on the expertise of the laboratory performing the test, which strain(s) of borrelia the patient was exposed to, and identifying the specific bands on the Western blot that reflect exposure to *Borrelia burgdorferi* or other borrelia species.

   Borrelia-specific bands reflect outer surface proteins (Osp) on the surface of the organism that are seen more often in Lyme disease than in other infections. These bands include the following five proteins, each with different molecular weights (in kDa): 23 kDa (Osp C, e.g., outer surface protein C), 31 kDa (Osp A), 34 kDa (Osp B), 39 kDa, and 83–93 kDa. If any of these bands are present on a Western blot, there is a high likelihood that you have been exposed to Lyme disease or another borrelia species, especially with the right clinical symptomatology. If two or more of these specific bands are present, the likelihood increases even further. We have found that a specialty lab, such as IGeneX, has a better chance of finding more borrelia-specific bands on the Western blot, because it uses different strains of *Borrelia burgdorferi* for its testing (both the B31 and 297 strains). While use of this laboratory often has been considered controversial among some IDSA physicians, many ILADS physicians find it to be a reliable resource. IGeneX has passed the strict testing guidelines of New York State and California, and is certified by the U.S. government via the Centers for Medicare and Medicaid Services (CMS). I perform a Western blot only through highly qualified laboratories, as there may be discrepancies in the testing, similar to the problems we face with the ELISA test.

6. Other tests: Polymerase chain reaction (PCR), a DNA test, is an important diagnostic tool for patients who have negative blood tests, but often require multiple samples over time, using specimens from different body compartments (such as serum, aspirated joint fluid, synovial tissue, urine, cord blood, placenta, and/or spinal fluid), and it must be performed at a reliable laboratory. The PCR has an overall sensitivity of around 30 percent on any individual specimen, with a specificity of over 99 percent (it is highly specific for the disease, with few false positive results). Advances in more sensitive PCR tests were reported in 2012; more recent tests for the direct molecular detection and identifying the specific species of borrelia have increased the sensitivity to 62 percent in early Lyme disease. In my practice, I may send off several sets of PCRs on blood or urine before getting back a positive result.

Culture of borrelia is the gold standard for testing, and it is universally accepted by the IDSA, ILADS, and the CDC. The successful culture of borrelia isolates in the laboratory, by using borrelia-specific Barbour-Stoenner-Kelly (BSK) media, even from confirmed Lyme disease cases, has been a challenging task because the organism grows slowly and is difficult to culture. Several of my patients have had this test performed by other physicians after treatment with extended courses of antibiotics for Lyme disease, and they returned with a positive culture from Advanced Laboratories, implying persistence of the organism. Results of the accuracy of this borrelia culture are pending publication in a peer-review journal, as the CDC has challenged the accuracy of the test. However, its accuracy was confirmed in a 2013 peer-reviewed study by Eva Sapi, PhD.

7. There are approximately one hundred strains of borrelia present in the United States and over three hundred different strains worldwide. In the Northeast, 10 percent to 20 percent of the borrelia presently in ticks are not *Borrelia burgdorferi*, the causative agent of Lyme disease, but they are genetically related to *Borrelia miyamotoi*, the agent of relapsing fever in Japan. These organisms will not test positive by ELISA, Western blot, or PCR assays for Lyme disease. A patient with a Lyme-like illness may therefore have been exposed to one of the other strains of borrelia, explaining seronegative test results for Lyme disease. Testing for *Borrelia miyamotoi* by antibody titer (not available in all states) and PCR may be helpful in determining whether other species are present. Other strains include:

- *Borrelia burgdorferi sensu stricto* (U.S., Europe, North Africa), a cause of EM rashes
- *Borrelia afzelii* (Europe, Asia), the cause of ACA skin rashes
- *Borrelia garinii* (Europe, Asia, North Africa), a cause of neuroborreliosis
- *Borrelia valaisiana*
- *Borrelia lusitaniae* (Portugal, Italy, North Africa)
- *Borrelia spielmanii* (Holland, Germany, Hungary, Slovenia), a cause of early skin disease
- *Borrelia burgdorferi sensu lato* (northern U.S.), a cause of STARI
- *Borrelia americanum* (northern U.S.)
- *Borrelia andersonii* (southern U.S.)
- *Borrelia bissettii* (western U.S., Europe, Asia)
- *Borrelia japonica, Borrelia turdi, Borrelia tanukii, Borrelia sinica* (Asia)

8. Other tick-borne diseases, such as Babesia (a malaria-like parasite) and Bartonella (cat scratch disease) can be transmitted by the

same tick that transmits Lyme disease. These diseases complicate the clinical presentation, often worsening the symptoms of Lyme disease. They are similarly difficult to diagnose reliably with standard screening procedures, using, for example, a Babesia smear (Giemsa stain) and Bartonella titer (immunofluorescent assay, or IFA), since like borrelia, there are multiple species, and testing must not only include antibody titers but also may need to include PCR (DNA testing) and FISH (RNA testing) assays as well.

9. Any positive titer for one tick-borne disease (TBD) suggests that other TBD's may be present, since ticks are often co-infected. This is especially true for patients who failed treatment regimens for any one specific disease process.

IDENTIFYING MULTIPLE SYSTEMIC INFECTIOUS DISEASE SYNDROME (MSIDS)

For every patient who comes into my office, I review the potential sixteen differential diagnoses against the results of the questionnaire and patient history. By doing so I can gather the most complete assessment of my patient's current health and what needs to be done regarding testing and treatment going forward.

Most of the disease processes that I am about to discuss are not new. But when healthcare providers can look at them together, the strength of using this system is that they will finally have a single tool that organizes the list of seemingly unrelated symptoms that a chronically ill person brings to the doctor.

Although the diagnostic process began with searching for answers for Lyme disease, I believe the MSIDS model is applicable to anyone with a chronic illness. All people with chronic diseases may have elements of MSIDS, and those with a chronic illness may benefit from using the sixteen-point differential diagnostic map described on the following page. Chronic inflammation lies at the heart of most chronic diseases, and addressing the underlying causes of inflammation, using the MSIDS map, has the potential to decrease inflammation and improve health. The initial inflammation may have developed as a direct effect of Lyme disease

and associated co-infections, or it could be a response to an overstimulated immune system, environmental toxins, food allergies, mineral deficiencies, imbalances of the microbiome, or an associated sleep disorder.

Another benefit of the MSIDS model is that even if you are having a
positive response to medications, you may have untoward long-term side
effects, and there may be ways of mitigating those side effects by finding
other treatable causes of your symptoms and the disease process.

This diagnostic tool can therefore serve as a map for clinicians evaluating not just a patient with Lyme disease and co-infections but anyone
with a chronic, unexplained illness. There may be disease processes that
we still don't completely understand, yet you can benefit clinically from
using this model. Understanding this syndrome is the key to gaining a
better understanding of chronic disease states as we uncover hidden
underlying factors driving your persistent illness.

MSIDS: Overlapping Factors Contributing to Chronic Illness

1. Lyme disease and co-infections
2. Immune dysfunction
3. Inflammation
4. Environmental toxins
5. Functional medicine abnormalities with nutritional deficiencies
6. Mitochondrial dysfunction
7. Endocrine abnormalities
8. Neurodegenerative disorders
9. Neuropsychiatric disorders
10. Sleep disorders
11. Autonomic nervous system dysfunction and postural ortho-
    static tachycardia syndrome (POTS)
12. Allergies
13. Gastrointestinal disorders
14. Liver dysfunction
15. Pain disorders/addiction
16. Lack of exercise/deconditioning

USING THE HOROWITZ SIXTEEN-POINT
DIFFERENTIAL DIAGNOSTIC MSIDS MAP

You can begin to use this system to determine if you are suffering from more than just Lyme disease. You may quickly find that you have MSIDS, and you then will be able to use this tool with your doctor to begin to improve your symptoms and overall health.

The first step is to get copies of all of your medical records. This may be difficult if you have been seeing many different doctors. However, it is your right as a patient to have access to your medical information. This information is essential so your current healthcare provider can review the scope of your testing and treatment and determine how best to proceed.

Once you have gathered your documentation, determine whether you have been appropriately and comprehensively tested for all of the conditions that comprise the sixteen-point differential diagnostic map. The following table can help you determine which tests to ask for, based on the results of your questionnaire. This list includes some of the most common differential diagnoses and medical conditions responsible for the associated symptoms. It is not intended to be a comprehensive differential diagnostic list or a comprehensive list of laboratory testing to consider. The most common testing panel for Lyme disease includes: Lyme ELISA, C6 ELISA, and IgM/IgG Western blots (through IGeneX Laboratories, which looks for borrelia-specific bands). PCRs, LTT (ELISPOT), and the Nanotrap test can also be included in the workup if the initial testing is negative or inconclusive. Culture tests and evaluating inflammatory chemokines in the Spirotest (i.e., CXCL9, CXCL10, CCL19) would be considered third-tier testing at this time, if available in your state. I refer to this testing panel in the chart below as "Suggested Lyme Panel." An * indicates a medical condition that is not generally part of the MSIDS map but is part of a differential diagnostic list that should be considered in a patient with those symptoms.

This list can help anyone who has failed multiple interventions to determine what is accounting for their symptoms. Healthcare providers can include a copy in patient charts to remind them of which approaches have been tried and where there have been successes and failures. I use the sixteen-point map to decide when to stop or rotate antibiotics if my patient has been through several rounds of medications and has not had

Table 2.1: Symptoms and Associated Medical Conditions on the Sixteen-Point MSIDS Map

Symptoms	Possible Related Medical Conditions	Laboratory Testing to Consider
Unexplained fevers, sweats, chills, or flushing	• Lyme disease (chronic and other bacterial, viral, parasitic, and fungal infections) • Babesiosis • Malaria • Brucellosis • Hyperthyroidism • Hormonal failure (early menopause) • Tuberculosis* • Non-Hodgkin's lymphoma* • Panic disorders • Autoimmune disorders • Inflammation	• CBC with a white cell count • CMP with liver functions • Lyme and co-infections • Giemsa stain and malarial smears • *Babesia microti* IFA • *Babesia* WA-1/*duncani* titers • Babesia FISH • Babesia PCR • Thyroid function tests (TFTs) • Sex hormone levels • Chest X-ray/PPD • Antinuclear antibody (ANA) • Rheumatoid factor (RF) • Erythrocyte sedimentation rate (ESR) • C-reactive protein (CRP) • Cytokine panel
Unexplained weight change, either loss or gain	• Lyme disease • Certain co-infections (brucellosis, among others) • Hormonal disorders (thyroid, adrenal, low sex hormones) • Metabolic syndrome with increased insulin secretion • Malignancy*	• Suggested Lyme panel • Co-infection testing, including Q fever, Bartonella species, Brucella species (antibodies/agglutination test), other infections, i.e., mycobacteria (QuantiFERON-TB testing) • TFTs • Sex hormones • DHEA/cortisol • HbA1c with insulin levels • Lipid profile • Appropriate cancer screening
Fatigue, tiredness	• Lyme disease and associated co-infections • Immune dysfunction • Inflammation • Environmental toxins and mold • Functional medicine abnormalities with nutritional deficiencies	• Suggested Lyme panel • Evaluate for Lyme specific bands, 23 [OspC], 31, [OspA], 34 [Osp B], 39, 83–93); consider LTT, Nanotrap test, culture, Spirotest • *Babesia microti* IFA • *Babesia duncani*/WA-1

Symptoms	Possible Related Medical Conditions	Laboratory Testing to Consider
Fatigue, tiredness *(continued)*	• Mitochondrial dysfunction • Endocrine abnormalities • Neurodegenerative disorders • Neuropsychiatric disorders • Sleep disorders • Autonomic nervous system dysfunction and POTS • Allergies • Gastrointestinal disorders • Liver dysfunction • Pain disorders/addiction • Lack of exercise/deconditioning	• Babesia FISH • Babesia PCR • Relapsing fever Borrelia (EIA, IFA, Western blots, culture, PCR) • *Ehrlichia* and *Anaplasma* titers • Bartonella species (IFA, PCRs), +/−FISH (through IGeneX) +/−Galaxy Lab testing • Mycoplasma species (IFA, PCRs, including *M. fermentans*) • *Chlamydia pneumonia* • RMSF, Q fever, typhus • tularemia • Brucella • Viruses (HHV6, EBV, CMV, West Nile) • CBC, CMP • ANA, RF • ESR, CRP • Ganglioside antibodies • Complement studies • CPK • HLA testing (DR2, DR4, B27) • GM1AB IgM/IgG, Mag IgM/IgG ABs, ASI GM AB IgM/IgG • Immunoglobulin levels (IgM, IgA, IgG) and subclasses • Cytokine panels • Six-hour urine DMSA challenge for heavy metals • Mineral levels (serum magnesium, RBC mag++, iodine, iron, serum and RBC zinc/copper) • Parasite studies (stool CDSA, blood) • Food allergy panel (IgE and IgG), histamine levels (blood, urine), DAO level, sIgA • Antigliadin ABs (i.e., Cyrex Labs), TTG • Hormonal studies (thyroid: T3, free T3, T4, reverse T3, TSH; DHEA/cortisol, salivary testing; sex hormone levels: estradiol, progesterone, testosterone, DHT, SHBG, pregnenolone; IgF1)

Symptoms	Possible Related Medical Conditions	Laboratory Testing to Consider
Fatigue, tiredness (continued)		• Five-hour glucose tolerance, with insulin levels • Tilt table with ANS evaluation • B_{12}, folate, MMA and HC levels • Mitrochondrial testing • Mold (Stachybotrys titers, mold plates, urine mycotoxin testing (Real Time Labs), and ERMI (Environmental Relative Moldiness Index) testing • Organix test (Genova Diagnostics) for E.I. • Lipid oxidation: thiobarbituric acid reactive substances assay (TBARS) and lipid peroxides • DNA oxidation (8-OhdG, autoantibodies to oxidized DNA, modified Comet assay) • Protein oxidation (protein carbonyls) • Sleep studies • Neuropsychiatric evaluation with SPECT scans • MRI brain scan
Unexplained hair loss	• Lyme disease and co-infections • Stress • Inflammation • Dermatological disorders* • Autoimmune disorders • Pregnancy* • Mineral deficiencies • Selenium toxicity • Hormonal disorders	• Infections • Mineral levels (serum and RBC) • Iron deficiency (Fe, TIBC, ferritin) • Thyroid deficiency • High Dihydrotestosterone (DHT) • ANA • ESR, CRP • Cytokine panel • Dermatological evaluation
Swollen glands	• Lyme disease and co-infections, especially Bartonella and tularemia if lymph nodes are significantly enlarged • Viruses such as mononucleosis/Epstein-Barr virus • Malignancy*	• Lyme and co-infections • Appropriate cancer screening

Symptoms	Possible Related Medical Conditions	Laboratory Testing to Consider
Sore throat	• Lyme disease (if symptom comes and goes in monthly cycles) • Strep* • Viral infections • Allergies	• Throat swab and/or culture for strep • Test for viruses • Lyme and co-infections • Allergy testing
Testicular pain (men), pelvic pain (women)	• Lyme disease • Epididymitis with or without orchitis* • Testicular torsion* • Endometriosis/ovarian cysts* • Urinary tract infection (UTI)*	• Lyme • Physical examination with urethral swabs • Abdominal/pelvic ultrasounds • Urinalysis and culture
Unexplained menstrual irregularity	• Lyme disease • Hormonal dysregulation, anorexia • Stress	• Female hormones and prolactin levels, check BMI (body mass index) • Lyme
Unexplained milk production, breast pain	• Lyme disease • Hormonal dysregulation· • Fibrocystic breast disease*	• Female hormones and prolactin levels • Serum iodine levels • Significant caffeine use? • Lyme testing
Irritable bladder or bladder dysfunction	• Interstitial cystitis, with or without Lyme disease and Bartonella • Dropped bladder* • BPH (benign prostatic hypertrophy with outlet obstruction)* • UTI (bacterial)* • Fungal infections • MS and diseases that affect nerve function	• Urinalysis (UA) • Culture and sensitivity (C+S) • Urological examination with scope and cystometric studies • Lyme and co-infections • Testing for MS (VEP, AEP, MRI, spinal tap checking for oligoclonal bands and MBP)
Sexual dysfunction or loss of libido	• Lyme with overlapping co-infections • Low sex hormones (testosterone, estrogen) • Vascular insufficiency* • Psychological factors • medication (i.e., SSRIs..)*	• Lyme and co-infections • Hormone evaluations: testosterone, free T, DHT, DHEA-S, SHBG, estradiol, pregnenolone and progesterone (women) • Check thyroid and adrenal if sex hormones normal • Vascular evaluation if ED • Psychological evaluation • Evaluation of side effects of medication

Symptoms	Possible Related Medical Conditions	Laboratory Testing to Consider
Upset stomach	• GERD with reflux* • *H. pylori* • Gallbladder dysfunction* • Food allergies • Histamine intolerance • Stress • Medications* • Lyme disease, co-infections	• GI testing: serum antibodies for *H. pylori* +/−breath test • Upper endoscopy • Gallbladder ultrasound/HIDA scan • Food allergy testing • Serum and urinary histamine levels, DAO levels • Evaluation of side effects of medications • Lyme, co-infections
Change in bowel function (constipation or diarrhea)	• Irritable bowel syndrome (IBS) • Small intestinal bacterial overgrowth (SIBO) • Inflammatory bowel disease (IBD) • Celiac disease • Gluten intolerance • Food allergies and intolerances • Stress • Dehydration* • Infections (*E. coli* 0:157, *Salmonella*, *Shigella*, *Campylobacter*, *Yersinia*, *Clostridium difficile*, rotaviruses, parasites) • Magnesium deficiency • Lyme disease • *Candida*	• CBC • CMP with electrolytes, BUN/creatinine, liver functions (LFTs) • Mineral levels • Antigliadin ABs (Cyrex Labs) and TTG levels • Food allergy panel • Breath test for small intestinal bacterial overgrowth (SIBO), leaky gut, fructose/lactose intolerance • Stool cultures: bacteria, parasites, *Candida* • Stool for *Clostridium difficile* toxin A&B, PCRs • Stool CDSA (comprehensive digestive stool analysis) • GI evaluation with colonoscopy • Lyme and co-infections
Chest pain or rib soreness	• Lyme disease • Costochondritis (inflammation in the ribs) • Coronary artery disease* • Fractures* • Pulmonary embolism*	• Lyme, co-infections • EKG and cardio-pulmonary evaluation (EST, D-dimer, CT pulmonary angiography) • Physical examination (pushing on the ribs is usually painful with costochondritis) • X-ray if suspecting fractures (pain, rub on auscultation)

Symptoms	Possible Related Medical Conditions	Laboratory Testing to Consider
Shortness of breath, cough	• Over 90 percent of coughs are due to allergic rhinitis with a postnasal drip, with or without asthma with reactive airway disease, and GERD with reflux* • Babesia presents with an atypical cough and "air hunger" • Bacterial and fungal infections (TB, chronic bronchitis, histoplasmosis, coccidiomycosis) • COPD* • Interstitial lung disease* • Malignancy in smokers* • Inflammation • Pulmonary embolism*	• *Babesia microti* and *duncani* IFA, FISH, PCR, Giemsa stain • QuantiFERON-TB, sputum samples/bronchoalveolar lavage (BAL), culture, antibody/PCR testing for fungal species (histoplasmosis, coccidiomycosis) • Allergy evaluation • Pulmonary function tests (PFTs) • Arterial Blood Gas (ABG)/oximetry • Diffusing capacity (Dlco) • Chest X-ray • Rapid CT scan chest • Doppler ultrasound/D-dimer test • Pulmonary evaluation with bronchoscopy if a cough persists without an obvious etiology • Cytokine panel
Heart palpitations, pulse skips, heart block	• Lyme disease, co-infections • Inflammation • Stress • Anxiety • Reactive hypoglycemia • Hyperthyroidism • POTS • Caffeine* • Medications* • Heart disease with arrhythmias* • Mitral valve prolapse (MVP)*	• Lyme disease and co-infections • Cytokine panel • EKG • Holter monitor and stress testing in appropriate clinical settings • Echocardiogram +/−transesophageal echocardiogram (TEE) • Five-hour GTT, with insulin levels • Thyroid hormones • Tilt table with ANS evaluation • Evaluate side effects of medications
Any history of a heart murmur or valve prolapse	• Q fever endocarditis • Brucella endocarditis • Bartonella endocarditis • Bacterial endocarditis* • Mitral valve prolapse* • Heart valve abnormalities* • History of rheumatic fever* • PFO (patent foramen ovale) * • Lyme disease	• EKG • Echocardiogram +/−transesophageal echocardiogram (TEE) • Cardiac evaluation • blood cultures • Lyme disease and co-infections • Q fever with phase I and phase II antibody titers • Brucella titers/agglutinating antibodies • Bartonella titers, PCRs

Symptoms	Possible Related Medical Conditions	Laboratory Testing to Consider
Joint pain or swelling	• Lyme disease and co-infections • Autoimmune diseases • Inflammation • Osteoarthritis (OA)* • Gout* • Acute bacterial infections (joint sepsis)* • Acute trauma* • Avascular necrosis (AVN)*	• Lyme disease and co-infections • ANA, RF • CCP • ESR, CRP • Autoimmune markers if appropriate (ss and ds-DNA, anti-RNP, etc.) • Cytokine panel • Uric acid levels • X-rays+/−bone scan if appropriate • MRI of the joint, if appropriate • Tap of joint to check for infection
Stiffness of the joints, neck, or back	• Lyme disease and co-infections • OA* • Autoimmune diseases • Muscle strain* • Trauma*	• Lyme disease and co-infections • X-rays • Autoimmune markers
Muscle pain or cramps	• Lyme disease and co-infections • Inflammation • Myositis • Trichinosis • Potassium and magnesium deficiencies • Dehydration* • Deep Venous Thrombosis (DVT)*	• Lyme disease and co-infections • Cytokine panel • CPK • Aldolase and LDH levels • Eosinophil count with *Trichinella* ELISA • Serum and RBC magnesium levels • K+ level • BUN/creatinine on CMP • Doppler/ultrasound, D-dimer test
Twitching of the face or other muscles	• Lyme disease • Bartonella • Magnesium deficiency • Mitochondrial disorders (i.e., MERRF) • Stress • Caffeine* • Sleep deprivation • Motor neuron diseases (ALS causes characteristic twitching in the extremities, tongue with loss of the muscles in the thenar eminence) • Myoclonus	• Lyme disease and co-infections • Bartonella: IFA, PCR, FISH • RBC and serum magnesium levels • EMG and nerve conduction studies (NCS) to rule out ALS and motor neuron diseases • Neurological evaluation • Mitochondrial evaluation/genetic testing

Symptoms	Possible Related Medical Conditions	Laboratory Testing to Consider
Headaches	• Lyme disease and co-infections • Food allergies • Reactive hypoglycemia • Migraines • Mineral deficiencies with environmental toxins • Mold • Tension headaches with stress • Inflammation/vasculitis • Caffeine withdrawal* • Medications* • Trauma* • CNS infections • Cerebral aneurysm* • Tumor*	• Food allergy panel (IgE, IgG), RAST testing • Serum/24-hour urine histamine levels, DAO levels • Five-hour glucose tolerance, with insulin levels • Serum & RBC mineral levels • Six-hour urine DMSA testing for heavy metals, and Organix, if environmental toxin exposure • *Stachybotrys*/mold toxins, ERMI • Lyme disease and co-infections • Cytokine panel • ESR • Psychological evaluation if history of trauma and PTSD • CT scan/MRI brain • Computed tomography angiography (CTA) • Magnetic resonance angiography (MRA)
Neck cracks, neck stiffness	• Lyme disease • Osteoarthritis* • Muscle strain* • Bacterial and viral meningitis (stiff neck, often with associated light and sound sensitivity, headaches, occasional vomiting, if meningitis. Meningococcal and other bacterial meningitis are often clinically more severe than the presentation with acute neurological Lyme disease)*	• Lyme disease • X-rays or MRI, if severe • Neurological evaluation with spinal tap, if clinically appropriate
Tingling numbness, burning or stabbing sensations	• Lyme disease • Bartonella • Autoimmune disorders • Carpal and cubital tunnel or any nerve entrapment syndrome (thoracic outlet)*	• Lyme disease and co-infections • GM1 AB IgM/IgG, Mag IgM/IgG ABs, ASI GM AB IgM/IgG, anti-myelin ABs • EMG

Symptoms	Possible Related Medical Conditions	Laboratory Testing to Consider
Tingling numbness, burning or stabbing sensations *(continued)*	• Diabetes* • Hypothyroidism* • Pregnancy* • Heavy metal toxicity (Hg, Pb, As) or other environmental toxins (TCE) • Vitamin deficiencies • Immune deficiency • Mitochondrial dysfunction • MS • Strokes or TIAs* • Anxiety, with hyperventilation	• Small fiber nerve biopsy +/− ANS evaluation • Hypothyroidism (T3, T4, free T3, reverse T3, TSH) • B-HCG • Blood sugar and HbA1c levels • B_{12}, folate • MMA and HC levels • Mitochondrial testing • Immunoglobulin levels with subclasses • Six-hour urine DMSA challenge for heavy metal burdens • Accuchem/PacTox laboratory evaluation for environmental toxin exposure, if appropriate (blood, fat biopsy) • Lipid peroxide levels and other markers of oxidative stress • MS (MRI, VEP, AEP, spinal tap for MBP, oligoclonal bands) • CT head or MRI, +/− carotid Doppler if suspecting acute stroke or TIA • Neuropsychiatric evaluation
Facial paralysis (Bell's palsy)	• CNS Lyme disease/other Borrelia species • CNS viral infections (herpes viruses) • Brain tumor* • Stroke* • Sarcoidosis* • Trauma*	• Brain CT scan or MRI • Lyme disease with lumbar puncture (LPs can be negative in early and late Lyme) • Other Borrelia species, i.g., *B. miyamotoi* • Spinal tap, rule out lymphocytic meningitis • Viral titers • Kveim test with ACE level and chest X-ray, if ruling out sarcoid
Eyes/vision: double, blurry, floaters	• Lyme disease • Co-infections, especially Bartonella	• Lyme disease and co-infections • Eye examination • Cytokine panel

Symptoms	Possible Related Medical Conditions	Laboratory Testing to Consider
Eyes/vision: double, blurry, floaters *(continued)*	• Inflammation • Environmental toxins • Functional medicine abnormalities • Concussion* • Trauma* • Stroke* • Brain tumor compressing the optic nerve* • Accommodation problems with aging*	• Brain CT scan or MRI • Organix/ION, with functional medicine workup
Ears/hearing: buzzing, ringing, ear pain	• Lyme disease • Co-infections • Heavy metal burdens (Hg) • Cerumen* • Medications* • Meniere's disease* • TMJ dysfunction/dental disorders*	• Lyme and co-infections • Six-hour urine DMSA challenge for heavy metals • Evaluate medication side effects (macrolides) • Audiometry, ENT/dental evaluation, MRI brain
Increased motion sickness, vertigo	• Lyme disease and co-infections • Viral infections (acute labyrinthitis) • Benign paroxysmal positional vertigo (BPPV)* • Environmental toxicity, including heavy metal burdens • Eighth nerve or cerebellar disorders • Meniere's disease*	• Lyme disease and co-infections • Dix-Hallpike test (BPPV) • Six-hour urine DMSA challenge for heavy metals • Organix/ION • Brain CT Scan or MRI • ENT evaluation with ENG
Light-headedness, wooziness, poor balance, difficulty walking	• Lyme disease and co-infections • Metabolic disorders • Environmental toxin exposure • Functional medicine abnormalities • Reactive hypoglycemia • POTS • Inflammation • Medication • Neurological diseases (MS, ALS) • Strokes*	• Lyme disease and co-infections • Blood alcohol and ammonia levels • Six-hour urine DMSA challenge • Organix/ION • Five-hour GTT with insulin levels • Tilt table, with ANS evaluation • Evaluate medication side effects • Cytokine panel • Brain CT Scan or MRI • Neurological evaluation

Symptoms	Possible Related Medical Conditions	Laboratory Testing to Consider
Tremors	• Lyme disease and co-infections • Mercury toxicity • Environmental toxins (pesticides) • Functional medicine abnormalities • Hyperthyroidism • Hypoglycemia • Anxiety • Caffeine* • Medication* • Parkinson's/Wilson's disease • Alcohol withdrawal*	• Lyme disease and co-infections • Six-hour urine DMSA challenge • Organix/ION • Accuchem/PacTox • Blood sugar (5-hour GTT) • Thyroid functions (T3, free T3, T4, TSH) • Blood alcohol/B vitamin levels • Evaluate medication side effects, withdrawal, and copper levels • Neurological evaluation
Confusion, difficulty thinking	• Lyme disease and co-infections • Viral encephalitis • Metabolic abnormalities • Inflammation • Reactive hypoglycemia • POTS • Strokes and neurological injury* • Hypothyroidism • Heavy metal burdens and other environmental toxins • Mold • Functional medicine abnormalities • Alzheimer's disease • Jacob-Creutzfeldt (prion disease)* • Vitamin deficiencies	• Lyme disease and co-infections • Blood alcohol and ammonia levels • Cytokine panel • Five-hour GTT, with insulin levels • Tilt table • Thyroid (T3, free T3, T4, TSH) • Six-hour urine DMSA challenge for heavy metals • Mold (Stachybotrys titers, mold plates, urine mycotoxin testing, ERMI) • Organix/ION testing, (Metametrix/Accuchem), PacTox, Great Plains Labs • Lumbar puncture with CT, MRI,+/−PET scan, with neurological consultation if appropriate for severe cases • Neuropsychiatric testing/Mini–mental state examination (MMSE) • Apo E positive • B_1, B_3, B_{12}/folic acid
Difficulty with concentration or reading	• Lyme disease and co-infections • Inflammation • ADD/ADHD* • Reactive hypoglycemia • POTS	• Lyme disease and co-infections • Cytokine panel • Five-hour GTT, with insulin levels • Tilt table, with ANS evaluation • Food allergies

Symptoms	Possible Related Medical Conditions	Laboratory Testing to Consider
Difficulty with concentration or reading (continued)	• Food allergies and intolerances • Heavy metals or environmental toxins (TCE, mold) • Functional medicine abnormalities • Sleep deprivation • Hypothyroidism • Metabolic abnormalities • Depression/anxiety • Vitamin deficiencies	• Six-hour urine DMSA challenge • Organix/ION testing • Testing for environmental toxin exposure (PacTox, Great Plains Labs) • Mold (Stachybotrys titers, mold plates, urine mycotoxin testing, ERMI) • Sleep studies • Thyroid function (T3, free T3, T4, TSH) • Blood alcohol and ammonia levels • Neuropsychiatric evaluation • B_1, B_3, B_{12}/folic acid
Forgetfulness, poor short-term memory	• Lyme disease and co-infections • Inflammation • Viral encephalitis • Metabolic abnormalities • Reactive hypoglycemia • POTS • Strokes and neurological injury* • Hypothyroidism • Heavy metal burdens and other environmental toxins • Mold • Functional medicine abnormalities • Alzheimer's disease • Jacob-Creutzfeldt (prion disease)* • Vitamin deficiencies	• Lyme disease and co-infections • Cytokine panel • Blood alcohol and ammonia levels • Five-hour GTT, with insulin levels • Tilt table, with ANS evaluation • Thyroid (T3, free T3, T4, TSH) • Six-hour urine DMSA challenge • Organix/ION • Testing for environmental toxin exposure (Metametrix/Accuchem, PacTox) • Mold (Stachybotrys titers, mold plates, urine mycotoxin testing, ERMI) • Lumbar puncture with CT, MRI, +/−PET scan, with neurological consultation if appropriate for severe cases • Neuropsychiatric testing/ Mini–Mental State Examination (MMSE) • Apo E positive • B_1, B_3, B_{12}/folic acid
Disorientation: getting lost, going to wrong places	• Lyme disease and co-infections • Inflammation • Viral encephalitis • Metabolic abnormalities	• Lyme disease and co-infections • Cytokine panel • Blood alcohol and ammonia levels • Thyroid (T3, free T3, T4, TSH)

Symptoms	Possible Related Medical Conditions	Laboratory Testing to Consider
Disorientation: getting lost, going to wrong places *(continued)*	• Dehydration • Strokes and neurological injury* • Hypothyroidism • Hypoglycemia • Heavy metals; environmental toxins • Mold exposure • Functional medicine abnormalities • Alzheimer's disease • Jacob-Creutzfeldt (prion disease)*	• Five-hour GTT with insulin levels • Six-hour urine DMSA challenge for heavy metals • Organix/ION • Environmental toxin exposure • Mold (*Stachybotrys* titers, mold plates, urine mycotoxin testing, ERMI) • Lumbar puncture with CT or MRI, with neurological consultation, if appropriate for severe cases • Apo E positive
Difficulty with speech or writing	• Lyme disease and co-infections • Inflammation • Viral encephalitis • Metabolic abnormalities • Reactive hypoglycemia • Strokes and neurological injury* • Parkinson's disease • Hypothyroidism • Heavy metals and other environmental toxins • Mold exposure • Functional medicine abnormalities • Alzheimer's disease • Jacob-Creutzfeldt (prion disease)*	• Lyme disease and co-infections • Cytokine panel • Blood alcohol and ammonia levels • Five-hour GTT with insulin levels • Thyroid (T3, free T3, T4, TSH) • Six-hour urine DMSA challenge for heavy metals • Organix/ION • Environmental toxin exposure • Mold (*Stachybotrys* titers, mold plates, urine mycotoxin testing, ERMI) • Lumbar puncture with CT or MRI, with neurological consultation if appropriate, for severe cases • Apo E positive
Mood swings, irritability, depression	• Lyme disease and co-infections • Inflammation • Heavy metal burdens • Environmental toxins • Mineral deficiencies • Functional medicine abnormalities • Mold • Sleep deprivation • Trauma* • PTSD • Depression • Medication*	• Lyme disease and co-infections • Cytokine panel • Neurotransmitter levels • Six-hour urine DMSA challenge for heavy metals • Serum mineral levels • Organix • Environmental toxins testing (PacTox, Accuchem) • Mold (*Stachybotrys* titers and mold plates, urine mycotoxin testing, ERMI) • Sleep evaluation

Symptoms	Possible Related Medical Conditions	Laboratory Testing to Consider
Mood swings, irritability, depression (continued)	• Food allergies and intolerances • Reactive hypoglycemia	• Food allergy profile, serum/urinary histamine levels • Five-hour GTT, with insulin levels • Evaluate medication side effects
Disturbed sleep: too much or too little or early awakening	• Lyme disease and co-infections • Inflammation with pain • Nocturia (urination several times per night secondary to bladder problems, BPH, ADH deficiency)* • Depression or anxiety • Medication* • Caffeine use late in the day* • GI reflux (GERD) • Reactive hypoglycemia • Endocrine disorders: hyperthyroidism, hypercortisolism, acromegaly, low sex hormones, low ADH • Obstructive sleep apnea (OSA)* • Restless leg syndrome (RLS)* • Shift worker syndrome	• Sleep study • Lyme disease and co-infections • Cytokine panel • Neurotransmitter levels • Urological evaluation, with urinalysis/culture and sensitivity • G.I./ENT evaluation (endoscopy, swallowing study) • Medication evaluation • Evaluate caffeine use • Five-hour GTT with insulin levels • Hormonal evaluation (thyroid, adrenals, sex hormones, growth hormone, ADH) • Neuropsychiatric evaluation
Exaggerated symptoms or worse hangover from alcohol	• Lyme disease and co-infections • Nutritional deficiencies • Functional medicine abnormalities	• Lyme disease and co-infections • Serum and RBC mineral levels • Organix/ION

*These medical conditions are not generally part of the MSIDS map but are part of a differential diagnostic list that should be considered in a patient with those symptoms.

adequate benefit, leading me to look at other approaches and see which points on the map have not adequately been addressed.

For example, if one of my patients has not gotten better, she may be suffering from adrenal fatigue with low cortisol levels, and if the antibiotics are not working, I will send her DHEA/cortisol adrenal test to the lab. The results will then indicate whether a patient needs adrenal supplements and/or hydrocortisone. Often people also have low blood pressure/POTS and/or low blood sugars (hypoglycemia) if they have resistant fatigue, or Babesia if they suffer from malarial-type symptoms. These require specific treatments based on the clinical history and proper testing. I might find that Lyme, Bartonella, B_{12} deficiency, and heavy metals like lead and mercury are contributing to neuropathy, and I prescribe antimicrobials, methylcobalamin, and oral chelation to treat the above overlapping factors. Or perhaps we are giving the correct antibiotics, the patient's cortisol levels are balanced, and heavy metals have been adequately removed, but the patient's sleep patterns are still poor, which is increasing chronic inflammation. The patient may require a medication that helps promote sleep, such as Lyrica, trazodone, Seroquel, Gabitril, or Xyrem, since the individual has failed standard sleep medications such as Ambien or Lunesta. Poor sleep can be the reason fatigue and memory and concentration problems persist. Or perhaps the patient has nutritional deficiencies in magnesium, iodine, copper, or zinc, which are needed for proper hormone production, controlling oxidative stress, detoxification, and immune function, and we have not run the appropriate blood and urine tests to check mineral levels and detoxification pathways (such as an Organix test, through Genova Diagnostics laboratories). Other possibilities include mitochondrial dysfunction from oxidative stress (free-radical damage to cells of the body), which has not been corrected, or perhaps patients have a parasite that has not yet been discovered on a Comprehensive Digestive Stool Analysis (CDSA), and they are deconditioned from a lack of exercise, which could account for their ongoing fatigue. The take home message: Most chronic disease manifestations have multiple overlapping etiologies which are found on the sixteen-point MSIDS map, so it is important to keep going back and checking Table 2.1 to establish a broad differential diagnosis if you have symptoms that are not getting better.

MOVING FORWARD

The testing and approaches that I will be describing throughout this book have been used in thousands of patients without ill effects, and where the benefit is outweighed by any possible risk. Furthermore, every part of the MSIDS protocols described in this book is based on published, peer-reviewed medical literature. It is my hope that this book, and each chapter, can serve as a road map of healing for healthcare providers and patients who have not found answers in the approach that modern medicine often uses in diagnosing and treating chronic illness.

THREE

Lyme Disease Specifics and Treatment Options

One of the many mysteries of Lyme disease is why some people do not get better using the same protocols that others respond to so well. Today we know that *Borrelia burgdorferi*, the etiologic agent of Lyme disease, can occur in different forms and hide in different locations in order to evade the immune system, the body's primary method of attacking intruding bacteria. The organism changes shape and moves into different tissues and compartments to adapt to its environment, and it can also change forms to evade killing based on both the antibiotic used (doxycycline versus a penicillin) as well as whether the environment contains adequate nutrition to support its growth.

The two major forms of *Borrelia burgdorferi* are:

- cell-wall forms
- cystic forms (also called cell-wall deficient forms, S-forms, L-forms, spheroplasts, or round bodies as defined by their shape)

The two major locations where borrelia are found:

- intracellular locations, where the mobile spirochete and/or cystic forms can be found within a host cell
- extracellular locations, such as biofilms, which are made up of cells and molecules found in the extracellular environment, creating a matrix, constituting a sheltered environment.

Lyme spirochetes and co-infections are carried by ticks, which are commonly found on mice, deer, foxes, raccoons, songbirds, chipmunks, and squirrels. They are transmitted in a zoonotic cycle, which means the ticks that have acquired the infection after feeding on an infected host (such as rodents and deer) then transmit it to humans. One notable exception to this rule is *Borrelia miyamotoi*, which is related to the relapsing fever group of spirochetes, in which the ticks do not always need to feed on an infected host and can transmit the infection directly to their offspring. This is particularly worrisome because it increases the risk of transmission of this borrelial species, and the common two-tiered diagnostic tests for Lyme will not pick up *B. miyamotoi*, which is rapidly spreading.

Lyme bacteria first enter the body during a tick bite in the classical corkscrew shape, which is the cell-wall form. There are anywhere from three to six flagella (a whiplike appendage that protrudes from the cell) at either end, allowing the bacterium to move spontaneously, propelling the organism through the body's tissues. In hostile environments of extreme temperature (heat or cold) or high or low acidity, the borrelia changes form, and a circular structure, or cyst, is created. This protects it from being killed off by the immune system and allows the organism to survive, dormant, for long periods of time. From its dormant state it can reactivate later, when circumstances are more favorable for its survival. The organism can also penetrate varied cells and enter the intracellular compartment, the area inside the cell wall that includes the nucleus and cytoplasm and contains all of the organelles that allow the cell to function metabolically. Like the cystic form, it allows the bacteria to hide from the immune system.

Finally, borrelia can form biofilm colonies: aggregates of bacteria (spirochetes and round body forms) in which the cells adhere to each other and are embedded in a slimy substance made up of extracellular material of DNA, proteins, lipids, and sugar molecules (polysaccharides) as well as other large molecules (macromolecules). Biofilms allow the bacteria to communicate among themselves, exchange DNA, and resist antibiotics through multiple mechanisms including efflux pumps (pumps that move antibiotics out of cells and biofilms). Scientific research by Johns Hopkins scientists in 2014 has also shown that borrelia forms "persister cells," which are a subpopulation of resistant cells that survive antibiotics (you'll learn more about persisters in Chapter 4), and biofilms have been shown to contain a higher population of dormant persister cells, contributing to antimicrobial resistance. These varied bacterial forms and locations occur as a dynamic process that is constantly going on in the body, and it is the basis for the therapeutic approaches for Lyme disease treatment that I have developed.

Regardless of the form, the disease can spread throughout the body from the site of the initial bite, and even within twenty-four hours can invade the central nervous system. The borrelia bacteria has a preference for certain areas, such as the eye, brain tissue and glial cells, the heart, collagen, skeletal muscle fibers, and the synovial membrane that surrounds the joints. This explains why the most common Lyme-related inflammation occurs in those tissues, causing arthritis, carditis (inflammation of the heart), optic neuritis (inflammation in the optic nerve), iritis (inflammation in the anterior chamber of the eye), meningitis, and encephalitis (inflammation in the sac surrounding the brain and in the brain tissue itself). Borrelia species (*B. burgdorferi* and *B. miyamotoi*) that invade the brain also are being found in biofilms in the central nervous system of those affected by Alzheimer's disease.

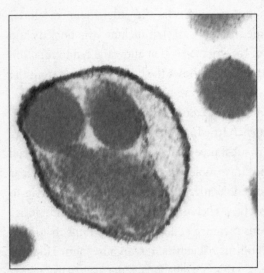

Cyst form of Borrelia burgdorferi *under the microscope.*

Electron micrograph: Cystic Borrelia form from culture of human blood in BSK 1987 Electron Microscopy at Stony Brook School of Medicine, Bernard P. Lane, Professor of Pathology. Photo final magnification 135,000×

REPRINTED WITH PERMISSION FROM THE PERSONAL COLLECTION OF ALAN B. MACDONALD, M.D.

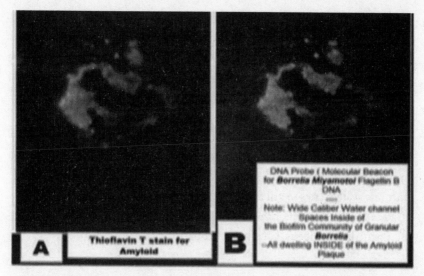

Amyloid stain (A) of an Alzheimer's plaque and the corresponding image of a Borrelia miyamotoi *biofilm inside of the amyloid plaque. From the personal collection of Alan B. MacDonald, M.D., 2016.*

REPRINTED WITH HIS PERMISSION

THE THREE I'S OF LYME DISEASE

The three I's of Lyme disease—infection, inflammation, and immune dysfunction—are the biological triad responsible for many commonly observed symptoms. Infections lead to inflammation that, when combined with genetics and environmental toxins, further contributes to inflammation, immune dysfunction, and illness. Inflammation can also be caused by the wrong kinds of intestinal bacteria in the microbiome, leaky gut syndrome (caused by long branches of yeast burrowing into the intestinal mucosa and damaging the intestines, so that macromolecules of food are able to pass across a damaged intestinal barrier), food allergies or sensitivities, nutritional deficiencies, sleep disorders, heavy metals, and environmental toxins.

Scientific research has shown that borrelia creates an inflammatory response in the body where molecules are produced, called inflammatory cytokines, such as interleukin-1 (IL-1), interleukin-6 (IL-6), tumor necrosis factor alpha (TNF-alpha), and interferon gamma. These can cause fatigue, pain, headaches, memory and concentration problems, and mood swings. Specialized signaling proteins, called chemokines, such as CCL-2 and CXCL-13, are also produced during an infection. These proteins recruit specialized immune cells such as B cells to make antibodies at the site of the infection, including the central nervous system, during neuro-inflammation. Cytokines and chemokines can both modulate immune activation and inflammation as they direct immune cells to the sites of tissue injury and infection. Some individuals who are genetically predisposed also develop autoimmune reactions during this inflammatory process due to a biological phenomenon called *molecular mimicry*. Our immune system tries to kill the bacteria, as borrelia-specific IgM antibodies attack the flagellar tail of the organism and, instead, cross-react with our own neuronal antigens, causing neuropathy.

TREATING LYME DISEASE BY TYPE AND STAGE

The ability to cure early Lyme disease and prevent it from progressing is essential in trying to control many of the extreme clinical manifestations that I unfortunately witness daily. In my medical practice we often treat simultaneously the cell-wall and cystic forms, as well as forms located in biofilms and inside the intracellular compartment. This is accomplished by rotating among different drugs and supplements to treat the various forms and locations of *Borrelia burgdorferi*.

We must take into account aspects of the biology of the organism, such as its long replication time, and that certain antibiotics that are bactericidal, like penicillins and cephalosporins, will only work when the organism is actively dividing and reproducing. This implies that several rounds of antibiotics may be necessary to cover the cycles of the organism. Other antibiotics, like tetracyclines, are primarily bacteriostatic: They inhibit the organism's growth (although higher doses may be bactericidal), so we must have a healthy immune system to kill borrelia. Unfortunately, borrelia and multiple co-infections can suppress the immune system, so we must take this into account when simultaneous infections need to be cleared.

Regimens must be individualized based on a history of allergies, tolerance to medications, positive or negative responses such as Herxheimer (JH) reactions, associated co-infections (like Babesia and/or Bartonella with other intracellular bacteria), and ongoing symptoms (i.e., peripheral and/or central nervous system symptoms).

We change antibiotics if patients do not improve after one or two months, and consider the use of IV antibiotics if central nervous system symptoms continue despite oral treatments or intramuscular shots, or if the initial presentation includes severe neurological symptoms (like optic neuritis, Bell's palsy, and/or a severe encephalitis). I've also found that my patients respond better when they follow a gluten-free, sugar-free, yeast-free diet, and take high-potency probiotics to balance the bacteria in their intestinal tract.

As I've said before, Lyme is best understood as a clinical diagnosis. Rule 1 in the Action Plan is that symptoms drive diagnosis and treatment, and reviewing the HMQ while performing a history and physical and creating a differential diagnosis will help you to determine which therapies are most appropriate early on in the course of treatment. What's more, testing is unreliable, and some laboratory results can take a long time to come back (especially if they are sent to a specialty laboratory), and by then you may lose your window of opportunity for catching the infection before it spreads. Discuss the risks and benefits of early treatment of tick-borne diseases with your healthcare provider.

UNDERSTANDING YOUR PRESCRIPTION

Ever wonder what your doctor's orders to the pharmacist mean? The letters "PO" mean taking medication orally. The frequency of use is described as:

- QD (once a day)
- BID (twice a day)
- TID (three times a day)
- QID (four times a day)
- QOD (every other day)
- QOweek (every other week)

In appendix A you will find a complete list of medications and appropriate dosages, and the most common side effects to watch for. When there are special considerations, I've included the dosages within the text.

Acute Lyme Disease: I have an EM rash with no systemic symptoms

According to the scientific literature, approximately 75 percent of patients are cured with the standard three-week course of doxycycline (100 mg PO BID) or Ceftin (500 mg PO BID). Some physicians may only prescribe a cephalosporin drug such as Ceftin when a patient presents with an EM rash. However, Ceftin or amoxicillin only treat the cell-wall forms and are therefore not routinely effective in treating all cases of Lyme disease. Dr. Gary Wormser published a study in the 1990s that compared doxycycline and Ceftin in treating early Lyme disease, which demonstrated that up to 20 percent of patients did not adequately respond to this treatment and went on to develop chronic symptomatology despite both medications. Doxycycline will primarily treat the intracellular forms (and is also useful for multiple intracellular co-infections). Neither of these two drug families treats the cystic forms or bacteria/persisters located in biofilms. Doxycycline and other antibiotics can also cause the organism to change forms, and not adequately address these forms and biofilm formation by *Borrelia burgdorferi*. This would explain why some people treated with doxycycline or Ceftin alone go on to develop chronic symptomatology.

If you have multiple EM rashes, or neurological symptoms such as a stiff neck, headache, dizziness, light and sound sensitivity and/or cognitive difficulties (central nervous system symptoms), or tingling/numbness/burning in the extremities (peripheral nervous system symptoms), then the organism has disseminated and one month of antibiotics is usually insufficient, since it is likely that you will develop persistent symptoms. Another explanation as to why a three-week course of doxycycline alone may be inadequate is that doxycycline alone does not address cystic forms, persister cells, and biofilms, allowing spirochetes to survive.

Although the standard treatment of doxycycline, or Ceftin, cures a significant percentage of all uncomplicated EM rashes, the biology of *Borrelia burgdorferi* suggests that it may be worthwhile to consider the following regimens for an uncomplicated EM rash. These protocols are based on average adult body weights and should be adjusted to your particular needs. Tetracyclines can cause staining of the teeth in children before the age of eight and are not generally used to treat EM rashes in children, and they should only be used in short courses (ten days) when other potentially life-threatening tick-borne infections such as Rocky Mountain spotted fever are suspected.

MONTH ONE: Plaquenil 200 mg, one PO BID; doxycycline 100 mg, two PO BID (with meals); nystatin tablets 500,000 units, two PO BID, with pulse Flagyl or Tindamax three days a week, based on body weight (body weight less than 120 pounds: 750 mg per day; between 121 and 150 pounds: 1,000 mg per day; greater than 150 pounds: 1,500 mg per day). The addition of the Flagyl or Tindamax eradicates some of the cystic forms that may arise during initial treatment. Grapefruit seed extract may be used as a natural supplement to address cystic forms in people who are allergic or cannot tolerate Flagyl/Tindamax. Serrapeptase (or similar enzymes that affect biofilms) with whole-leaf Stevia extract (Nutramedix) should be used concurrently since Stevia has significant effect in eliminating *B. burgdorferi* spirochetes, biofilms, and persisters. Monolaurin, a coconut oil extract, has also recently been shown to have the ability to significantly affect three morphological forms of *Borrelia burgdoferi* and *Borrelia garinii*: spirochetes, latent round body forms, and borrelia biofilms, while simultaneously decreasing yeast overgrowth in the GI tract. It can be used in combination with the above protocol, especially in patients prone to yeast infections. Although these combinations address the different forms of borrelia from a biological perspective, we still need controlled scientific trials to show improved efficacy as compared to standard treatment protocols.

MONTH TWO: Even if a patient has adequately responded to doxycycline with Plaquenil, with or without pulse Flagyl or Tindamax, combined with biofilm busters like Stevia/Serrapeptase/monolaurin for the treatment of acute Lyme disease, then after one month we will often rotate to a cell-wall, cystic, and intracellular protocol with biofilm busters for an additional month (unless there was a significant improvement in the first month without side effects). This protocol would include a combination of:

- cell-wall drugs: cephalosporins such as Omnicef, Ceftin, or penicillins such as amoxicillin;
- cystic drugs: Plaquenil and/or grapefruit seed extract (GSE), occasionally combined with Flagyl or Tindamax;

- intracellular drugs: Zithromax or Biaxin, and occasionally Bactrim (sulfamethoxazole/trimethoprim, a persister drug), rifampin, and/or tetracyclines like doxycycline or minocycline. These can have an effect on overlapping co-infections (Bartonella and/or associated parasitic infections like Babesia). The rule is that two intracellular drugs generally work better than one in chronic disease. I have seen many relapses (proven by positive polymerase chain reaction, i.e., PCR, for Lyme, Bartonella, Mycoplasma, and Babesia) using single-drug therapy, and in some cases, triple or even quadruple intracellular therapy is necessary for treating the most severe cases. These can be pulsed to keep down side effects. Dapsone, which is the newest persister drug proven to work in our office for chronic Lyme disease and babesiosis, will be discussed in Chapter 4, with explanations on how to combine it in chronic resistant cases;
- nystatin: to prevent yeast infections associated with antibiotics;
- biofilm busters: Stevia plus Serrapeptase, and/or monolaurin. Once you become asymptomatic for two months on treatment, stop the antibiotics and consider an herbal protocol with biofilms busters like monolaurin for several months to ensure that there are no new or relapsing symptoms.

Every person is unique, and general guidelines may not be applicable. For example, a patient presenting with early neuropathy, or with a history of severe candida, may not be an ideal candidate for Flagyl or Tindamax, as these drugs have the potential of increasing those symptoms. However, these medications play an important role in clearing complicated infections and may help prevent you from going on to the chronic form of Lyme disease with the inherent suffering and disability that often ensues.

I have an EM rash with systemic symptoms, or multiple EM rashes:

Typically, acute Lyme disease without any other co-infections will resolve in approximately 75 percent of patients with the above treatment protocol. Yet I have also found that many of my patients need a longer course of antibiotics than simply the two-month regimen, especially if they are presenting with a stiff neck, headache, and/or tingling and numbness of the extremities or with multiple EM rashes. If they have one of these presentations, this implies that they have disseminated Lyme disease: that it has spread throughout the body. Multiple EM rashes means that the organism has spread, which requires longer and more aggressive treatment to try and prevent chronic illness. A stiff neck and headache with an EM rash implies that the organism has effectively penetrated into the central nervous system early on in the disease, where antibiotics may not penetrate well. Tingling, numbness, and/or burning of the extremities with an EM rash imply that the organism has penetrated into the peripheral nervous system (PNS). In these cases, thirty to sixty days of antibiotics may not cure the disease. This may be due in part to biofilms protecting dormant persister cells.

Since a single tick bite may transmit multiple co-infections, the most effective drugs and herbal combinations must provide good central nervous system penetration (e.g., doxycycline, minocycline, Flagyl, Tindamax, high-dose amoxicillin, and IV Rocephin), and treat all forms of *Borrelia burgdorferi*, including cystic and biofilm forms, and possible associated co-infections. The most common parasitic co-infection is babesiosis, and if you suffer from day and/or night sweats (which can be mild or drenching), chills, and flushing, with an unexplained cough and shortness of breath ("air hunger") after a tick bite, that implies Babesia may be present if other etiologies have been ruled out. Babesia makes all of the underlying Lyme symptoms worse and is often a cause of inadequate responses to antibiotics. Bartonella and other intracellular bacteria (i.e., Mycoplasma, chlamydia, Q fever, tularemia, and Brucella) also are responsible for chronic persistent symptoms, and often require between two to four intracellular drugs in the most resistant cases. Treatment until the patient is several months' symptom free is essential, or the risk of relapse is high.

When using several drugs at the same time, pulsing antibiotics can minimize side effects. Pulsing regimens can include using a cephalosporin like Ceftin, 500 mg twice a day, three days a week (e.g., Monday, Wednesday, Saturday); pulsed high-dose rifampin (300 mg, two capsules twice a day) one to three times per week, or QOD; and long-acting macrolides like Zithromax (250 mg, twice a day), four days in a row per week. Significantly impaired individuals with multiple chronic intracellular infections (i.e., borrelia, with Bartonella, and/or Mycoplasma, Q fever, tularemia, Brucella) may require multiple intracellular antibiotics simultaneously (combining two to four medications, like doxycycline, rifampin and Bactrim) with pulse Ceftin in order to have a sustained positive clinical response.

Blood work should be done regularly to make sure that there are no side effects from the antibiotics. Follow a complete blood count (CBC) and comprehensive metabolic profile (CMP) monthly (or more often if on IV therapy or starting the Dapsone protocol we will discuss in Chapter 4).

I'm not getting better: Treatments for the cystic forms of Lyme

There are now four separate treatment options to kill the cystic forms of Lyme disease, all of which have been published in the scientific literature. These include the use of three drugs: Plaquenil, Flagyl, and Tindamax, as well as the nutraceutical grapefruit seed extract.

We regularly use a cyst-buster medication like Plaquenil in combination therapy, which alkalizes the intracellular compartment, making certain intracellular antibiotics more effective. It also affects DNA gyrase, an enzyme responsible for bacterial replication, and regulates immune dysfunction. Plaquenil is contraindicated for persons with psoriasis and retinal problems. Although eye exams are required once a year on Plaquenil, we have never seen Plaquenil-induced retinopathy.

Since patients can have strong reactions to cystic drugs like Flagyl or Tindamax, we will often pulse these medications. This means that we use them for several days in a row, then take a break for several days. I have found that this method keeps down flares and the worsening of symptoms. These drugs also have the potential to cause increased yeast problems, as well as the unwanted side effect of neuropathy (increased tingling, numbness, or burning sensations). These side effects can be minimized by using pulse therapy and combining the medications with high doses of B vitamins. Alcohol must be avoided to prevent nausea and vomiting (an Antabuse type reaction). Despite possible side effects (primarily with Flagyl and Tindamax), many patients improve resistant symptoms after their use (including neuropathy), and the use of cystic drugs may help to lower the bacterial load of borrelia in the body.

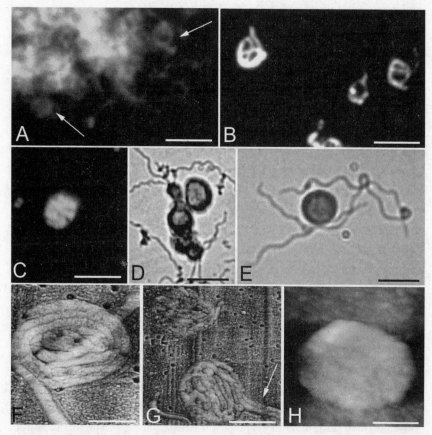

Persisting atypical and cystic forms of Borrelia burgdorferi *in neurological Lyme disease.*

Rolled and cystic forms of Borrelia burgdorferi *spirochetes observed after one week of culture in medium to which Thioflavin S had been added. A: Observation by Thioflavin S fluorescence. Arrows point to rolled cystic forms at the periphery of an agglomerated mass of spirochetes from strain B31. Rolled (B) and cystic (C) forms observed by dark field microscopy (strain B31). D and E: Cyst forms of* Borrelia burgdorferi *(strains ADB1 and B31, respectively) following immunostaining with the monoclonal anti-OspA antibody. F and G: Atomic force microscopy (AFM) images of Borrelia cysts. Rolled spirochetes are clearly visible in F (strain B31) and G (strain ADB1). Arrow in G shows that the cyst is formed by two spirochetes rolled together. H: The cystic form is entirely covered by a thickened external membrane masking the content of the cyst. Photos obtained with permission from Dr. Judith Miklossy. Initially published in "Persisting atypical and cystic forms of* Borrelia burgdorferi *and local inflammation in Lyme neuroborreliosis," J. Miklossy et al., Journal of Neuroinflammation 2008, 5:40.*

My doctor says I have biofilms

Borrelia in biofilm colonies have been found in various areas of the body, including the skin, and my colleague, Dr. Steven Fry, has found biofilms in the blood using microscopic analysis. In 2016, Dr. Herbert B. Allen and colleagues at Drexel University also discovered biofilms containing spirochetes in the plaques of patients with Alzheimer's disease (AD), hypothesizing that the neuroinflammation associated with the disease are due to the immune system's reaction to the bacteria in biofilms. Prior published research by Dr. Judith Miklossy and Dr. Alan MacDonald showed that Lyme spirochetes were found in the brains of those with AD, and recently discovered biofilms of other borrelia species, like *Borrelia miyamotoi*, in those with AD. Does this mean that if you have Lyme you will get AD? No, but as you will see in Chapter 13, there may be multiple causes of Alzheimer's, and addressing infections, toxins, and factors on the MSIDS map that increase inflammation may be a key to prevention.

Eminent researchers like Dr. Kim Lewis at Northeastern University claim that "all bacteria form persisters," so we should not be surprised that biofilms containing dormant persister cells are known to exist in many diseases, ranging from Alzheimer's to chronic otitis media (inner ear infections) in children, to patients with osteoarthritis and prosthetic joints. Biofilms, cystic forms, immune evasion by regularly changing outer surface proteins, long replication times, hiding in the intracellular compartment or going deep in tissues where antibiotics don't penetrate well, are all reasons that help explain why borrelia can survive after seemingly adequate antibiotic therapy, and why some clinical treatment trials for Lyme disease, even with several months of antibiotics, showed only temporary benefit.

There are several mechanisms to prevent the formation of borrelia biofilms as well as aid their destruction. Rifampin (with or without Dapsone), as well as natural enzymes such as nattokinase, lumbrokinase, and Serrapeptase, plus Stevia and monolaurin, have all been shown to affect borrelia biofilms, decreasing their formation, and monolaurin affects all forms. We generally use at least two biofilm busters simultaneously, including whole-leaf Stevia extract (Nutramedix). Some patients have had a worsening of symptoms using Stevia, consistent with a JH reaction, so we usually increase the dose slowly over several weeks.

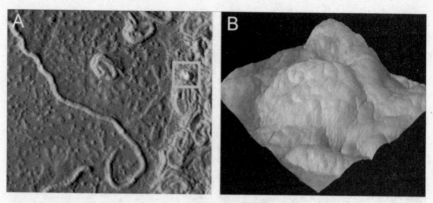

Cyst forms of Borrelia burgdorferi *embedded in borrelia biofilms.*

Atomic Force Microscopy images of Borrelia burgdorferi *B31 strain at the edge of a biofilm (**A**), with a small round body (cyst form) indicated (in the box), and a higher magnification of a small round body/cyst form (**B**). Luecke D. F. and Sapi E., University of New Haven, Lyme Disease Research Group (unpublished data 2013).*

Other biofilm busters include ethylenediaminetetraacetic acid (EDTA), Boluke, and aminoglycosides (like gentamycin), as well as newer ones such as Oxantel (an antiparasitic drug), and herbal extracts (pomegranate, maple syrup extract, and cinnamon/peppermint "nanobombs"). Recent research published in 2016 in *Frontiers in Microbiology* showed that the combination of daptomycin, cefuroxime, and doxycycline completely eradicated biofilm-like structures with no visible bacterial growth after one week and three weeks. Clinical studies still need to be performed to evaluate the efficacy of this combination of a persister drug (daptomycin) with an active drug (cefuroxime), as well as the efficacy of single or combined biofilm busters in chronic disease.

Table 3.1 on page 81 illustrates the different drugs and nutraceuticals used in combination therapies to treat the different forms and locations of borrelia.

A Word About Antibiotic Resistance

Drug regimens usually include several antibiotic combinations to help address the different forms and locations of Lyme disease, and also to help prevent antibiotic resistance that could arise from single-drug therapy. Although we have not seen antibiotic resistance clinically in our

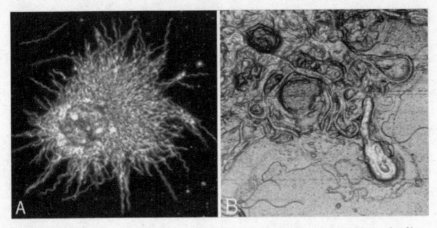

Dark field image of a small developing in vitro Borrelia burgdorferi *B31 strain biofilm* (**A**); *spirochetes at the edge of the biofilm can be easily identified but not the other alternative forms such as the cystic forms. Atomic Force microscopy image of a similar biofilm* (**B**); *several alternative forms, such as the cystic forms, become readily apparent. Photo courtesy of David Luecke and Dr. Eva Sapi, University of New Haven, Lyme Disease Research Group (unpublished data, 2013).*

practice, it is a theoretical concern and should always be on the minds of healthcare practitioners prescribing long-term antibiotics.

RECOGNIZING AND TREATING JARISCH-HERXHEIMER REACTIONS

Jarisch-Herxheimer (JH) flares are a temporary worsening of the symptoms of Lyme disease that occur when the Lyme spirochete is being killed off by antibiotics, creating inflammation. This common reaction was first described in the medical literature in relation to syphilis—a spirochetal cousin of Lyme disease. These JH reactions produce cytokines (TNF-alpha, IL-6, and IL-8), which then create inflammatory symptoms, including increased fever, muscle and joint pain, headaches, cognitive impairment, and a general worsening of the underlying symptomatology. This is a major reason why so many people with Lyme disease seem to temporarily get worse—and not better—when they are taking antibiotics.

Unfortunately, when I take my chronically ill patients experiencing JH reactions off antibiotics, although their symptoms may temporarily

Table 3.1: Combination Treatment Therapies for Lyme Disease

Cell-Wall Form	Cystic Forms*	Intracellular Forms	Biofilms*
Penicillins: Amoxicillin, Augmentin, Moxatag ER Bicillin LA (intramuscular benzathine penicillin)	Plaquenil	Macrolides: Zithromax Biaxin Roxithromycin (Europe)	Stevia, Serrapeptase, monolaurin, Biocidin* (my first-line choices)
Cephalosporins: oral Ceftin Omnicef Cedax Suprax	Grape fruit seed extract	Quinolones: Cipro, Levaquin, Avelox Factive*	Others: Nattokinase, Lumbrokinase, Boluke, EDTA
IV Cephalosporins: IV Rocephin IV Claforan IV Teflaro* (ceftaroline)	Flagyl Tindamax	Tetracyclines: doxycycline, minocycline, tetracycline HCL	
Other IV Medication: IV vancomycin* IV Primaxin*		Mycobacterium drugs: Rifampin, Dapsone*, Pyrazinamide*	Rifampin*
		Sulfa drugs: Bactrim	
Other IV Medication for "persisters": IV Daptomycin*		Other IV medication: IV doxycycline IV Zithromax IV gentamycin (aminoglycosides) IV Levaquin/Avelox IV rifampin	Others: IV Daptomycin+ IV Rocephin+ doxycycline*

*These have shown to be effective in retrospective clinical studies and laboratory studies.

subside, they often return. This creates a difficult situation: The antibiotics are making the patient better while they temporarily make them feel worse. In some people, pushing through the flare helps them to feel much better afterward. In others, the JH reaction won't end until the treatment protocol is changed. The way to tell whether you are having a "good" Herx or a "bad" Herx is that when you come out of a flare with a good Herx, you are better than before you started, that is, at a higher level of functioning (implying effective lowering of the bacterial load). With a bad Herx, you flare and then go back to your prior baseline functioning.

The only way to break the cycle is to either hold off using the antibiotics for a period of time until the symptoms die down, rotate to a different antibiotic protocol (and/or use lower doses) that doesn't cause severe JH reactions, and/or to use intermittent flare protocols that decrease the production of inflammatory cytokines (i.e., "shut off the faucet") while removing them from the body ("open the drain"). This involves using various medications such as low-dose naltrexone (LDN), non-steroidal anti-inflammatory drugs (NSAIDs), or COX-2 inhibitors (Celebrex) with high-dose nutraceuticals like omega-3 fatty acids found in fish oils (including krill with astaxanthin), curcumin, green tea extract, resveratrol, and broccoli seed extract (sulforaphane glucosinolate), each of which have been scientifically proven to decrease inflammation.

I have found a five-step approach to be effective in up to 70 percent of my Lyme disease patients who suffer from JH flares:

A. Alkalize: During Jarisch-Herxheimer reactions, as well as in severe illness in general, the body can get acidic. This is detrimental to health, as the enzymatic processes of the body function best at a neutral pH of around 7.4. We therefore want to shift the acid/base balance and balance the pH if we become acidic, using Alka-Seltzer Gold or an equivalent medication, such as sodium bicarbonate tablets. Other effective methods include buffered Vitamin C and lemon-lime water.

I presented an abstract at the International Lyme and Associated Diseases Conference in 2003 on the use of "lemon-lime" therapy for the treatment of Herxheimer reactions. We know that alkaline reserves act as buffers to maintain a pH balance in the blood, which is essential to proper metabolic functioning.

During periods of inflammatory responses, acid by-products are produced that may deplete alkaline reserves with a corresponding increase in free-radical production, damaging tissues. Lakesmaa and colleagues published in the *Journal of Infectious Diseases* that the effects of these tissue and circulating cytokines can explain many of the symptoms and inflammatory reactions seen with Jarisch-Herxheimer (JH) reactions. The study we performed was designed to observe whether antioxidant supplementation and increasing the alkaline reserves during the JH flare would have an appreciable effect on symptoms in a cohort of Lyme patients during antibiotic therapy. The methodology involved patients squeezing one to two fresh lemons or limes in a glass of water and drinking it over several minutes at the onset of a JH flare. Among thirty patients surveyed, 70 percent reported mild to moderate improvements in symptoms within several hours, including fatigue, muscle and joint pain, fever, sweats, hot flashes, muscle spasms, and paresthesias (tingling, pricking, or burning of the skin), with several patients reporting an improvement in overall wellness within minutes.

Fruits and vegetables are generally alkaline-containing foods. Lemon and lime juice, although tasting acidic, are converted to alkaline ash in the body, thereby temporarily raising alkaline reserves. These will buffer acid by-products of infection and provide an increase in water-soluble antioxidants that are available to counter increased free radical production. Alkalinization can also augment the effect of certain antibiotics in killing intracellular bacteria. These results imply that in certain Lyme disease patients depleted alkaline reserves and increased free radical damage with oxidative stress may be temporarily responsible for increased symptoms during Jarisch-Herxheimer reactions, apart from intermediary cytokines and their overall metabolic effects on the body.

Another study, published in the *American Journal of Epidemiology*, reported on data from the thirty-thousand-subject Iowa Women's Health Study. Results indicated that beta-cryptoxanthin, a substance present in citrus fruit, helped decrease the incidence and risk of developing rheumatoid arthritis. It is therefore possible that other substances in citrus fruits are playing a beneficial role apart from increasing the alkaline reserves.

B. Support the elimination of toxins: Other supplements that support liver detoxification aside from glutathione include milk thistle, ellagic acid (in raspberries), N-Acetylcysteine (NAC), alpha lipoic acid, B vitamins, watercress, dandelion, and phosphatidylcholine. There are also different methods of intestinal detoxification, including charcoal, bentonite clay, zeolite, Questran (cholestyramine), Welchol (colesevelam), or occasionally enemas.

C. Shut down the production of cytokines: LDN and antioxidants can decrease the stimulation of NFKappaB, which is a switch in the nucleus of the cell that increases inflammatory cytokines. These antioxidants include alpha-lipoic acid, glutathione, resveratrol, curcumin, broccoli compounds like [DIM], and broccoli seed extracts such as glucoraphanin/sulforaphane.

D. Supplement with minerals used in the detoxification reactions: These include magnesium (used in more than three hundred detox enzymes), zinc (needed in phase I liver detoxification and alcohol dehydrogenase), and copper (used in superoxide dismutase, or SOD), which can be found in a good multimineral supplement.

E. "Open up the drain": There are different nutraceutical remedies available, such as ones that work on lymphatic drainage (Itires, Pekana drainage remedies), or general drainage formulas, such as the herbs parsley and burbur found in the Cowden protocol (NutraMedix). Taking in extra fluids and getting adequate sleep, combined with a mild exercise program and infrared saunas for further elimination of toxins, can also be helpful.

Other Treatments for Pain and JH Reactions:

TRANSDERMAL PAIN MEDICATIONS: Some patients have pain localized over one or two areas and do not require oral medications. The benefits of topical treatments include delivering higher drug concentrations at the site than can be achieved through oral delivery, while significantly reducing or eliminating GI, hepatic, and systemic side effects. One readily available example is Voltaren gel, which is mainly used for osteoarthritis and is usually applied up to four times a day to the affected site.

HERBAL THERAPIES: The herbs most commonly used in our practice for patients with Lyme disease and pain are Andrographis, Polygonum (a form of resveratrol), Stephania root, Smilax, redroot, and boneset. These all have strong scientific support and can be useful for those with ongoing symptoms and inflammation. These herbs can be added to any regimen to help decrease inflammation and pain. Herbal protocols made by Greenwood Herbals and Researched Nutritionals combine several of these herbs: Smilax, redroot, and boneset for Herxheimer (JH) reactions. Patients have reported that this combination has been effective in decreasing pain associated with JH flares.

CHRIS HAD ONGOING JH REACTIONS

Chris is a twenty-eight-year-old male who came to see me for the first time in 2009. He had a past medical history significant for food allergies, exercise-induced asthma, temporal mandibular joint (TMJ) dysfunction, peptic ulcers, hypoglycemia, and Lyme disease. Chris may have been exposed to Lyme five years before a diagnosis had been made. He was asymptomatic until he sustained a concussion in the tenth grade and then developed forgetfulness, joint pain, headaches, light sensitivity, dizziness, and significant insomnia. He suffered until he was correctly diagnosed with Lyme disease. His blood tests came back with a positive ELISA and IgM Western blot, and he was treated for the next three years with oral antibiotics. These included antibiotic rotations of amoxicillin, Zithromax, Biaxin, doxycycline, tetracycline, and Flagyl. He had gradual improvement in his symptoms, and treatment was stopped. He contracted the Epstein-Barr virus the next spring, which led to a diagnosis of chronic fatigue syndrome.

By the time he came to see me he had been without any treatment for eight or nine years. He complained of moderate to severe fatigue; joint pain in his toes, knees, ankles, and fingers that migrated around his body; mid- to low-back pain; tingling and numbness of his extremities; muscle pains; weight loss; decreased libido; testicular pain; constipation alternating with loose stools; occasional shortness of breath; twitching of his eyes; blurry vision; ringing in his ears; light-headedness and balance problems; tremors in his hands; mild to moderate memory, concentration, and word-finding problems; and irritability, anxiety, and depression, all of which would come and go, with good and bad days. Chris had swollen mucosa inside the nasal passages consistent with his allergies; a small axillary lymph node, approximately half a centimeter in size, which was mobile and slightly tender; and a decreased vibratory sensation in his extremities. The lack of perceived vibration in his extremities was consistent with Lyme neuropathy, where the nerves are often affected. Chris was very discouraged; due to his declining health, he had to quit his job.

His prior physician had done a good job of ruling out many different diseases to explain his symptoms, but there were still several tests that had not yet been done. These included a more extensive endocrine evaluation, with different tests for thyroid function for his severe fatigue (free T3, T3, T4, and reverse T3); a DHEA/cortisol test to rule out adrenal fatigue; and an insulin-like growth factor 1 (IgF1) level to rule out growth hormone deficiency. We also sent off for Vitamin D levels; a MTHFR test, to check for methylation/detoxification problems; a B_{12}, methylmalonic acid, folate and homocysteine levels for B vitamin deficiencies, and immunoglobulin levels, to evaluate his immunity. I also ordered an expanded food allergy panel, given his history of allergies and asthma; an *H. pylori* test, given his history of peptic ulcer disease; and an expanded tick-borne co-infection panel, including testing for viruses (human herpes virus 6 or HHV-6, Epstein-Barr, cytomegalovirus, and West Nile), Mycoplasma, chlamydia, Rocky Mountain spotted fever, Brucella, and Q fever, as well as repeat testing for Lyme disease and Bartonella. He was also sent for a neurological evaluation for his peripheral neuropathy, with an electromyogram (EMG) nerve conduction test, a small-fiber biopsy, and an autonomic nervous system evaluation. Lyme disease can cause a small-fiber peripheral neuropathy, which affects the skin, peripheral nerves, and autonomic nervous system, leading to paresthesias, temperature dysregulation, and abnormal sweating. A small-fiber skin biopsy helps establish the diagnosis.

Chris's testing came back positive for Lyme disease. His adrenal testing showed very low cortisol at 8:00 A.M. (1.2; the normal range is between 3 and 6 ng/ml) and high levels at night (5.7; normal range is 0.15 to 0.5 ng/ml), which would explain in part the severe fatigue in the morning and problems falling asleep at night. His food allergy panel returned positive for dairy, wheat, and eggs, with a low serum IgA, often seen in patients with multiple food allergies. These could have contributed to his allergic symptoms as well as his fatigue and muscle and joint pain. His EMG (electromyelogram, a nerve conduction test) showed a sensory polyneuropathy (abnormal nerve conduction), with a small-fiber biopsy confirming a small-fiber neuropathy. The combination of the adrenal problems, food allergies, detoxification problems, and Lyme disease could have been responsible for the neuropathy, joint and muscle pain, insomnia, and cognitive difficulties. The testing of his autonomic nervous system, which controls temperature regulation, was also abnormal, showing moderate effects of the Lyme disease on his sympathetic nervous system. All in all, Chris had MSIDS: multiple abnormalities responsible for his chronic symptoms, which explained his resistance to simple Lyme treatment.

We gave Chris IV glutathione for his resistant fatigue and neuro-cognitive deficits. He noticed an improvement in his symptoms almost immediately, before leaving the office, and his energy and concentration improved significantly. We therefore suggested he take N-Acetylcysteine (NAC) and alpha-lipoic acid, supplements that support glutathione production, as glutathione also helps detoxify neurotoxins from the body. He also was told to avoid his allergic foods.

Over the next two years Chris rotated through multiple Lyme regimens. He would improve temporarily, but would often relapse each time he was taken off of the drugs and herbs. He had extremely severe Jarisch-Herxheimer reactions. His fatigue, muscle and joint pain, cognitive difficulties, depression, anxiety, and sleep problem would worsen. We would therefore have to stop the drugs to let the JH reaction die down. Yet every time we stopped the drugs, although his symptoms had temporarily gotten better, he would relapse and feel worse again within days.

Sleep disorders increase inflammation in the body, and some of the same inflammatory molecules produced from sleep deprivation (interleukin-6, or IL-6) are also produced during Jarisch-Herxheimer reactions. We therefore gave Chris several sleep medications and herbs to help him go to sleep and stay asleep, since sleep deprivation makes all of the Lyme symptoms worse. We tried Ambien, Lunesta, Flexeril, Remeron, Restoril, Gabitril, and trazodone as well as nutraceuticals, including valerian root, melatonin, and phosphatidylserine. He was only able to tolerate Remeron (an antidepressant with sedating effects at the lowest dose), as it did not cause side effects and helped him to stay asleep. This helped decrease the severity of the flares. He was also given low-dose naltrexone (LDN) with herbs such as curcumin and green tea extract to decrease inflammation. He took oral liposomal glutathione every day, since he had had a positive response to IV glutathione, and this was used in higher doses with Alka-Seltzer Gold when he had a Herxheimer flare. This would also give him some relief from his symptoms.

Yet every time we tried to reintroduce his cystic drugs or intracellular medications, he had severe reactions with a worsening of his symptoms. We therefore switched him over to intramuscular shots of Bicillin, a long-acting penicillin that is particularly effective in treating persistent Lyme disease and MSIDS. He did notice marked improvement with the addition of Bicillin and with pulsing the intracellular medications. In fact, he said he felt "awesome" after four weeks, the best he had felt in the previous two years. The combination of the IV glutathione and years of attacking the Lyme disease were finally showing considerable progress.

Chris returned a month later. He had had an amazing response to the new regimen. His energy was improving, his libido was finally improving (his wife, sitting next to him in the room, smiled slyly), the dizziness was better, and there was less peripheral nerve pain. Yet Chris still had an occasional significant Herxheimer flare while on these drugs. We therefore stopped all of his antibiotics and placed him on a traditional Chinese herbal protocol from Dr. Zhang instead (Coptis, HH, Circulation P, and AI#3).

At the next follow-up visit Chris felt the best he had in the last fifteen years. His only residual symptoms were a headache, which he attributed to his TMJ, and his good days were up to 90 percent of normal with only occasional mild fatigue. He no longer had any of his severe Herxheimer reactions when he was off the antibiotics. We therefore discussed a diet and exercise program in order to build him back up, and we kept him on his adrenal and detox supplements, mitochondrial support, sleep medication, and the traditional Chinese herbal protocol, which was clearly helping him.

The keys to getting Chris better were aggressive treatment for the Lyme disease, getting him to sleep, treating his low adrenal function, avoiding the food allergens, stopping blood sugar swings with a hypoglycemic diet, mitochondrial support, detoxing him properly, and shutting down the production of inflammatory cytokines responsible for the Jarisch-Herxheimer flares. The MSIDS approach was the key for helping Chris get his life back.

LYME, CO-INFECTIONS, AND PREGNANCY

Borrelia burgdorferi may be transmitted transplacentally to the fetus, as may associated co-infections like *Borrelia miyamotoi*, Babesia, and Bartonella. *Borrelia burgdorferi* has also been isolated from breast milk. Although the incidence of transmission through breast-feeding has been debated in the scientific literature, there is nevertheless a potential risk. An open and informed dialogue with expectant mothers regarding the risks and benefits of antibiotics during pregnancy and breast-feeding should routinely take place.

Antibiotics such as penicillins, cephalosporins, and macrolides like Zithromax are considered to be safe in pregnancy. Flagyl is potentially safe in late pregnancy, but trimester and population-specific risks exist and it should not be routinely used unless clinically indicated. Dosages, side effects, and contraindications are the same as previously discussed. Clindamycin (Cleocin) can be used when there are co-infections, including babesiosis, but first-trimester studies are unavailable and should therefore primarily be used in the second and third trimester. I have safely used combinations of Cleocin, Mepron (atovaquone), and Zithromax for third-trimester babesiosis (in two cases), where the babies were healthy at birth with no evidence of parasitemia or hemolytic anemia. Clindamycin and Quinine have also been used safely in third-trimester pregnancy, but due to potential side effects of Quinine (nausea, vomiting, rashes, and/or ringing in the ears), it is not my first choice. Ob-gyns and primary care doctors need to be asking women with a history of Lyme disease and co-infections if they have any specific symptoms of Lyme (like migratory pain) and symptoms of babesiosis (i.e., unexplained day and night sweats, which can be drenching) so that appropriate diagnostic and treatment regimens can be instituted as early as possible to prevent complications. Bartonella can only safely be treated with cephalosporins and Zithromax. Other drugs like tetracyclines, quinolones, and Bactrim are contraindicated during pregnancy.

Examples of antibiotic regimens used in pregnancy include oral cell-wall antibiotics such as amoxicillin, Omnicef, or other oral cephalosporins such as Ceftin. Intramuscular injections of Bicillin LA are also very effective, and they are useful in women with severe symptoms unresponsive to oral medication, and/or significant nausea. The long-acting effect of Bicillin may also potentially decrease the risk of maternal-fetal transmission, as regular injections avoid some of the variations seen in peak and trough levels with oral medications. We have, however, seen positive polymerase chain reactions (PCRs) for *Borrelia burgdorferi* on specimens of the placenta and/or cord blood postpartum, as well as Mycoplasma PCRs being positive in amniotic fluid, despite women remaining on oral antibiotics like Zithromax, although the babies were healthy at birth. Macrolides such as Zithromax do not penetrate well into the placenta but may be useful for controlling symptoms in the mother. Rarely IV medication like Rocephin is needed for maternal neurologic and/or cardiac involvement, or will be considered in the first trimester when the fetal organs are forming, especially if a woman has a history of frequent miscarriages associated with Lyme disease.

Pregnant women with active tick-borne infections should be managed in conjunction with a high-risk OB-GYN, and all medication and nutritional regimens should be coordinated with a gynecologist. Polymerase chain reaction specimens should be sent off at birth for Lyme (placenta, amniotic fluid, cord blood) and suspected co-infections. Lyme antibody testing in the baby can be done after six months, when maternal antibodies have declined.

MARY WAS TRYING TO GET PREGNANT

When Mary first came to see me, she was beside herself. Mary sat across from me at my desk. "Dr. H, what else can we do?" she asked. "I really want another child."

Mary had been my patient for two years and initially presented with symptoms of constant fatigue, migratory joint pain, intermittent tingling and numbness of her extremities, headaches, chest pain, palpitations, and memory and concentration problems. Her prior physicians had given her multiple diagnoses for her illness, including chronic fatigue syndrome, fibromyalgia, and even something called "stressed mommy syndrome." She had a two-year-old child who was still keeping her up at night, and

Mary's doctor suggested that her active child might be one of the main causes for her symptoms.

Her initial history and physical were unremarkable, but her Western blot was positive. Her clinical course was fairly typical. Her symptoms would come and go, and some symptoms would flare up temporarily with Jarisch-Herxheimer flares, requiring either stopping the antibiotics or rotating the regimen. She improved month after month, and after two years of treatment she reported being back to 100 percent of normal functioning. This was a tremendous improvement from her baseline functioning of 50 percent normal. I decided to continue her treatment for two more months to prevent a relapse. It was then that she told me she wanted to have another child.

Mary seemed well enough to get pregnant once she finished the antibiotic regimen. She returned six weeks later, feeling great, although she complained of fleeting joint pain in her hands one time over the past two months. There were no other symptoms. "Let's take you off the antibiotics and see how you do," I told her, and six weeks later she returned and announced that she was pregnant, and feeling "great."

"Excellent," I said. "Let's follow up in several months and see how you are doing."

Mary came back six weeks later, brokenhearted. She had just miscarried. I ordered PCR tests on the fetus and placenta just to be sure that Lyme disease wasn't involved in the miscarriage. Unfortunately, the results came back positive; borrelia was found in both the placenta and the fetus. It appeared that Mary was still infected with Lyme disease, despite two years of treatment, which she had passed on to her unborn child.

The next time I saw her, Mary told me again that she wanted another child more than anything in the world. I turned to her slowly and said, "OK, Mary. Let's put you back on antibiotics." Although she still couldn't pinpoint any active symptoms, the Lyme was clearly present. I reviewed the OB-GYN literature, which did show evidence of occasional maternal-fetal transmission of Lyme. I therefore placed Mary on Ceftin and Zithromax with meals, which were antibiotics shown to be safe in pregnancy for the fetus. The Ceftin would cover the cell-wall forms of borrelia, and the Zithromax would cover the intracellular forms (although Zithromax doesn't cross the placenta readily). I also ordered a low-carbohydrate diet with lots of fruits and vegetables and told her to take frequent doses of acidophilus, a probiotic used to replace the good bacteria killed by the antibiotic treatment, and which helps to prevent diarrhea. I really hoped that this treatment course would allow her to carry her next pregnancy to term.

Mary was doing fine at her next six-week follow-up. She had no Lyme symptoms, and her complete blood count and liver-function tests were normal while she was on the antibiotics. However, the same dreaded scenario played out sixteen weeks later. We again sent off PCR testing on the placenta and fetus. Both were again PCR positive for Lyme disease.

Mary had gone back to her OB-GYN in between our appointments and he reported that he could not find any other cause for her miscarriages. All of her hormone levels were normal, and there were no antiphospholipid/antilupus antibodies. It had to be the Lyme disease that kept showing up in her unborn baby that was causing the miscarriage.

When she came back to my office, tears were flowing down her cheeks. Mary and I had a long discussion of the pros and cons of her continuing to get pregnant, including the psychological burden it was placing on her and her family.

"I'm up for it, Dr. H," she said. "Just tell me what to do."

After extensive discussions, we decided that we needed to be as aggressive as we could be to prevent borrelia from being transmitted again to the fetus. I decided on using IV Rocephin during the first trimester of her pregnancy, when the baby was most at risk. Mary understood the possible gallbladder complications that are already inherent in pregnancy due to normally high estrogen levels and the fact that there are reports of patients having gallbladder problems while on Rocephin. She understood the possible complications of IV access, including phlebitis and infection, since the drug is given by a peripherally inserted central catheter (a PICC line, which is a stationary IV line that remains in the arm).

Once she knew she was pregnant, we would begin treatment. Eight weeks later, Mary started on IV Rocephin for the cell-wall forms of borrelia, and Zithromax for the intracellular forms. We scheduled monthly follow-ups, and she also saw her high-risk obstetrician on a regular basis.

There were no problems at month one. No problems, month two. No problems, month three. A sonogram was scheduled for week sixteen. We held our breath waiting for the results. I got a call from her after the sonogram.

WHAT KIND OF DOCTOR SHOULD I BE SEEING?

Your primary care physician is the best first resource. If you are not getting better despite several months of treatment, seek out a physician who specializes in Lyme disease in your area. You can find one on the following Web sites: http://ilads.org/ilads_media /physician-referral/ or www.lymediseaseassociation.org. Also, functional medicine trained healthcare practitioners who are familiar with treating Lyme and co-infections can help you with the protocols described in this book.

"So far, so good, Dr. H. All is well."

Once we got past the sixteen- to twenty-week mark I removed the IV line and put her back on oral antibiotics. I prayed that she would have a continued healthy pregnancy. I didn't know if her family or I could take another fetal loss. Fortunately, the rest of the pregnancy was uneventful. She gave birth to a healthy eight-pound baby boy that June. I received a letter in the mail from her with a picture of her new baby. It said, "If it wasn't for you, Dr. Horowitz, none of this would have been possible."

When my wife, Lee, read this card, she wanted to know just how much of a role I had actually played in this pregnancy! You learn over time not to push the limits of comedy with a potentially jealous Sicilian wife. "Oh, honey, come on. He barely looks like me. Except for maybe that nose. Does his nose look a little big to you?"

I have now treated approximately one hundred pregnant women with antibiotics classified as safe for the fetus. We have found that the women with active Lyme symptoms had an easier time during their pregnancy on antibiotics, and the babies were all healthy at birth. A few of the babies were, however, PCR positive for borrelia or Mycoplasma in the placenta, cord blood, or amniotic fluid despite maternal therapy. They are being followed carefully by their pediatricians to determine if further therapy is needed, and hopefully these children will not turn into future patients with persistent Lyme disease. In Chapter 4, you will learn about the new research on pulsing and "persisters" that gives hope to those with chronic symptoms unresponsive to prior therapies.

FOUR

"Persisters" and Pulsing for Treating Resistant Lyme Disease

"Let no one who has the slightest desire to live in peace and quietness be tempted under any circumstances to enter upon the chivalrous task of trying to correct a popular error."

—WILLIAM THOMS, 1873

"To persist, or not to persist, that is the question."

—DR. RICHARD HOROWITZ, 2016

The question of whether Lyme disease can persist after administering standard courses of antibiotic therapy for three to four weeks remains a hotly debated topic. We know that short-term antibiotics fail in 25 percent to 71 percent of patients with late-stage disease, and that treatment relapses are common. Despite dozens of peer-reviewed scientific studies illustrating persistence of borrelia by both PCR and culture (our gold standard), some physicians deny the evidence that Lyme persists, and that prolonged antibiotics resolve symptoms.

In 2014, researchers at Johns Hopkins University and Northeastern University showed that borrelia was able to form persister bacterial cells. Persisters are a subpopulation of resistant cells that can survive antibiotics or other medications. These cells can lay dormant (either non-growing or slow growing), and can reactivate when conditions are favorable. Certain chronic infections like tuberculosis and leprosy that are slow-growing intracellular infections (like Lyme) can take up to one year or longer to treat, and they illustrate the issues of persisters and relapse. For these conditions, we combine drugs that hit the different bacterial forms. Some of the antibiotics used to treat TB, like isonizide (INH) and rifampin, kill growing bacteria, but pyrazinamide (PZA) is needed at the same time to kill persisters. Persisters not killed by antibiotics can revert to active bacteria and cause a relapse. That is why three- and even four-drug regimens (adding ethambutol) are necessary, with INH being continued longer term to treat active bacteria that arise from reverting persister cells.

Persisters have been recognized for other chronic bacterial infections like syphilis (a spirochetal cousin of Lyme disease), as well as bacteria involved in chronic heart valve infections (endocarditis), brucellosis, and Q fever (another tick-borne infection, *Coxiella burnetii*). Many persistent infections also involve biofilm formation, as is the case with chronic gum infections (periodontitis), chronic otitis media (inner ear infections with multiple bacteria, including *S. pneumoniae*, *Haemophilus influenzae*, and *Moraxella catarrhalis*), prosthetic devices (valve and joint replacements), and Lyme disease.

THE FORMATION OF PERSISTER CELLS AND BIOFILMS

Dr. Kim Lewis and colleagues published in *Antimicrobial Agents and Chemotherapy* in May 2015 that borrelia is able to form drug-tolerant persister cells. In this study the authors examined the ability of *B. burgdorferi* to form persisters, and they found that the killing of growing cultures of *B. burgdorferi* with antibiotics had two distinct phases, during which some bacteria were actively dividing and able to be killed, but there was a small subpopulation of surviving cells that were not as metabolically active (dormant persisters), which survived the initial antibiotic challenge. Upon regrowth, these cells formed a new subpopulation of antibiotic-tolerant cells, some of which were able to be killed by reintroducing the antibiotics, indicating that these cells are persisters rather than resistant mutants. The level of persisters increased sharply as the culture transitioned from an actively dividing phase (exponential) to a stationary phase (dormant or less metabolically active), and combinations of antibiotics did not improve the rate of killing. Further research at Hopkins by Dr. Ying Zhang and colleagues in 2016 showed that Daptomycin plus doxycycline plus cefuroxime eradicated biofilm-like structures and persisters with no growth of bacteria in culture, however we need clinical studies to confirm the efficacy of this regimen. According to Dr. Zhang, "Persisters underlie persistent and latent infections and post-treatment relapse, posing significant challenges for the treatment of many bacterial infections."

Persister cells and biofilms help us understand some of the mechanisms behind relapses in Lyme disease. Lyme bacteria can withstand some of the strongest antibiotics, forming persister bacteria, which can then reactivate under favorable conditions (when antibiotics are stopped). Biofilms—the protective coating these cells form—might also be playing a large role in contributing to borrelia's persistence.

Biofilms create a matrix, which provides a physical barrier for antibodies and antibiotics, and shields persisters from the immune system. It helps explain in part the persistence of other bacterial infections. Examples of other well-known biofilm infections that persist include *Clostridium difficile*, salmonella, *Candida albicans* (yeast), staphylococcus, Klebsiella, and *Porphyromonas gingivalis* (the bacteria that hides under the plaque on our teeth, causing chronic gingivitis). Dr. Eva Sapi and colleagues published in 2012 and again in 2016 that borrelia are found in biofilms, protecting the organism from the effects of antibiotics.

More Evidence That Lyme Persists

Despite prior published research showing positive PCRs and cultures of borrelia after standard courses of antibiotics, scientists at the NIH set out to study whether chronic persistent infection with *Borrelia burgdorferi* really exists. They attempted to answer this question by conducting a study using a new technique called "xenodiagnostics." Live, disease-free ticks were placed on patients with a history of Lyme disease who were treated with several weeks of antibiotics. Both the ticks and the patients were tested to see whether there was evidence of persistent infection. The results of the study, published in 2014 in *Clinical Infectious Diseases*, found that the DNA from *Borrelia burgdorferi* could still be found in patients previously treated for Lyme disease.

The same results were replicated in a 2014 NIH animal xenodiagnostic study, which found that Bb could not be cultured from tissues after antibiotic treatment for Lyme, yet low numbers of borrelia DNA were detectable in tissues up to eight months after completion of treatment, and RNA transcription of genes was seen with visualized spirochetes. RNA transcription is only possible with viable DNA. That same year, Dr. S. H. Lee reported that spirochetemia (spirochetes in the blood) and positive PCRs were seen in previously treated patients with Lyme during winter months, again implying persistence of the bacteria. These results join numerous other peer-reviewed scientific studies showing evidence of persistence of Lyme disease by both PCR and culture, despite "seemingly adequate" antibiotic therapy. Should we therefore be surprised that several months of antibiotics in the recent Persistent Lyme Empiric Antibody Study Europe (PLEASE) trial helped patients but did not fully resolve infection? They did not treat all the different forms of Lyme (or adequately screen and treat for associated co-infections), nor use biofilm busters, or newer "persister" drugs identified in the scientific literature. As per recent NIH studies, borrelia can persist by PCR, and only live borrelial DNA can turn on genes and transcribe RNA and proteins.

Naysayers have claimed that these multiple scientific studies showing positive PCRs for borrelia after standard treatment represent dead DNA. Can the dead DNA of bacteria exist in tissues eight months after therapy and turn on genes? The scientific literature says no. Prior studies show that DNA is rapidly cleared from the system, and in the mouse model, unprotected, foreign DNA is excreted by the body within forty-two hours. Similarly, studies in 1997 found that dead spirochetes should not be able to turn genes on or off, which is a property of living cells. The finding of persistent borrelial DNA in patients with ongoing symptoms in this NIH study, as well as other published studies showing positive PCRs and cultures for borrelia after treatment, joins numerous peer-reviewed, published scientific studies showing evidence of persistence of Lyme disease despite "months" of antibiotic therapy.

Other published studies have confirmed persistence of Lyme, as well as other borrelia species, after standard therapy. Dead spirochetes in the circulating blood left over from an acute infection would be quickly removed by the spleen, and both spirochetemia and positive PCRs post antibiotics point to persistence. Identification of positive PCRs helps medical doctors to detect and diagnose other active infections such as viral infections (like HIV and hepatitis) and evaluate the efficacy of therapies by looking at the viral load (quantitative PCR). It also permits identification of non-cultivable or slow-growing bacteria like mycobacteria. Positive PCRs in the blood in these and other diseases means the infections are active and alive. Although these are highly sensitive tests, where laboratories need strict controls to prevent contamination, multiple authors over the years are finding positive PCRs for Lyme and other borrelia species post-treatment, indicating that the bacteria persist after standard antibiotic therapies.

The new research coming out of Hopkins and Kim Lewis's lab on persisters, and Dr. Eva Sapi's and Alan MacDonald's lab on biofilm colonies protecting the Lyme bacteria, all point in the direction of a solution not just for Lyme but for many chronic bacterial infections. When these studies are combined with prior research showing PCR and culture positivity for borrelia after both short-term and long-term antibiotics, we are poised to institute new therapies using novel drugs and pulsing regimens to find cures.

We know that borrelia can change shape once it is introduced into the human body, and that certain forms, known as cyst forms (also known as S-forms, L-forms, spheroplasts, round bodies, and CWD/cell wall deficient forms), allow borrelia to persist under adverse circumstances. As we learned in Chapter 3, these cyst forms can go dormant and later transform into mobile spirochetes under proper conditions. Older research implicated cystic forms as one of the primary reasons that Lyme persists. The new research shows that borrelia also persists because it has additional strategies to evade the immune system: immune evasion, persisters, and biofilms all help explain post-treatment relapses.

Immune Evasion

Borrelia has been shown to be capable of affecting our immune system, preventing it from having a long-lasting, functional antibody response. This is another reason why some people living in endemic areas who are continually exposed to spirochetes do not clear the infection. Normally, IgM antibodies are created early on in an infection and then disappear, and are followed by the creation of IgG antibodies, which are more effective than IgM antibodies in combatting infections. However, a 2015 study found spirochetes that accumulate in the outside part of lymph nodes created more IgM antibodies than IgG antibodies, and therefore impede the clearance of the infection. This finding is confirmed by laboratory results. We see many more CDC-positive IgM antibody responses in chronic Lyme patients, and not IgG responses (although borrelia-specific bands on the Western blot oftentimes change over time, indicating persistence and recognition of the bacteria by the immune system).

Prior scientific studies showed that borrelia is able to kill important immune cells in our body such as lymphocytes, and that some serum-resistant strains of borrelia evade the complement pathway, which is another way our immune system helps to clear pathogens from the body. Although this mechanism was known to exist for *Borrelia burgdorferi*, a recent article showed that the relapsing fever spirochete *Borrelia miyamotoi* is also resistant to human complement mediated killing, and may help explain persistent symptoms.

Besides hiding from the immune system, borrelia goes deep into tissues where antibiotics can't penetrate well. Despite the use of seemingly "adequate antibiotics," published scientific research has shown that borrelia can hide and persist in the eyes, central nervous system (i.e., glial cells in the brain), joints, ligaments, and fibroblasts of the skin. Borrelia can also hide in the intracellular compartment, and intracellular infections can be difficult to completely eradicate. Co-infections also contribute to chronic illness.

I have treated patients with tick-borne co-infections, such as Babesia and Bartonella, and found that they play an important role in keeping patients ill, yet these co-infections are often not included in research exploring the persistent symptoms of Lyme. Borrelia, Bartonella, Mycoplasma, and chlamydia species can all hide within the intracellular compartment and act synergistically to increase inflammation and cause resistant illness. We find a high infectious burden (IB) of multiple intracellular infections in patients who are the sickest. Intracellular Mycoplasma can persist and stimulate autoimmune reactions and increase inflammatory cytokines in people with arthritic symptoms. Intracellular borrelia secretes particles of DNA, called blebs, which are highly stimulatory to the immune system, and when these blebs are inside our cells they can convert our own host cells into targets for the immune system, contributing to autoimmunity. Intracellular chlamydia species have extrapulmonary manifestations, and they can be a causative agent of reactive arthritis and undifferentiated oligoarthritis (where arthritic symptoms are worsened by heavy metal exposure, which is common in Lyme patients). Bartonella species increase symptoms, are known to persist, and bacteremia (infection in the blood stream), potentially spanning decades in duration, have been shown in people with normal, healthy, functioning immune systems.

All these infections can be present in Lyme patients, along with heavy metals contributing to their illness, and we have seen evidence of positive PCRs for Lyme, Babesia, Bartonella, and Mycoplasma infections using single intracellular long-term antibiotic therapy. The failure of single intracellular therapy for Lyme, Bartonella, and Mycoplasma requires double, triple, and even quadruple intracellular antibiotic therapies if we are to get our sickest patients better. The failure of standard Babesia regimens (Clindamycin and Quinine, and/or Mepron and Zithromax) oftentimes requires simultaneous use of multiple antiparasitic drugs and herbs if we are to improve our sickest patients with persistent babesiosis. These chronic infections represent "persister" bacteria and "persister" parasites that require new, innovative therapies. Our Action Plan for getting resistant patients better therefore includes not only longer-term combination antibiotic therapy but the use of newer persister drugs and biofilm busters in patients with multiple intracellular infections. We are finding these novel regimens are working for a large percentage of patients who have failed prior therapies.

The majority of our patients who are chronically ill have parasitic infections like Babesia, which you will learn more about in Chapter 6. If you just treat Lyme and intracellular bacteria but do not adequately treat the parasites, you will not achieve optimum results. In the United States, the parasites are usually *Babesia microti* or *Babesia duncani* (WA-1), with some showing evidence of toxoplasmosis (a close genetic cousin of Babesia that can be transmitted by cats), FL-1953 (*protomyxoa rheumatica*), and/or associated intestinal parasites. In Europe, we generally see *Babesia divergens*, but other species like *B. microti*, *B. duncani*, EU-1, and Therelia species are also now being found. Babesia can significantly increase Lyme symptoms, making you three times sicker while suppressing the ability of the body to fight and eliminate other parasitic infections. In 2014 Dr. Eva Sapi discovered filarial parasites (nematodes, i.e., worms) inside *Ixodes scapularis* ticks in Connecticut, while Dr. Alan MacDonald has been finding larval forms of these filarial nematodes in patients with MS. Although we do not understand the full significance of these findings, there are patients with Lyme and/or Morgellons disease (a skin disorder known to be related to *B. burgdorferi*) whose Lyme symptoms sometimes respond to antiparasitic drugs like Ivermectin, Biltricide, Pin-X, Alinia, and Albenza, where no clear parasite apart from Babesia and/or an intestinal parasite can be identified. Recent laboratories studies by Dr. Shah at IGeneX have identified Bartonella species in some with Morgellons, apart from borrelia species. We are therefore often dealing with multiple bacteria and parasites at once, which is an important lesson to remember if you suffer with resistant, unexplained symptoms.

What's more, *B. burgdorferi*, through gene recombination, can also modify its surface antigens, helping it to avoid immune recognition, which is the same mechanism relapsing fever borrelia uses to persist in the body. Lastly, borrelia can go dormant for long periods of time. Some antibiotics (penicillins and cephalosporins) only work with actively replicating bacteria.

THE DAPSONE AND PYRAZINAMIDE STORY: A TALE OF TWO MYCOBACTERIUM DRUGS

Although the MSIDS model helps the vast majority of people who come to me for treatment, there is always a small population of resistant patients. These are usually my "Herx kings and queens," whose JH reactions flare during treatment (especially with intracellular medications) and never completely improve.

Based on the new research that borrelia is a "persister" bacteria and that pulsing antibiotics may help improve the efficacy of treatment, I developed a protocol with new combinations of antibiotics that can address cell-wall and cystic forms, forms inside biofilms as well as bacterial persisters in the intracellular compartment for those failing traditional therapies. These intracellular drug combinations are similar to what is used to kill mycobacteria like TB and leprosy. Mycobacteria share certain similar biological characteristics to those of Lyme: They are both persister bacteria that are slow growing, located inside cells, and are resistant to many common antibiotics, causing chronic disease. At least a year of treatment is required to treat leprosy, and anywhere from six to eighteen months of treatment is required to treat tuberculosis (for multidrug resistant TB and/or central nervous system involvement the length of time to treat is even longer).

The newest protocol we use features the medication Dapsone, which is already approved for a number of diseases, including toxoplasmosis (genetically related to Babesia), malaria prophylaxis (Babesia has malaria-like properties), and several dermatological conditions, including dermatitis herpetiformis (a disease associated with celiac disease), Behçet's syndrome (an autoimmune disease), and acne. Dapsone is also an intracellular medication used for persister bacteria like leprosy, with antimalarial properties. This led me to examine whether it would be useful for Lyme, an intracellular persister bacteria, and Babesia, a persistent parasitic infection that is present in the majority of my Lyme patients, contributing to their illness.

Since the Johns Hopkins studies have classified borrelia as a persister bacteria, it made sense to look at the pharmacological literature to see what was available to treat persisters. I already had some success using double intracellular drugs such as doxycycline and rifampin in patients with Lyme and Bartonella (which are causes of chronic neuropathy and neurocognitive symptoms), but symptoms would oftentimes persist and relapse when these drugs were stopped. I therefore decided to try triple or quadruple intracellular regimens, like the ones used to treat tuberculosis and leprosy, and see if adding a mycobacterium persister drug like Dapsone to the regimen would make a difference. It did, helping many patients with resistant symptoms that were never helped by any other treatments. Dr. Phyllis Freeman and I published our results in the scientific literature in April 2016, where we demonstrated statistically significant improvement with Dapsone in 100 patients who had failed classical treatment protocols for Lyme and Babesia. This was the first published scientific study of an effective oral "persister" drug protocol for resistant Lyme disease and babesiosis. Fatigue, joint and muscle pain, neuropathy, sleep disorders, memory and concentration problems, difficulty with speech and writing, and malarial-type Babesia symptoms (day sweats, night sweats, chills, and flushing) all significantly improved (with the exception of headaches). Adding a novel "persister" drug to rifampin, tetracyclines, and/or macrolides with a cell-wall drug (cephalosporins), as well as treating biofilms, made the difference among patients for whom all prior therapies had failed. Dr. Eva Sapi recently confirmed our results with an in vitro study at the University of New Haven. She showed that Dapsone with either doxycycline or cefuroxime decreased biofilms by 40 percent, and when Dapsone was combined with doxycycline and rifampin (a triple intracellular combination), it significantly reduced borrelia biofilm mass by 50 percent after only three days! This was confirmed by live and dead microscopic analysis. The effectiveness of the protocol may therefore be secondary to its ability to both affect biofilms and address persistent intracellular infections.

We also tried using rifampin and pyrazinamide, another tuberculosis drug, in a small group of patients who were sulfa sensitive, unable to use Dapsone, and whose prior classical protocols had failed. We found that rifampin and pyrazinamide were also effective in some of these patients, illustrating the usefulness of older, established persister drugs for novel uses in Lyme and co-infections. Rifampin is usually part of a TB or leprosy regimen, so it has overlapping properties against mycobacteria as well as Lyme and intracellular co-infections like Bartonella and tularemia. In a case study that I published in 2016 in the *Journal of Arthritis and Rheumatism*, Dr. Freeman and I demonstrated that pyrazinamide, combined with a tetracycline and rifampin, helped a patient with Lyme and a resistant autoimmune disease, Behçet's syndrome, who failed twenty years of standard anti-rheumatic drugs, with severe rheumatologic manifestations. Dapsone has been proved to help patients with Behçet's, an autoimmune dermatological condition with multisystemic symptoms, and although Dapsone was superior to prior regimens for some of her Lyme and co-infection symptoms, it did not significantly help treat her Behçet's disease. Only adding pyrazinamide to doxycycline and rifampin was effective in treating her chronic ulcerations and skin changes (granulomas) associated with Behçet's and Bartonella.

Apart from Lyme, this patient also had evidence of persistent Bartonella and tularemia that relapsed during treatment on immunosuppressive therapy (she was on intermittent prednisone and chronic Imuran therapy for sero-negative rheumatoid arthritis from her rheumatologist). She had failed multiple combinations of intracellular drug therapy (two- and three-drug combinations), and was effectively treated with a four-drug intracellular antibiotic regimen for relapsing Bartonella and tularemia, including a tetracycline (doxycycline), rifampin, Dapsone, and a quinolone (Avelox). Intracellular persister bacteria in chronically ill, debilitated patients with Lyme, associated co-infections and/or autoimmune disease may require multiple intracellular drugs, including the addition of persister drugs (Dapsone and Pyrazinamide), used in novel ways to obtain positive clinical results.

For my most resistant patients I now use several different combinations of intracellular drugs, including combinations of tetracyclines (minocycline and/or doxycycline), rifampin, macrolides (Zithromax or Biaxin), and Dapsone (two to three intracellular drugs, occasionally four), combined with Plaquenil and grapefruit seed extract (two cyst-busters), pulsed cell-wall drugs (Ceftin, Omnicef, penicillins or IV Rocephin), nystatin (for preventing yeast), biofilm busters (like Serrapeptase, Stevia, and mono-laurin, which is a coconut oil extract), with extra folic acid to help prevent side effects of Dapsone. I use Leucovorin, a pharmaceutical folic acid, and a nutraceutical high-strength activated folic acid from Xymogen called 5-MTHF-ES (5-methyltetrahydrofolate extra-strength) or Folify-ER. A total of at least 30 mg of folic acid a day must be used (sometimes higher, i.e., 45 to 60 mg/day) to minimize the anemia associated with Dapsone. Average decreases in hemoglobin of about 2 to 3 grams can be expected with Dapsone using the above doses of folic acid, which stabilizes over time. Deplin (L-methyl folate) can also be included in the protocol.

Although Dapsone can be effective, it is not a benign drug without side effects, and the risks/benefits must be discussed with the patient. There are four main potential side effects—Herxheimer reactions, Anemia, Rashes and Methemoglobinemia—that can be remembered with the acronym, Do No "HARM."

Herxheimer (JH) reactions are seen in the majority of patients using Dapsone, and they can be severe, in which case the dose will need to be temporarily decreased or held for several days, especially if the JH reactions persist despite using LDN, high-dose glutathione with NAC, alpha-lipoic acid, alkalizing the body and drainage remedies. Some patients take months to get to the full Dapsone dose secondary to severe JH reactions, but they still improve significantly over time. Although the full dose (100 mg per day) was the most effective dose in our studies to date, severe Herxheimer reactions with other intracellular medications may require starting at a low initial dose (25 mg every other day), and slowly increasing the dose (i.e., 25 mg/day for one to two weeks, then 50 mg alternating with 25 mg for one to two weeks, then 50 mg/day for one to two weeks (the minimum effective dose), until slowly getting to the full dose.

Another side effect is anemia, secondary to Dapsone interfering with folic acid synthesis. This will cause the size of red blood cells to increase, causing a macrocytic (large cell) anemia, which is the most common form of anemia seen with the drug. Rarely, Dapsone can cause a hemolytic anemia (where the red blood cells burst). You will need to initially have blood drawn every two to three weeks on the protocol (CBC, CMP, occasionally checking a Coombs direct antibody for hemolytic anemia) and consider getting checked for G6PD (glucose 6 phosphate dehydrogenase) deficiency, which can be an overlapping cause of hemolytic anemia. Certain antibiotic/antimalarial medications as well as ingestion of fava beans can cause anemia in people who are G6PD-deficient. Even though hemolytic anemia is possible with Dapsone, we have not witnessed it in over four hundred patients on the protocol. Once patients stop Dapsone, the anemia usually reverses and goes back to baseline levels within a month, as long as folic acid supplementation continues and there are no overlapping causes of anemia.

I also suggest treating iron deficiency anemia before starting Dapsone, and following iron levels (iron, TIBC [total iron binding capacity], and ferritin) in women of childbearing age, since heavy menstrual periods and iron loss will worsen anemia. Any woman prone to heavy menses must be on iron and contact her healthcare provider if there is any heavy bleeding, which may require stopping Dapsone, increasing folic acid, and increasing iron intake. Since Dapsone will cause on the average a 2 to 3 gram drop in hemoglobin (rarely more), women should aim to have an initial starting hemoglobin of at least 13 grams/dL, so as to not drop below 10 grams/dL. Despite the anemia, many women report that their energy level is significantly better!

Another side effect of Dapsone is rashes. It is a sulfa drug, and may cause a rash in those who are sulfa sensitive, although we have seen patients who can't tolerate Bactrim, another sulfa drug, who can take Dapsone without any side effects. If you are sulfa sensitive, and the risk/benefit ratio requires doing a trial of Dapsone due to having failed multiple other antibiotic protocols, discuss with your healthcare provider using an H1 blocker (Zyrtec and/or Benadryl) with an H2 blocker (Zantac) prior to starting treatment, which may keep down side effects of rashes and itching. If, however, there is a history of severe sulfa allergies, it may be best to avoid the drug.

The last, significant side effect of Dapsone is methemoglobinemia. This is where the hemoglobin in our red blood cells, which carries oxygen, is exposed to increased oxidative stress and oxidizes the iron molecules so that they can't effectively release oxygen to the tissues. This can rarely cause a "blue man/woman syndrome" where the lips and extremities turn blue due to low oxygen levels (hypoxia), with shortness of breath. This will usually not happen with methemoglobin levels below 10 percent, although levels between 5 and 10 percent can occasionally cause symptoms of fatigue, dizziness and shortness of breath. Levels below 5 percent are usually asymptomatic. Methemoglobinemia can resolve rapidly within twenty-four hours of stopping the drug and increasing folic acid with antioxidants. A pulse oximetry checking oxygen levels is a good screening test, and methemoglobin levels should be checked periodically during treatment. I therefore recommend high-dose antioxidants (like resveratrol, and/or curcumin), with liposomal glutathione, NAC and alpha-lipoic acid, since glutathione has been shown to be an alternative pathway to reverse met-hemoglobin. In severe cases, supplemental oxygen with a methylene blue 1 percent solution (10 mg/ml, at 1 to 2 mg/kg intravenously slowly over five minutes) can be used to quickly reverse methemoglobinemia. Tagamet (yes, the H2 blocker) can also be used to treat elevated methemoglobin levels. We have fortunately only seen high methemoglobin levels in a handful of patients (especially if they were using oxidant therapies on their own, such as ozone), and stopping Dapsone and reintroducing it at lower levels when the methemoglobin returns to normal, while avoiding pro-oxidant therapies with more glutathione support, has generally prevented a recurrence.

Despite the potential side effects, we have found Dapsone to be safe and effective. We don't yet know if 50 mg versus 100 mg of Dapsone per day is superior when used in long-term combination therapy (higher doses of Dapsone usually have greater efficacy in our clinical studies), or the length of time of treatment required to effect a "cure" (if it is possible), or which combination of meds will produce the best long-term results. We are also not sure about the success rate once the drug is stopped at twelve months (which is the time frame of our ongoing study). This is the same length of time required to treat other persister bacteria like leprosy with rifampin and Dapsone. Why did we choose twelve months? We tried stopping Dapsone at two months, but symptoms relapsed. We tried again at four and six months, but the same thing happened, although symptoms were clearly better than when they started, with some patients getting neurological improvements not seen with other drugs. One woman could text and use her thumbs, which had been almost paralyzed from Lyme and Bartonella; another had been sick for twelve years, and her brain fog, joint, and muscle pain improved as she went from 20 percent to 80 percent of normal within a few months. One man with severe neuropsychiatric symptoms (psychosis) who failed all antibiotics and antipsychotic medications after taking Dapsone at 25 mg QOD for two weeks, woke up and started speaking normally after a severe Herxheimer reaction. Unfortunately, the beneficial effect didn't last when the drug was stopped, and we are re-evaluating using Dapsone at higher doses with more detox support. Clearly, mycobacterium "persister" drugs like Dapsone are acting differently than other intracellular antibiotics I have used.

We have had some patients relapse at six months using lower dosages, and others who took it for seven months with other intracellular drugs who remained symptom-free. Some patients had greater clinical improvements with the Dapsone protocol than with any other drug regimen, but had PCR evidence of Lyme and Bartonella midway during therapy. We are therefore evaluating different dosages, combinations, and lengths of therapy. The combinations that seem to be the most effective usually involve taking Dapsone with a tetracycline and macrolide (Zithromax or Biaxin) or a tetracycline with rifampin, but there are some severely ill patients who failed multiple protocols who are on four-drug intracellular regimens (pulsing rifampin and Zithromax, with regular use of minocycline or doxycycline with Dapsone) who are doing extremely well. All of these patients were on Plaquenil and grapefruit seed extract (GSE) for cyst forms, pulsed cell-wall drugs (Ceftin or Omnicef) three days a week (Monday, Wednesday, Saturday) with nystatin BID (for yeast), and biofilm busters (Serrapeptase, Stevia, and/or Lauricidin).

By following this protocol, many of my sickest patients, as well as my Herx kings and queens, have started to improve. We have enrolled over four hundred patients on the Horowitz Dapsone protocol, and the vast majority are improving. Patients who have been sick for many years (five to forty) have reported that this was the best regimen they had ever taken. If you have failed classical protocols and you are disabled from tick-borne disorders, with chronic fatigue, pain, neuropathy, and memory/concentration problems, as well as sweats and chills (chronic babesiosis), then have an informed conversation with your healthcare provider. If you follow the above recommendations, Dapsone may help you.

LINDA SAW PROGRESS AFTER TWELVE YEARS OF LYME TREATMENT

Linda was forty-six years old with a past medical history of breast cancer, high cholesterol (hyperlipidemia), irritable bowel syndrome, reactive hypoglycemia, migraines, ADHD, and depression. She first came to our office after experiencing three years of an undiagnosed illness, which began with flulike symptoms several days after she had spent time in her garden, where she got over a hundred pricks from pruning her rosebushes. There was no evidence of a tick bite, but she lived in a Lyme-endemic area in the northeastern United States.

Linda complained of drenching night sweats with chills and flushing, which was interfering with her sleep. She saw her gynecologist, who told her that she was not yet in menopause, as she still had regular periods with a normal follicle-stimulating hormone (FSH), luteinizing hormone (LH), and estrogen levels. She then experienced a twenty-pound weight gain and noticed that she had debilitating fatigue that worsened whenever she ate lots of sugar. She also had hair loss, swollen glands, and a sore throat that would come and go; decreased libido; occasional right lower pelvic pain; an unexplained cough and shortness of breath; joint pain and stiffness in her fingers, knees, and hips that would migrate and come and go; migratory muscle pains of the lower extremities that would come and go; facial twitching; headaches; tingling of her nose; blurry vision with episodes of double vision; tinnitus (ringing in the ears); balance problems with dizziness; and severe memory and concentration problems, where she would get disoriented from time to time. She had previously consulted a neurologist, who told her that her symptoms were most likely psychiatric in origin as he could not find anything "organic" in nature. Her dermatologist had the same response when Linda started noticing lesions on her face, arms, legs, nose, and abdomen, with colored filaments and fibers coming out of the lesions. The dermatologist told her that she was suffering from "delusional parasitosis," confirming her fears that she suffered from a psychiatric condition and that her health complaints were "in her head."

When I met Linda, I noticed right away that she was a highly intelligent and articulate woman, albeit extremely anxious. Her blood pressure was 170/100 with a pulse rate of 104 BPM. She had a history of hypertension that had never been treated, as it was attributed to stress induced by doctors—who would have thought? My physical exam only revealed red swollen nasal turbinates suggestive of allergies and fibrocystic breasts, with some healing lesions of her skin. She had been a frequent smoker and had significant exposure to inks, dyes, and different chemicals, as she had worked in a paper mill in California for several years before returning to Connecticut. She was on Neurontin at bedtime for her neuropathy, Lunesta for sleep, and Adderall for her ADHD. Her mother had been diagnosed with MS, her father died of a stroke with hypertension, and one brother had a stroke at forty-two years old. No wonder Linda hated to see doctors!

Her past laboratory results were positive for inflammation, hyperlipidemia, toxoplasmosis exposure, and herpes virus exposure. Based on her exam and her responses to the MSIDS questionnaire, we sent off a full blood workup for tick-borne infections, chlamydia and Mycoplasma exposure; viral infections (Epstein-Barr, cytomegalovirus, human herpes virus-6, and West Nile); an autoimmune panel (including dsDNA, ssDNA, SM Ab, ssA/ssB [Sjögren's antibodies], rheumatoid factor, and anticardiolipin antibodies); vitamin and mineral levels (B_{12}, folate, MMA, HC/magnesium, iodine, selenium, and zinc); a food allergy panel (IgE, IgG) with an antigliadin antibody and TTG (for gluten sensitivity/celiac disease); a hormone panel (adrenal, thyroid, and sex hormones, especially checking the 2/16 OH estrogen ratio with her history of breast cancer); a 1,25/25 OH Vitamin D ratio (for inflammation), lipid peroxides, sulfates, and nitrates (checking for oxidative stress and detoxification problems); immunoglobulin levels and subclasses; and a HbA1c, VAP lipid profile, and PLAC test to further evaluate her cardiovascular risk with hypertension and a family history of strokes.

Her tests returned positive for Lyme disease, Babesia, toxoplasmosis (IgG positive), Mycoplasma, and chlamydia, and were suggestive of Bartonella. There was old exposure to Epstein-Barr virus and human herpes virus-6. There was significant inflammation with a sedimentation rate of 39 (normal less than 20), a HS-CRP of 19.8 (normal less than 1), and an elevated 1,25/25 OH Vitamin D ratio, with a low 25 OH Vitamin D at 28 (normal greater than 30). She was antigliadin positive, TTG negative (gluten sensitive), had a mildly elevated HbA1c and lipids (suggestive of metabolic syndrome, which, with her hypertension, increased her future risk of cardiovascular complications), had elevated heavy metals (lead 39, normal less than 5; mercury 7, normal less than 4), and severe adrenal deficiency (low DHEA and very low cortisol levels, close to zero).

I told Linda in her follow up consultation that I thought that she had Lyme-MSIDS. I also told her that her skin disorder with colored fibers coming out of the skin was Morgellons disease, known to be caused by borreliosis, reassuring her that except for perhaps bacteria, parasites, and neurotoxins in her brain, her symptoms were not "in her head."

We began a low-salt, low-carbohydrate, gluten-free, anti-inflammatory diet (for her elevated BP and pre-diabetes, avoiding trans fats, and keeping down meat, dairy, and grains with increased fresh fruits, vegetables, and olive oil), with PT/exercise (for her dizziness and balance problems) combined with a series of rotating antibiotic regimens and hormonal/detoxification support. Although she would improve from time to time with double or triple intracellular antibiotics as well as Babesia/Bartonella treatment, she kept relapsing every time she was taken off antibiotics and tried on herbal protocols. This went on for eleven years, although her Morgellons skin lesions cleared up and never returned. We did a mold test for her resistant symptoms, which came back positive from Real Time Labs in Texas for trichothecene (0.57, normal up to 0.2 ppb) and we discussed increasing her detoxification with far infrared saunas, using an oral mold detox protocol with phosphatidylcholine, glutathione, alpha-lipoic acid, NAC, and N-butyrate. Both Linda and I were frustrated but committed to getting her better.

In April of 2015 I had just begun using Dapsone as a "persister regimen." After explaining the possible side effects, I discussed with Linda going onto my new protocol. This regimen involved three intracellular drugs, one of which she had never previously taken. She remained on hydrocortisone (Cortef) in the morning for her low adrenal function with DHEA (sublingual), and high-dose probiotics to prevent yeast and diarrhea.

Linda returned two months later. She had been on Dapsone for five weeks and was feeling the best she ever had felt in the past twelve years! Her cognitive difficulties had resolved, and her brain function felt almost 100 percent normal. She reported improvements in her joint and muscle pain as well as stamina and overall energy, with improved moods and decreased depression. Her resistant Babesia symptoms also improved as she had significantly less heat intolerance, temperature dysregulation, day and night sweats, and chills. She went from feeling 20 percent of normal to 75 to 80 percent of normal. Clearly this protocol was highly effective for Linda, and the best she had taken, but when we tried stopping or lowering the dose of Dapsone, Linda started to relapse, although she still was significantly better than when we started.

Pulsing Medication for Borreliosis

The idea of pulse-dosing to eradicate bacterial persisters came from Joseph Bigger in 1944, when he first demonstrated the eradication of persisters by pulse-dosing with penicillin in test tubes. However, this therapy had never been used to treat any persistent infection in patients. In 2015, Northeastern University researchers Drs. Sharma and Lewis found that pulsing may kill borrelia, as they examined the ability of pulse-dosing an antibiotic to eliminate persisters. In their experiment, after treating borrelia in culture with Rocephin and washing it away, surviving persisters resuscitated, and Rocephin was added again. Four pulse-doses of Rocephin eventually killed persisters, eradicating all live bacteria in the culture. Drs. Monica Embers and John R. Caskey evaluated a different pulse regimen for persisters using doxycycline, published in *Antimicrobial Agents and Chemotherapy* in July 2015, and found that it was not effective in killing off borrelia in the stationary phase, nor effective in pulse-dosing, as was Rocephin. How do we interpret these different results between Dr. Sharma's group and Dr. Embers's group?

Doxycycline prevents bacteria from reproducing, but it needs the help of our immune system to remove the bacteria from the body. This would not happen in vitro in a culture medium. The recent study using Rocephin, a bactericidal antibiotic that kills growing bacteria and even some stationary phase cells of borrelia, showed lack of regrowth even after four pulse-dosing treatments. These studies, however, were not done in humans, where patients may have cystic and biofilm forms, intracellular forms, and associated co-infections with multiple abnormalities on the sixteen-point MSIDS map. It is therefore difficult to generalize the results.

Pulse-dosing may not work well if the bacteria are in different growth phases or metabolic states. Depending on each person's immune system, the persisters may not relapse or come back easily or simultaneously, and the pulse-dosing may not work, or may work only partially or imperfectly. One way to avoid that obstacle may be to pulse antibiotics based on an individual's cyclical symptoms. A simple example can be seen with women who feel clinically well most of the month (implying a low load of borrelia in their body) after undergoing effective treatment, yet who relapse with mild symptoms right around their menstrual cycle. It would therefore make sense to pulse antibiotics just when the symptoms appear and the bacteria are active (either every day, or possibly every other day for four cycles). If we don't account for individual variations in symptoms, there are many uncertainties that we face in pulsing, such as how long the antibiotic-free period should be, and when the antibiotic pulse should be given again. If one waits too long, we may have a relapse, but if the pulse is too short, the persisters that are heterogeneous may not fully come back to become susceptible to the antibiotic treatment. Each patient is unique, with different bacterial infections and metabolic states, so pulse-dosing may not be able to completely cure persistent infection(s).

Dr. Ying Zhang follows a model that combines persister-active drugs with drugs that target growing organisms. He found that combining daptomycin (a persister drug), with cefoperazone (a drug targeting active bacteria) with doxycycline completely eradicated even the most resistant form of borrelia (biofilm-like microcolonies). We used that model in our published Dapsone study. Our persister drug was Dapsone, and the active drug was a cephalosporin, usually combined with a tetracycline and rifampin (and/or other biofilm busters).

Pyrazinamide and Persistent Intracellular Infections

Another persister drug used to treat mycobacterium, and particularly mycobacterium tuberculosis, is pyrazinamide. I first used a combination therapy of INH, rifampin, and pyrazinamide when I was in residency almost thirty years ago, treating HIV patients who suffered from tuberculosis. I was now curious if pyrazinamide would also be an effective persister drug for Lyme patients. It wasn't until Dr. Zhang's research showing borrelia to be a persister bacteria, with prior scientific research showing mycobacterium drugs to be potent candidates against persisters, that I was willing to try these medications in my sickest patients who had run out of options, since they can have adverse side effects, including elevations in liver functions. As we discussed, I did see significant improvements in a small cohort of patients on pyrazinamide.

Pyrazinamide has to be used correctly to avoid antibiotic resistance (that is why triple-drug regimens are used for TB). It is normally only used for two months in TB regimens, as it helps to decrease the length of treatment required. Whether it could do the same for Lyme disease needs to be explored further. Both Dapsone and pyrazinamide enter into the intracellular compartment and act as persister drugs, and pyrazinamide has been shown to be very effective against bacteria located in acidic environments and inside immune cells called macrophages. The Lyme spirochete has been shown to persist in macrophages like TB. Dapsone, however, has certain advantages for those who have failed classical therapies and do not have a significant sulfa sensitivity: It can be used for longer periods of time than pyrazinamide, and side effects are manageable when used in conjunction with very high-dose activated folic acid and antioxidants like glutathione.

PYRAZINAMIDE WAS THE ANSWER FOR BARBARA

Barbara had been very healthy, running marathons until October 2000, when she became ill with flulike symptoms and started feeling light-headed, at times nearly passing out. Barbara went from doctor to doctor without getting a firm diagnosis. She went to a cardiologist, who found multiple pauses on a twenty-four hour Holter monitor, with occasional low blood pressure. She was tried on Florinef for dysautonomia, otherwise known as autonomic neuropathy. It is a condition frequently seen with Lyme, where the part of the nervous system that controls our blood pressure, heart rate, bladder, and bowels is adversely affected (see Chapter 15). She then developed chest pain with increased heart palpitations, sweating, nausea, and tremors, accompanied by a blood pressure of 190/100 with a heart rate of 125 beats per minute. She went to the ER, where they gave her nitroglycerine for chest pain. She promptly passed out and became unresponsive, with a blood pressure of 80/40, needing oxygen. When she woke up, they did a full cardiac workup. No clear cause was found, and she continued to deteriorate with constant chest pain.

Over the next few weeks, Barbara lost her appetite and developed muscle-twitching all over her body, with Parkinsonian-like tremors. Her doctors tried her on metoprolol (a beta-blocker to control her heart rate and tremors). Then she was given an antidepressant, Lexapro, and had a seizure-like episode, with an EEG showing some abnormal activity. A neurologist recommended antiseizure medication, which caused headaches, weakness, and excessive yawning, and she then developed severe short-term memory loss and brain fog. An MRI of the brain showed white-matter hyperintensities, which were nonspecific.

In April of 2010, ten years after her initial diagnosis and disabled with severe cardiac and neurological symptoms, Barbara found another doctor to review her case. He felt that she had Lyme disease and placed her on Ceftin, Plaquenil, and Biaxin for one month. She finally improved for one week to about 80 percent of normal but then crashed. Her neurological symptoms were so severe that she went for a spinal tap, which was negative. The physician felt that she still had Lyme and placed her on a series of antibiotics including rifampin and Biaxin, then amoxicillin and Biaxin, and finally, IV Rocephin with pulse Flagyl and Zithromax with Mepron. There was a slight improvement, but the medications increased her liver functions and needed to be stopped. After ten weeks on Rocephin, she was switched to oral Omnicef with Flagyl and Zithromax without any further improvement, so he rotated her onto Bactrim and Ciprofloxacin, and for the first time her brain fog started to improve. Unfortunately, she plateaued and relapsed again. Since intracellular drugs were proving to be helpful, she was rotated to IV doxycycline with Zithromax, rifampin, and pulse Flagyl (a triple intracellular combo), but there was no shift, and she was taken off IV and retried on Bactrim and Cipro, the only regimen to significantly help. There was a significant improvement and she started running again, but then she developed tendonitis and stopped the Cipro. (It wasn't clear whether it was from running or the quinolone drug, but since tendinopathies are a well-known side effect of quinolones, it was the prudent thing to do.) Unfortunately, she backslid and was placed on a different intracellular combo with Zithromax, rifampin, and Bactrim, but her liver functions increased again and she had to stop the antibiotics.

By this point everyone felt desperate. There were windows of improvement, but Barbara was unable to sustain a response. A final attempt was made to place her back on Bactrim and Cipro, but she did not improve this time and developed an allergic rash. She was now functioning at 40 percent of normal and came to see me.

We sent off tick-borne titers that returned positive for exposure to Lyme and multiple co-infections, including *Borrelia hermsii*, Babesia, Ehrlichia, Mycoplasma, and *Chlamydia pneumonia*, and she was also positive for human herpes virus-6 (HHV6) and Epstein-Barr (EBV) exposure with a low-positive tularemia titer, which did not increase over time. Although it is possible that she had tularemia and was treated unknowingly with her doxycycline and rifampin regimens, we see low-level, false-positive tularemia titers in patients with other intracellular infections, consistent with her response to quinolone drugs, which are intracellular antibiotics. Other testing revealed a low zinc level, low iodine, low iron saturation, low Vitamin D, and a slightly high IgM immunoglobulin level occasionally seen with infections (although we oftentimes see low IgM levels in chronic Lyme-MSIDS).

Because Barbara had failed many different antibiotics, including IV therapies, we tried multiple herbal and integrative approaches over the next several years, including detoxification for her severe cognitive issues, but none were helpful. In the beginning of 2015 I put her back on antibiotics with Bicillin injections, combined with doxy/minocycline and Zithromax, and there was a slight improvement in her energy, migratory joint pain, palpitations, twitching, and insomnia. Her cognitive issues, however, were worse. She complained of severe short-term memory loss, an inability to concentrate, and brain fog. I discussed with Barbara the new research on persisters, and specifically, pyrazinamide. I placed her on Plaquenil, Doryx (a long-acting tetracycline, easier on the stomach), rifampin and pyrazinamide, with a sugar-free, yeast-free diet with high-dose probiotics, as well as Serrapeptase and Stevia for biofilms. She had signed an informed consent, and I explained the possible side effects, giving her extra liver support with N-Acetylcysteine (NAC), alpha-lipoic acid, glutathione, and milk thistle, as she had occasionally bumped up her liver function tests (LFTs) in the past. We discussed following LFTs carefully and had her return to the office in one to two months' time.

Barbara returned in June of 2015 feeling good. She hadn't felt any difference during the first two weeks on the protocol, but by the third week she started to improve. Her energy was moderately better, her joint pain disappeared, the twitching was gone, and her cognitive function was the best it had been in a long time (from 40 percent of normal to 80 percent).

Could initial use of pyrazinamide, as in TB, shorten the treatment course for chronic Lyme? While pyrazinamide for several months does not appear to be a cure, it proves that bacterial infections hiding inside the intracellular compartment are playing a large role in keeping patients like Barbara ill, and that lowering down the bacterial load (infectious burden) by using multiple intracellular medications (three antibiotics, one being a persister drug) helps to improve resistant symptomatology.

WHY ISN'T MY DOCTOR ON BOARD WITH THIS NEW RESEARCH?

The research in the past two years is nothing less than groundbreaking, yet many doctors continue to use outdated Infectious Disease Society of America (IDSA) guidelines as a basis to forego long-term antibiotics. Their decisions are based on three NIH-funded trials regarding the treatment of chronic Lyme disease. Unfortunately, in each of these treatment trials the sample sizes were extremely small, ranging from thirty-seven to seventy-eight patients. Critics have pointed out that studies this small lack sufficient statistical power to measure clinically relevant improvement. Nevertheless, two of the three clinical trials demonstrated that retreatment improved some patients' measures, such as fatigue and pain, as well as improving cognitive function in those with Lyme encephalopathy.

A 2016 European Lyme study published in the *New England Journal of Medicine* showed the same results. Statistically significant results were seen early on when all patients were on Rocephin, but patients did not see continued improvements when they took orals (doxy and/or macrolides) and stopped the antibiotics. Shocking. The authors used the same study design as prior NIH trials and did not incorporate any of the new scientific data on persisters, pulsing, and biofilm forms, nor did they treat associated tick-borne co-infections even though they are the rule in ticks, not the exception, in Europe. Why is new published research using old paradigms?

The politics surrounding the diagnosis and treatment of Lyme disease have hampered effective research and treatment for the last several decades. Federal funding for Lyme disease has lagged behind that of other infectious diseases. In August 2015 CDC researchers stated that chronic Lyme sufferers have been shown to be as sick as patients with chronic congestive heart failure. Many patients become disabled if not treated early on in the course of illness, yet we do not have a scientific consensus as to the cause of ongoing symptoms after more than thirty-five years of medical research. The problem is compounded by insurance companies that deny treatment for chronically ill patients, basing their decisions on the same outdated IDSA guidelines.

While there is a real concern about antibiotic resistance that may accompany misuse of antibiotics, and that concern is an argument used as a barrier to adopting long-term antibiotic strategies, we now know that a large part of the problem comes from overuse of antibiotics in animal feed, not in humans. What's more, research from Northeastern University shows that borrelia forms antibiotic-tolerant cells, not resistant cells, and resistant strains have not been proven to date. We would never imagine denying effective treatment to a person with a life-threatening chronic infection like TB, leprosy, Q fever, or brucellosis (another persister bacteria) with long-term antibiotics because of a concern with resistance. We use combination drug regimens in these diseases to prevent resistance, and we know that some of these infections persist in part because of biofilms. Many of my chronically ill patients who failed classic combination therapies are improving with persister drugs like Dapsone, and new scientific research on pulsing, persisters, and biofilm busters are giving us renewed hope in finding answers for those disabled from chronic Lyme and associated co-infections.

What Else Is Hampering My Recovery?

In the following chapters you will learn exactly how other illnesses and medical problems on the sixteen-point MSIDS map can impact Lyme disease, and how Lyme bacteria can affect other medical problems you may have. First, we will explore bacterial infections that can occur simultaneously with Lyme disease, as we are finding that many ticks are carrying much more than just Lyme bacterial spirochetes.

PART II

Lyme and MSIDS

FIVE

Ticks Can Carry More Than Lyme: Associated Bacterial Infections

icks are often carrying multiple infections inside of them, which can all be transmitted simultaneously to a host at the time of the tick bite. These include a broad range of bacterial, parasitic, and viral infections.

You may also unknowingly be carrying other bacterial, parasitic, viral, and fungal infections that are completely unrelated to the tick bite. These infections may be so minute that they don't affect your daily life. However, they can be reactivated or exacerbated by Lyme bacteria and associated tick-borne co-infections, or when your immune system is suppressed (i.e., using drugs like prednisone, other immunosuppressive drugs, or having another type of immune deficiency like chronic variable immune deficiency [CVID] or adrenal insufficiency). I have found that the sickest patients are usually the ones who have Lyme along with multiple other infections, because these co-infections can increase the severity of symptoms in Lyme-MSIDS, in part through suppressing the immune system and preventing the body from properly fighting off these and other unrelated infections, and also because they can increase underlying inflammation.

The following is a list of the most common bacterial co-infections we find with Lyme disease.

EHRLICHIA/ANAPLASMA

Many of my patients test positive for Ehrlichia or Anaplasma. These bacteria, along with babesiosis (which is a parasite we will discuss in the next chapter) and relapsing fever borrelia, are some of the most common tick-borne co-infections.

Ehrlichiosis comes in many forms, including:

- *human sennetsu ehrlichiosis*
- *human granulocytic anaplasmosis*
- *human monocytic ehrlichiosis*
- *human ewingii ehrlichiosis*
- *human Wisconsin-Minnesota ehrlichiosis*

Most of these organisms are transmitted by a specific species of hard-bodied insects called *Ixodes scapularis* ticks, but *Ehrlichia chaffeensis* is transmitted by the lone star tick, *Amblyomma americanum*. This tick has also been associated with bacterial infections such as tularemia, and Southern tick associated rash illness (STARI), and as per the Centers for Disease Control and Prevention (CDC), it is also now thought to carry a novel viral infection known as the Heartland virus. In a 2012 article published in the *New England Journal of Medicine*, the Heartland virus was found to cause an illness clinically similar to ehrlichiosis, but it was unresponsive to antibiotics. Two years later in 2014, the Bourbon virus, another viral tick-borne illness found in the Midwest, again caused hematological abnormalities resembling anaplasmosis, ehrlichiosis, and rickettsial infections that were unresponsive to tetracyclines.

One new emerging infection that also resembles anaplasmosis, but is responsive to tetracyclines, is the relapsing fever bacteria, *Borrelia miyamotoi*. It can cause leucopenia (low white cell counts), thrombocytopenia (low platelet counts), and transaminitis (elevated liver functions). False positive tests for ehrlichiosis can also be seen with common viral infections like EBV, as well as rickettsial infections (RMSF, typhus, Q fever), and brucellosis. All of these should be considered in the differential diagnosis.

Novel tick-borne infections are being discovered almost every year, and Anaplasma is no exception. *Anaplasma capra*, a new species found in China in 2015 by University of Maryland researchers, was found in

6 percent of Chinese subjects in an area with greater than 1 billion people (potentially over 60 million people infected) because there was no simple blood test for this species. Anaplasma rates are rising, and emerging tick-borne infections are the rule, not the exception.

The most common symptoms of ehrlichiosis are a high fever accompanied by severe headaches, flulike symptoms, muscle pains, and fatigue in the spring, summer, or fall. Anaplasmosis can also rarely cause GI manifestations like diarrhea. It is important to clinically suspect and treat for Ehrlichia and Anaplasma in the very young and in the elderly, as it can be fatal in individuals who are immunocompromised.

Most patients who tested positive for Ehrlichia or Anaplasma when we tested for Lyme disease were completely unaware that they had ever had a tick bite. HGA, due to *Anaplasma phagocytophilum*, can also be transmitted by a blood transfusion (along with other tick-borne infections like Bartonella and Babesia). This is particularly problematic in the very young or elderly with suppressed immune systems who receive a tainted transfusion, as the infection can be fatal. Always ask if the blood used for a transfusion is Red Cross–screened blood to help ensure safety.

When properly diagnosed and treated, Ehrlichia or Anaplasma do not appear to cause the same severe chronic clinical manifestations that we see with other organisms such as Bartonella, Mycoplasma, or Babesia. Ehrlichia or Anaplasma can be diagnosed through a combination of blood tests, including antibody titers, a complete blood count, and liver functions. The HME and HGA titers are antibodies that can be seen early on (IgM) and later in the illness (IgG). A complete blood count is especially useful in diagnosing Ehrlichia/Anaplasma, as there are specific abnormalities that can alert the clinician to the presence of Ehrlichia species, including a low white cell count (leukopenia), low platelet counts (thrombocytopenia), as well as elevated liver functions (AST, ALT). Intracellular colonies, called "morulae," can also be visualized under the microscope when examining white blood cells, bone marrow, and the cerebral spinal fluid (CSF) of cells infected with Ehrlichia. Rarely a macular (flat) or maculopapular (flat+/−raised) rash can be present, with petechiae (red, broken blood vessels).

Treatment of Ehrlichiosis/Anaplasmosis

The CDC recently revised their guidelines for using doxycycline in children with potentially life-threatening infections, like rickettsial infections such as Rocky Mountain spotted fever, which presents with the same early nonspecific symptoms and hematological abnormalities as Ehrlichia/ Anaplasma (leucopenia, thrombocytopenia, and elevated liver functions). The new research shows that it is safe to use short courses of doxycycline in children without risk of tooth staining, and it is "first-line care for the treatment of suspected rickettsial infections at any age."

Doxycycline for seven to ten days is usually adequate to treat Ehrlichia and Anaplasma. If there is an allergy, intolerance, or contraindication to using tetracyclines, then rifampin can be used instead.

JENNIFER'S WALK IN THE WOODS

Jennifer was seventeen years old, with no significant past medical history, and she went to camp for the first time to work as a counselor. I received a panicked call from her parents three days after she left. Jennifer was complaining of the worst headache of her life, had flulike symptoms, severe muscle aches all over her body, overwhelming fatigue, and a fever. She had not noticed a tick bite or thought to look for a rash, but she was working in wooded areas.

I advised Jennifer's parents to take her to the local emergency room and have them specifically check a CBC to see if she had a low white cell count and platelet count, as well as to check her liver functions. I also advised them to test her for tick-borne diseases, such as Lyme disease, but explained that these tests might return negative. Jennifer was experiencing symptoms after being in a wooded area for only three days, which is typically shorter than the usual time it takes to mount an antibody response.

Because of the wooded location of the camp, along with her very severe headache, severe muscle and joint pains, and high fever—flulike symptoms that are uncommon in the summertime—I strongly suspected a tick-borne bacterial illness such as ehrlichiosis, and suggested a course of doxycycline if any of the laboratory values were abnormal, even if no other immediate cause could be found.

I got a phone call from the parents the next day. They were amazed when the blood tests came back exactly as I had predicted. The ER doctor was also surprised that Jennifer had a low white cell count (2.9; normal is between 4 and 10), low platelet count (113,000; normal is 145,000 or higher), and elevated liver functions (AST 62, ALT 76; the normal range is below 40). Jennifer had ehrlichiosis. The ER doc agreed with my suggestion and placed her on doxycycline. Within twenty-four hours her fever broke, and she was feeling much better. Jennifer has remained well, without any evidence of chronic tick-borne illness. Ehrlichia and Lyme disease can both be cured if caught early.

BARTONELLA

Bartonella species are important emerging bacterial pathogens with varied manifestations. *Bartonella henselae*, or cat scratch disease, usually presents as a rash or papule (a small, red, raised bump on the skin) that progresses to a vesicular, or blistery, crusty stage, and within one to two weeks causes the regional lymph nodes to swell. Seventy-five percent of cases are thought to be mild. Several other species of Bartonella, such as *Bartonella quintana*, are transmitted by human lice, which are responsible for trench fever. *Bartonella bacilliformis*, which is transmitted by sand flies and fleas as well as ticks, can cause Carrion's disease. There are over thirty different species/subspecies of Bartonella, and seventeen have been associated with human infections. New Bartonella species (*B. koehlerae*) have recently been identified, and antibodies against *Bartonella henselae, B. koehlerae*, or *B. vinsonii subsp. berkhoffii* were found to be high in patients with Lyme disease (46.6 percent), arthralgia/arthritis (20.6 percent), chronic fatigue (19.6 percent), and fibromyalgia (6.1 percent), implying a possible causal role. There are numerous overlaps with the symptoms of Lyme disease and the clinical manifestations of bartonellosis, and Bartonella species like *B. vinsonii subsp. berkhoffii* have been shown to induce immunosuppression in animals and successfully evade the immune system, implying a causal role for the organism in those with persistent Lyme symptoms.

Doctors used to think that Bartonella could only be transmitted to humans through the bite (or scratch) of a cat, fleas, lice, biting flies, or sand flies. It was not until the late 1990s that Bartonella was considered to be a tick-borne co-infection associated with symptoms in persistent Lyme disease. However, the typical manifestations of Bartonella taught in medical school are not the same as we usually see in patients with MSIDS. Patients with Lyme disease and overlapping Bartonella infections can have unusually severe neurological manifestations, including meningitis;

new episodes of seizures and ophthalmological problems; severe cardiac problems like infections of the heart valves (endocarditis), heart muscle (myocarditis), and sac surrounding the heart (pericarditis); and they may even resemble other medical illnesses, such as sarcoidosis (with inflammation of the lymph nodes).

One unusual presentation is stretch marks found on the abdomen, flanks, thighs, breasts, and upper shoulders, which are often mistaken for stretch marks due to weight loss. This presentation was originally described by Dr. Martin Fried at a Lyme Disease Association conference, where he reported that the rash was found in patients who tested positive for Bartonella. I tried biopsying the same lesions on my own patients but have never been able to get positive polymerase chain reaction (PCR) results for Bartonella or *Borrelia burgdorferi*, although other medical practitioners have frequently reported the same findings. Regardless of whether they are due to Lyme disease itself, with borrelia burrowing through the subcutaneous fat, and/or to Bartonella, they appear to be indicative of tickborne infections.

Another classic dermatological manifestation of Bartonella is granuloma formation in various regions of the skin (bacillary angiomatosis), which can appear as painful red nodules. These granulomas can also appear in the liver (peliosis hepatis), or in the spleen (peliosis splenitis). Pharyngeal crescents (red crescent-shaped lesions in the back of the throat) and pain in the soles of the feet, with an occasional positive vascular endothelial growth factor (VEGF) blood test, have similarly been reported in Lyme disease patients co-infected with Bartonella.

Bartonella can also be transmitted from a mother to a fetus. This, unfortunately, adds one more organism to the long, growing list of infections that we must pay attention to in women of childbearing age. By becoming cognizant of these infections we have the opportunity to prevent miscarriages and possible disabilities.

Symptoms suggestive of Bartonella include resistant neurological issues, such as headaches, encephalopathy with severe cognitive dysfunction, seizures, radiculitis, myelitis, or vasculitis (inflammation in the nerves coming out of the spine, spinal cord, or inflammation in the blood vessels), as well as ophthalmological manifestations such as a neuroretinitis (inflammation of the retina) and vision loss, branch retinal artery occlusions, an oculoglandular syndrome with preauricular lymph nodes (inflammation of the eyes and lymph nodes in front of the ears), and conjunctivitis (pinkeye). In 2014 Bartonella was linked to cataracts and inflammatory breast cancer. Systemic inflammatory disorders resembling sarcoidosis with associated painful red nodules (erythema nodosum), arthritis, osteolytic lesions (destruction of the bones), and a lymphoma-like pathology (hard, swollen lymph nodes) can also be present.

Bartonella testing is known to be unreliable, as Bartonella can evade the immune system and hide intracellularly where antibodies cannot recognize the bacteria. Studies have shown that up to 85 percent of chronically infected individuals may test negative for antibodies through immunofluorescent (IFA) serology, and blood smears (Fry test), sensitive PCRs (DNA testing), and/or Bartonella FISH testing (IGeneX, RNA testing) may be necessary to find the bacteria. In my own clinical practice, *Bartonella henselae* immunofluorescent assay (IFA) and ELISA testing were positive in less than half of the patients who had evidence of Lyme disease and associated Bartonellosis. Polymerase chain reaction (PCR) testing was able to detect Bartonella in 53 percent of those patients who were seronegative in our office, and several patients had positive PCR results despite months of classical Bartonella antibiotic treatment regimens. Bartonella is a known "persister" bacteria, having been published in the scientific literature to cause chronic bacteremia (infection in the blood) in immunocompetent individuals. It joins the ranks of other bacterial persisters like Borrelia, Coxiella (Q fever), and Mycoplasma species. Bartonella has persisted despite medication courses of tetracyclines (doxycycline and minocycline), macrolides (Zithromax and Biaxin), IV cephalosporins such as Rocephin, and quinolones (Cipro, Levaquin, or Avelox).

Therefore, we can't always rely on antibody testing, and long-term therapy with combinations of intracellular antibiotics may be necessary. If you suspect Bartonella, I suggest checking antibodies against different species as well as PCR testing for multiple species (in several sets), especially for patients failing treatment. Scientists at North Carolina State University, working with Galaxy laboratories, have shown that an enrichment blood culture is needed to grow Bartonella to detectable levels for PCR to overcome the risk of a false negative result. A Bartonella FISH assay (RNA) is also available through IGeneX laboratory, which can be positive when antibody and PCR testing is negative.

Treating Bartonella Species

We can't rely on a single-drug regimen to treat Bartonella. A combination therapy with at least two intracellular antibiotics for several months is preferable. Treatment regimens include rotations of intracellular antibiotics using dosages previously described (see Chapter 3) for the treatment of Lyme disease. Two intracellular drugs such as doxycycline and rifampin or Zithromax and rifampin are preferred, with Bactrim being helpful in combination therapy, but three- or four-drug regimens and/or IV gentamycin and IV Rocephin may be necessary in some severely ill, treatment-resistant individuals with Lyme and Bartonella (i.e., Bartonella endocarditis) and associated intracellular co-infections. In the case study we published in *The Journal of Arthritis and Rheumatism*, we needed to use pyrazinamide in combination with Plaquenil, minocycline, and rifampin (a triple intracellular antibiotic protocol) to effectively treat the signs and symptoms (i.e., pain and granulomas) of Bartonella, after the patient failed multiple other intracellular drug regimens. Although Bartonella is an intracellular pathogen, extracellular forms are found where broad-spectrum cephalosporins can also have an effect on the organism. Drugs such as chloramphenicol and a beta lactam antibiotic (cephalosporin) or streptomycin may be necessary in Bartonella species like *B. bacilliformis* (Carrion's disease) that can cause life-threatening septicemia (an infection in the blood) and hemolytic anemia.

Combination Antibiotic Regimens for Bartonella and Other Intracellular Organisms

- Plaquenil/doxycycline/rifampin/nystatin+/−macrolide (Zithromax). Use two- or three-drug combinations, i.e., a tetracycline/rifampin, macrolide/rifampin, or tetracycline/rifampin/macrolide with Plaquenil and nystatin.
- Plaquenil/doxycycline/rifampin/nystatin+/−quinolone (Levaquin, Avelox, Factive). Higher generation quinolone drugs (avoiding Cipro) may be preferable due to possible bacterial resistance, but mean inhibitory concentrations (MIC) of the drugs vary within species.
- Plaquenil/doxycycline/rifampin/nystatin+Septra. This can be an effective combination in other severe intracellular infections apart from Lyme and Bartonella, such as Brucella.

- Plaquenil/Zithromax/rifampin/nystatin+Septra. Two-drug antibiotic combinations such as Zithromax and Septra, Zithromax and rifampin, or doxycycline and Septra can be effective in certain individuals, and Septra can also be used effectively in three- or four-drug regimens, adding it to doxy, rifampin, with Zithromax or quinolones, in severely ill, resistant patients.
- Plaquenil/rifampin/doxycycline (or Minocin)/Dapsone, or Plaquenil/rifampin/Zithromax/Dapsone with or without either a pulsed or daily cell-wall drug like a cephalosporin (Ceftin or Omnicef). These regimens were particularly effective in our pilot study treating 100 patients with chronic Lyme disease and co-infections like babesiosis, as Dapsone is a powerful intracellular killing agent with antimalarial activity. We don't know how many patients had overlapping Bartonella due to the insensitivity of testing, but many showed serological evidence of prior infections with *Mycoplasma pneumoniae* and *Chlamydia pneumonia*.

MYCOPLASMA

Thanks to the work of Dr. Eva Sapi at the University of New Haven, there are now several species of Mycoplasma identified in the same ticks carrying Lyme. We are now finding ticks containing *Mycoplasma pneumoniae*, *Mycoplasma genitalium*, and *Mycoplasma fermentans*, the latter organism being the one responsible for Gulf War syndrome. Occasionally these organisms are also found in patients with Lyme-MSIDS.

It is difficult to know the exact role that Mycoplasma species are playing in these patients with Lyme disease, since the blood tests are unreliable and the signs and symptoms overlap those of other diseases. Therefore, we may perform both immunofluorescent antibodies (IFA) and serial PCR (polymerase chain reaction) blood tests to check for different Mycoplasma species. Mycoplasma may be exacerbating the symptoms of MSIDS, especially for patients who present with autoimmune manifestations. Mycoplasmas have been shown to interact with B-lymphocytes (as does Bartonella), one of the primary immune cells in the body, which secretes antibodies in response to infection.

There are five different types of immunoglobulin-antibody molecules produced by plasma cells and B-cells: IgA, IgM, IgG, IgD, and IgE antibodies. Mycoplasma may cause these B-cells to be overstimulated, promoting autoimmune reactions and rheumatoid diseases. This subsequently leads to symptoms of increased fatigue with joint and muscle pain. Mycoplasma infections have also been shown to persist despite long-term antibiotic therapy, and can increase the production of proinflammatory cytokines such as Il-1, Il-2, and Il-6, leading to chronic fatigue, with musculoskeletal and/or neuropsychiatric symptoms. Lyme disease and other intracellular co-infections may synergistically work with Mycoplasma to increase the inflammatory response and drive autoimmune reactions, and it should be considered as an overlapping cause of autoimmune manifestations, in combination with environmental toxins like mercury and small-particle pollution.

Treating Mycoplasma

We have had patients test positive for Mycoplasma infections such as *M. fermentans* with single-drug therapy after almost one year of continuous treatment (rotating between macrolides, tetracyclines, and quinolones). One of my pregnant patients with Lyme disease also recently tested positive for Mycoplasma species by PCR in her amniotic fluid (at birth), despite taking Ceftin and a macrolide (Zithromax) for nine months. Although the baby was healthy, one intracellular antibiotic is usually inadequate to eradicate Mycoplasma, and combination therapy with at least two intracellular antibiotics is preferable when there is proof of active Mycoplasma infection. This is, however, difficult to do during pregnancy, since Zithromax and Ceftin are some of the few drugs that are proven to be safe. Use the same type of combinations described for treating Bartonella and other intracellular infections (when not pregnant). The choice of antibiotics depends on your present or prior response to the medications (positive response, neutral, or negative, i.e., Herxheimer reaction), as well as potential side effects (i.e., QT interactions with macrolides and quinolones, and/or any history of tendonitis with quinolones), interactions with other drugs (rifampin can lower doses of other medications), as well as whether overlapping co-infections are present. The idea is to create a protocol that simultaneously addresses as many bacterial and parasitic infections as possible with the least side effects, while also treating overlapping etiologies on the sixteen-point MSIDS map.

CHLAMYDIA

Chlamydia is an intracellular infection like Mycoplasma and is treated with similar intracellular drugs. Ticks aren't known to carry chlamydia, and not all chlamydia is sexually transmitted. There are other forms of chlamydia, such as chlamydia TWAR, which causes upper respiratory infections, and dormant chlamydial infections can be reactivated when Lyme and other tick-borne co-infections are present. Chlamydia is associated with oligoarthritis (arthritis in multiple joints), and *Chlamydia pneumonia*, like Mycoplasma species, has been reported in the medical literature as having a possible link to autoimmune diseases like MS. Chronic fatiguing illnesses, such as CFS/SEID, fibromyalgia, and certain autoimmune illnesses, such as rheumatoid arthritis, have also been reported to have a link with multiple intracellular infections like Mycoplasma and/or chlamydia, which are either causative or a cofactor for the illness, aggravating symptoms.

Other factors that can increase the adverse effect of these infections are environmental toxins. The combination of heavy metals with intracellular bacteria, such as chlamydia, may be contributing to the severe arthritis seen in MSIDS patients. Heavy metals such as mercury have been reported in the scientific literature to cause arthritis, increase autoimmune reactions, and create free radicals and oxidative stress that can turn on nuclear-factor kappa B (NFKappaB), a switch in the nucleus of the cell that creates cytokines, the inflammatory molecules. Heavy metals similarly increase arthritis in patients co-infected with chlamydia. Both our own clinical experience and the scientific literature support testing and treating Lyme patients for multiple intracellular co-infections such as chlamydia and detoxing them for environmental pollutants like heavy metals.

Treating Chlamydia

Chlamydia is an intracellular bacteria, so the same treatment regimens apply as with Bartonella and Mycoplasma.

RICKETTSIAL INFECTIONS

Rickettsia are bacteria that live within host cells like chlamydia and Mycoplasma, but some rickettsial organisms (*R. typhi* and *C. burnetii*) can also survive for extended periods of time outside the host and remain extremely infectious. The most common rickettsial infections are Rocky Mountain spotted fever (*R. rickettsii*), typhus (*R. typhi*), and Q fever (*Coxiella burnetii*). New species of rickettsia have appeared in the past four years, such as *Candidatus Rickettsia tarasevichiae*, a member of the spotted fever group, and *Rickettsia sibirica*, both of which were found in China. In 2016, researchers identified another new rickettsial species in the United States, related to a European pathogen, *Rickettsia slovaca*.

Rickettsia such as Rocky Mountain spotted fever (RMSF) are transmitted by several different species of ticks, including the lone star tick (*Amblyomma americanum*), the wood tick (*Dermatocenter andersoni*), and the dog tick (*Dermatocenter variabilis*). Although transmission of Lyme disease from a tick bite is normally believed to take a minimum of twenty-four hours (it has been reported to take place within several hours if spirochetes were in the tick salivary glands prior to feeding), transmission of rickettsial diseases like *Rickettsia rickettsii* by Amblyomma ticks can occur in as little as ten minutes.

Unfortunately, the early clinical presentations of this bacterial infection can be nonspecific. You may have fever, nausea, vomiting, severe headaches, and muscle pains, which can be commonly mistaken for a flulike syndrome. The classic red-spotted petechial rash—tiny red hemorrhagic spots from blood vessels that have broken—that can appear on the palms and soles of the feet are only present 50 percent to 80 percent of the time, and may not be present until after the sixth day of exposure. Therefore, finding the rash as a means to diagnose RMSF is not a reliable clinical sign. The CBC may present with some of the same abnormalities seen in ehrlichiosis, such as low white-cell counts, low platelet counts, and elevated liver functions, which is fortunate since both bacterial infections, although caused by different organisms, are treated effectively with tetracyclines. Most spotted fever rickettsia present with similar hematological abnormalities (leukopenia, thrombocytopenia, and/or elevated liver functions) and a rash, but there are exceptions. The appearance of the rash differs among species. *Rickettsia sibirica* can have confluent pale pink maculae (a flat rash) widely distributed on the trunk and limbs, not the classic red-spotted petechial rash seen in Rocky Mountain spotted fever. Also, *Candidatus Rickettsia tarasevich-*

iae does not have a rash, and the white cell counts can be elevated. This can lead to misdiagnosis, improper treatment, and increased morbidity, as several patients developed a coma, with renal and respiratory failure, and died.

Coxiella burnetii (Q fever) is another rickettsial infection. It can similarly present with nonspecific symptoms, and in 50 percent of the cases there are no signs of an acute clinical illness. You might present with symptoms that could be confused with an acute viral illness, such as high fevers, chills and sweats, severe headaches, and muscle pains. However, Q fever can also present with myriad diverse symptoms, and therefore could be considered as one of the great imitators like Lyme disease, Bartonella, and syphilis. Coxiella can present as hepatitis, with associated nausea, vomiting, and diarrhea; pneumonia, with a nonproductive cough; meningoencephalitis, with confusion; myelitis, with an inflammation of the spinal cord; and even as Guillain-Barré syndrome. One of the most troubling symptoms is that it can cause a chronic endocarditis, an infection of the heart valves, which can occur one to twenty years after the initial infection. Anyone with unresolved Lyme disease who presents with any of the above symptoms and has associated elevations in liver functions and/or a heart murmur must be checked for Q fever (i.e., antibody titers +/− an echocardiogram/transesophageal echocardiogram).

Q fever is commonly transmitted from domestic animals, especially cattle, sheep, and goats. Coxiella can produce a mild infection in these animals, and the organisms can infect the placenta and mammary glands, transmitting the organism in infected milk and meat products. Coxiella can also survive in the environment in dust and soils on animal farms, so that a highly infectious aerosol can be found around infected animals. To make matters worse, Q fever is also a bioterrorist agent. I have had many conversations with various state and local health departments regarding Q fever titers that have come back positive for my patients: We needed to quickly determine whether these results were the first sign of an impending bioterrorist threat, or if the patient had been on an animal farm and/or drank unpasteurized goat milk, or simply received a tick bite. The implications are obviously quite different!

Any high clinical suspicion (tick bite or exposure in a highly tick-endemic area) and laboratory testing showing an abnormal white blood cell count, thrombocytopenia, and/or elevated liver functions (similar to abnormal laboratory testing seen with Ehrlichia/Anaplasma) should prompt immediate treatment. The diagnosis of Q fever is made using blood antibody testing, called phase I and phase II titers. These are compared in a ratio: High phase I : phase II titers indicate an acute infection; high phase II : phase I titers indicate a chronic infection, which is seen in patients with chronic Q fever and especially in chronic Q fever endocarditis, where Coxiella has infected the heart valves. Over the years we have had at least two hundred positive Q fever titers, and several of them did show a four-fold rise in the phase II titers consistent with possible chronic Q fever and a chronic endocarditis. Therefore, Q fever joins the ranks of intracellular co-infections that are classified as "persisters" and long-term, double intracellular antibiotic therapy may be necessary in severe infections. Q fever titers are not specific, and false positives can be seen with other rickettsial infections and viruses.

Treating Rickettsial Infections

Rocky Mountain spotted fever, typhus, and Q fever are all gram-negative intracellular bacteria and are treated effectively in the acute stages with tetracyclines such as doxycycline. As RMSF can be fatal in the very young or the very elderly, who are immunocompromised, it is essential to immediately start on a tetracycline, such as doxycycline, if there is any clinical suspicion of acute exposure to rickettsia. Children are no exception.

Neither tetracyclines nor chloramphenicol (second-line therapy) are rickettsicidal, so an adequate immune system is required to use them effectively. Chronic Q fever endocarditis requires long-term treatment with antibiotics. Several regimens that have been published in the medical literature include the use of doxycycline and Plaquenil for up to three years and doxycycline and quinolones (or rifampin) for several years. Use the same dosages previously described for Lyme disease and associated co-infections. These cases are best managed in conjunction with a cardiologist and infectious disease specialist.

TICK-BORNE RELAPSING FEVER: *BORRELIA HERMSII* AND *BORRELIA MIYAMOTOI*

Up until now we have been discussing tick-borne diseases transmitted by hard-bodied ticks (family: Ixodidae), but there are also tick-borne infections in the United States like Tick-Borne Relapsing Fever (TBRF) that can be caused by both hard- and soft-bodied ticks (family: Argasidae). These tick-borne relapsing fever spirochetes are a broad group of spirochetal infections that are closely related cousins to the Lyme disease spirochete, *Borrelia burgdorferi*. Tick-Borne Relapsing Fever in the United States that is transmitted from the bite of the fast-feeding soft tick, genus Ornithodoros, is usually caused by one of three species, *Borrelia hermsii*, *Borrelia turicatae*, and *Borrelia parkeri*. In other countries like Africa, *B. duttoni* and *B. crocidurae* are responsible. Since soft ticks remain attached for only fifteen to twenty minutes while feeding and the bites are usually painless, most people are unaware of ever having been bitten. Infection can also take place from contamination of the wound or skin by tick secretions or from exposure to body lice that carry the organism (known as louse-borne relapsing fever, with *B. recurrentis*). Soft ticks are infectious for life and can transmit the spirochete quickly while a person is sleeping (possibly within thirty seconds), so they win the race among tick-borne transmitted pathogens like Lyme disease and rickettsia.

Tick-Borne Relapsing Fever is found throughout most of the world but is endemic in Colorado, California, and the Pacific Northwest as well as in parts of Central and South America, Asia, and most of Africa. These soft ticks may survive for twenty years without feeding, and infected ticks pass the spirochetal organism onto their offspring, as do some rickettsial species.

Just as one of the hallmarks of Lyme disease is that the symptoms tend to come and go, the natural course of TBRF is that there are periods of high fevers (101.3 to 104 degrees Fahrenheit), with drenching sweats and shaking chills and an associated headache, fatigue, and joint and muscle pains that can last for several days (with associated large numbers of spirochetes found in the blood). It can then resolve, only to return in a relapsing fashion every several days. Associated symptoms can include a loss of appetite, dry cough, abdominal pain, nausea, vomiting, neck stiffness (meningismus), light sensitivity (photophobia), and neurological complications, including confusion with an encephalitis, facial nerve palsy, unilateral hearing loss, iritis (inflammation in the iris of the eye), peripheral neuropathy, and neuropsychiatric disturbances. These symptoms will relapse as spirochetes like *B. hermsii* rearrange its DNA on its outer surface. This creates different antigenic markers known as "variable major proteins," which allows it to evade recognition by the immune system. This antigenic variation allows it to hide in different organs of the body during periods without a fever, and relapse occurs in a cyclic fashion when the new serotype (bacteria with new cell surface antigens) reenters the bloodstream and causes bacteremia (bacteria in the bloodstream).

Clinical signs that accompany the infections with relapsing fevers (which may last from twelve hours to seventeen days) may include a variety of skin rashes. These can include a flat reddish rash (macular eruption), diffuse petechiae throughout the body (small red spots due to minor hemorrhaging in the skin), or *erythema multiforme* (target-shaped lesions, not to be confused with the bull's-eye rash in Lyme disease). The liver can be enlarged as well as the spleen, and liver functions could be elevated, including signs of obstruction with jaundice secondary to liver congestion. Severe complications include potentially fatal disseminated intravascular coagulation (DIC), when blood coagulation factors and platelets are used up, occasionally causing the patient to hemorrhage (including strokes with cerebral hemorrhage) and become hypotensive (low blood pressure), with cardiac dysfunction and arrhythmias secondary to injury to the myocardium (myocarditis). In rare cases, acute respiratory distress syndrome (ARDS) has been reported, which also can be fatal.

Like Lyme disease, Tick-Borne Relapsing Fever (TBRF) can affect pregnant women, and it can result in fetal death and spontaneous abortion, or premature birth with perinatal sickness. Fetal death is probably caused by DIC, due to the low platelet counts and hemorrhage in the uterus resulting from the infection.

The diagnosis of TBRF is confirmed by a Wright-Giemsa stain, with paired acute and convalescent antibody titers by EIA and IFA (i.e., we compare the enzyme immunoassay/indirect immunofluorescent antibodies in early and late stages of the disease). Western immunoblots, culture, and PCRs as well as monoclonal antibodies may also help in establishing the diagnosis. We have had many patients in our practice with Lyme disease from *Borrelia burgdorferi* test positive for antibodies against *Bor-*

relia hermsii. Since many patients recover from TBRF either with or without antibiotic treatment, this may indicate either a larger spread of the illness than has been recognized or false-positive titers for relapsing fever, as these patients often do not present with the appropriate clinical picture.

Patients with symptoms of a meningitis or encephalitis should use IV Rocephin (ceftriaxone), as in Lyme disease, as the brain may serve as a reservoir for borrelia.

Other relapsing fever spirochetes, such as *Borrelia miyamotoi*, which are found in hard-bodied ticks, can also present with similar signs and symptoms with a Lyme-like illness, and *B. miyamotoi* will not test positive using the standard ELISA and Western blot for Lyme disease. *Borrelia miyamotoi* has been reported to cause relapsing fever and Lyme disease–like symptoms in Russia, Western Europe, and the United States: a meningoencephalitis (inflammation in the brain and meningeal sac surrounding the brain and spinal cord), possibly with an erythema migrans (EM)–type rash in up to 9 percent of patients. Since *B. miyamotoi* infection is now found in 1 percent to 16 percent of ticks worldwide (*Ixodes persulcatus* in Russia, *Ixodes ricinus* in Western Europe, and *Ixodes scapularis* in the United States), patients with the appropriate clinical picture need to be considered for relapsing fever.

There is no standard diagnostic testing for *B. miyamotoi.* Imugen Laboratory has a new antibody test, but it is not available where I practice, although IGeneX laboratory has PCR testing approved for relapsing fever borrelia in New York. Dr. S. H. Lee also recently designed a pair of genus-specific PCR primers to detect all pathogenic spirochetes, including *Borrelia burgdorferi*, *Borrelia miyamotoi*, and other related borreliae, and he has been finding the ratio of *B. burgdorferi* to *B. miyamotoi* infections to be as high as 3:1. I have been finding the same ratio among patients tested at Quest laboratories for a cousin of *B. miyamotoi*, *B. hermsii*, relapsing fever. Relapsing fever borrelia like *B. miyamotoi* are transmitted transovarially to larvae (6 percent to 73 percent of the time), increasing its prevalence. Many patients with presumed Lyme disease who test negative on standard tests may be infected with either *B. miyamotoi* alone, or co-infected with multiple bacterial species.

TICK PARALYSIS

Tick paralysis (TP) is a rare and potentially lethal tick-borne bacterial infection. It can be caused by some four hundred different tick species, including the same ticks that transmit Rocky Mountain spotted fever, such as the Rocky Mountain wood tick, the American dog tick, and occasionally the lone star tick, the Eastern black-legged tick, and the Western black-legged tick.

Symptoms can include a nonspecific viral-like illness with malaise and weakness, followed by a neurotoxic phase in which the one who is affected will be unable to sit up and walk without help (an acute ataxia, the lack of coordination of muscular movements), with the paralysis progressing upward from the lower extremities, causing the muscles to lose function. These symptoms are caused by salivary neurotoxins secreted by the ticks leading to a paralysis of the muscles that starts with the lower extremities yet leaves sensory functioning (feeling) intact.

Unfortunately, this clinical presentation is most often confused with Guillain-Barré syndrome (GBS), which can be a complication of vaccinations or viral infections like the Zika virus. This confusion may lead to unnecessary therapies, such as plasmapheresis (a plasma exchange, which removes the patient's plasma from their blood, treats it, and returns it to the circulation) that is commonly used in GBS. However, this will not be effective in tick paralysis.

Instead, the first line of treatment is to remove the tick from the body (often found in children on the head and scalp). If the tick is not removed, the patient may die from respiratory complications. Proper and prompt tick removal is therefore necessary, as the fatality rate for TP has been reported to be up to 6 percent in retrospective case studies. When properly diagnosed and treated, full neurological recovery can take place within one to two days.

STARI (SOUTHERN TICK-ASSOCIATED RASH ILLNESS) AND OTHER BORRELIA SPECIES AND RASHES

Although most EM and bull's-eye–type rashes are due to the bacteria causing Lyme disease, *Borrelia burgdorferi sensu stricto*, there are other rashes that resemble Lyme disease that are caused by other species, as we saw with the relapsing fever spirochete, *Borrelia miyamotoi*. Southern tick-associated rash illness (STARI), also known as Master's disease, can cause a rash that is indistinguishable from the ones seen in early Lyme disease. There has been controversy as to whether STARI can lead to the same chronic arthritic and neurological complications as Lyme, but long-term follow-up of patients is lacking in the published scientific studies.

There are patients who complain of long-term symptoms after getting the diagnosis of STARI, and Masters published evidence that sequelae including arthritis and carditis occur. Despite this evidence, some infectious disease doctors choose not to treat STARI and published a study in 2013 advising physicians to only treat if disseminated Lyme disease occurs, because they felt that only the northeastern form of Lyme disease, caused by *Borrelia burgdorferi sensu stricto*, could cause long-term disease manifestations. Carditis is a potentially life-threatening cardiac complication from Lyme disease, and the CDC reported in that same year that there were three sudden cardiac deaths from Lyme carditis. Why was the evidence ignored?

The bacterial etiology of STARI was first identified in 2013 by Dr. Kerry Clark from the Department of Public Health, University of North Florida. He discovered another species of borrelia, *B. burgdorferi sensu lato*, by PCR in the blood and skin of patients with STARI and in lone star ticks. The species of borrelia causing STARI was previously unknown, and this was the first report that some cases of Lyme-like illness with STARI in the southern United States may be attributable to previously undetected *B. burgdorferi sensu lato* infections. Two years later, Dr. Clark published in *Clinical Microbiology and Infection* that he succeeded in cultivating live *B. burgdorferi sensu lato* spirochetes from samples of humans who suffered from not only STARI but also undefined disorders, with symptoms not typical for Lyme borreliosis. He also cultivated a live *Borrelia bissettii*–like strain causing illness, which had been implicated in 2011 as a human pathogen in Mendocino County, California.

Fifteen other borrelia species have since been discovered. These include *B. americanum* and *B. carolinensis* (in the south), *Borrelia kurtenbachii* species, as well as the recent discovery of *Borrelia mayonii* by Mayo Clinic researchers. In many of these spirochetal infections, like *Borrelia mayonii*, the standard two-tiered testing for Lyme disease failed consistently to pick up evidence of the spirochete, and there were atypical symptoms such as a diffuse or focal rash instead of the classic EM rash. Other skin rashes that can appear with borrelia are *Borrelia lymphocytomas* (purplish lumps on the earlobe, nipple, or scrotum) and a violaceous skin rash of the extremities called acrodermatitis chronica atrophicans (ACA), which is due to a European strain of borrelia called *Borrelia afzelii*. This rash is rarely seen in the United States, as it is caused by European strains in ticks.

Recent scientific studies have proven that we have underestimated the role of borrelia infections not only in Lyme but also in other chronic-fatiguing, musculoskeletal illnesses, and involvement of new spirochetal species in Lyme borreliosis changes our understanding and recognition of clinical manifestations of Lyme and other chronic disease. Some of these borrelia species are transmitted by *Ixodes scapularis* ticks, but others can be transmitted by the bite of the lone star tick, *Amblyomma americanum,* causing STARI. Many patients improve with a tetracycline antibiotic, but IV Rocephin should be considered for those with severe neurological involvement.

There is no reliable blood test for STARI to aid in the diagnosis (including the newer C6 Lyme ELISA test), so patients should be treated clinically as if they have contracted early Lyme disease to prevent any possible long-term complications. A review of the medical literature has shown that borrelia-specific bands may be present on a Western blot for STARI, which can help confirm exposure to a borrelia species.

TULAREMIA

This expanding tick-borne illness can also be acquired through the bite of a deerfly, by inhaling aerosolized bacteria, or by exposure to infected rabbits (including ingesting contaminated rabbit meat). Tularemia is caused by an intracellular bacteria, *Francisella tularensis*. The symptoms may vary in severity and presentation, based on the virulence, dose, and site of contact. Nonspecific initial symptoms are reminiscent of a viral-type illness, as with other tick-borne infections, such as fevers, chills, body aches, runny nose, sore throat, and headache. As with Q fever, it also can present with atypical symptoms reminiscent of pneumonia, or mimic a gastrointestinal infection (the typhoidal form), with nausea, vomiting, and diarrhea. Several tick-borne infections like *Borrelia hermsii* (relapsing fever), Lyme disease, ehrlichiosis, and Rocky Mountain spotted fever can also cause diarrhea (with other GI manifestations), acting as "great imitators," so healthcare providers need to be on the alert for atypical manifestations of tick-borne illnesses. It can even occasionally present with sepsis, a potentially fatal blood-borne infection. Some of the most classical presentations of tularemia, however, are the ulceroglandular form (ulcers on the skin, with enlarged lymph nodes) and oculoglandular presentations (eye symptoms such as conjunctivitis with enlarged lymph nodes). The ulceroglandular form may happen when tularemia is contracted handling an infected animal, and an ulcer forms on the hands where the animal was touched, also causing regional lymph nodes to enlarge. The oculoglandular form can occur when the patient touches an eye with a contaminated finger. Ten percent of nationally reported cases come from Cape Cod and Martha's Vineyard, and Colorado health officials reported in 2015 that tularemia cases were on a record-breaking pace.

Treating Tularemia

I have had patients test positive for tularemia over the years, and it presents a significant clinical dilemma when the test returns positive, since IV gentamicin and IV streptomycin are some of the drugs of choice, which can have significant side effects, such as ototoxicity (hearing loss), if not used correctly. Testing includes performing IFAs, ELISAs, immunoblotting, antigen detection assays, and PCRs, but due to the highly infectious nature of this organism, cultures and/or immunohistochemical stains of secretions, exudates, and biopsies are only performed in experienced laboratory facilities. Many patients with other intracellular infections like Bartonella or Brucella return with low-positive tularemia titers, which is not indicative of an active infection with tularemia, and follow-up titers are necessary. An antibody titer of more than 1:160, or detection of a four-fold increase in blood samples taken at different times (at least two weeks), and presence of clinical findings consistent with tularemia suggest an acute infection.

Treatment regimens for Lyme-MSIDS patients infected with tularemia include IV/PO doxycycline, quinolones (such as IV/PO Cipro), with other quinolones like Levaquin showing some efficacy in case studies, IM/IV streptomycin, IV gentamycin, and rarely, chloramphenicol in treatment-resistant cases. Resistant patients often require combination therapy such as doxycycline or chloramphenicol plus streptomycin or (gentamycin treatment), or IV gentamycin alone for seven to ten days. *F. tularensis* strains are sensitive to rifampin, but it is unclear in clinical studies whether it is effective, and there have been treatment failures reported with beta lactam antibiotics, and with intracellular antibiotics, including ciprofloxacin, tetracyclines, and macrolides used alone. A case report that I recently published in the journal *JSM Arthritis* highlighted an immunosuppressed patient with relapsing tularemia who responded positively to a four-drug intracellular antibiotic regimen, including Plaquenil with Avelox (a higher generation quinolone than Levaquin), doxycycline, rifampin, and Dapsone. Further studies are needed to confirm the long-term efficacy of this novel protocol for tularemia.

BRUCELLOSIS

Human brucellosis is an intracellular bacterial infection caused by various strains of Brucella (*Brucella melitensis*, *Brucella abortus*, *Brucella suis*, and *Brucella canis*), although most human disease is due to *B. melitensis*. It has been found in ticks, but human infection most commonly results from the ingestion of infected animal tissue or milk products, or through skin wounds during contact with freshly killed animal tissues. Brucella is another intracellular "persister" bacteria that can cause a chronic illness if not caught early.

Brucellosis is a rare infectious disease that can present with nonspecific symptoms such as fever, sweats, headaches, cough, and arthralgias (joint pain), and GI symptoms that include diarrhea and constipation. Over 90 percent of patients will experience chills, drenching sweats, and fevers, along with weakness and general malaise. The most distinguishing characteristic is that over half the patients experience significant weight loss, usually averaging up to fifteen to twenty pounds. The most common signs, apart from high fevers, are lymphadenopathy (swollen lymph nodes) and hepatosplenomegaly (an enlarged liver and spleen), which we can also see in severe cases of babesiosis. Some Brucella cases present with significant fatigue, headaches, joint pain, and memory/concentration problems, which are clinically indistinguishable from other severe cases of Lyme disease with co-infections, so keep it on your list of differential diagnoses if you are not getting better with standard therapy.

Brucella can present as one of the great imitators, as it can also cause multiple pulmonary complications, a chronic osteomyelitis (infection of the bones), urinary tract infections, optic neuritis (inflammation of the optic nerve) with multiple eye complications, including keratitis, uveitis, and retinopathy (inflammation of the cornea, iris/uvea, and retina). It can even present with a meningitis, encephalitis, or endocarditis, as we have seen with Q fever. According to Dr. Garth Nicolson's 2005 study in the *Journal of Chronic Fatigue Syndrome*, Brucella infections have been found to occur in up to 10 percent of chronic fatigue syndrome patients, especially those living in rural areas, and in some patients Brucella infections occur simultaneously with Mycoplasma infections, increasing the severity of the illness. I have been seeing increasing numbers of positive Brucella titers in the past several years, but false-positive tests are possible, indicative of other intracellular infections. A fourfold rise in titers from serum drawn up to four weeks apart is indicative of true exposure, as well as positive IgM and IgG agglutinating antibodies (which are the most reliable tests). Retest positive antibody titers and negative agglutination tests intermittently to be sure the tests do not turn positive.

Treating Brucellosis

Treatment for Brucella lasts for a minimum of six weeks, and relapses are common if it is not caught early. Tetracyclines or doxycycline plus streptomycin help to decrease relapse rates. IV gentamycin has also been effective in decreasing relapses, as has the addition of Bactrim, or rifampin to a tetracycline regimen, especially in patients with central nervous system (CNS) involvement (meningoencephalitis). In the case of Brucella endocarditis, triple-antibiotic regimens (doxy, rifampicin, and streptomycin; or doxy, rifampicin, and cotrimoxazole) are recommended for at least six months, until titers decrease to a minimum of 1:160. We have had some success treating patients with the latter regimen (doxy, rifampin, and Bactrim DS) in cases where patients were chronically ill, and Brucella agglutination testing turned positive.

Combination Antibiotic Regimens for Lyme and Multiple Intracellular Bacterial Infections

The treatments for most intracellular bacterial infections are similar to the ones we discussed for treating persistent Lyme and Bartonella, with the exception of tularemia and Brucella, which occasionally require stronger drugs like chloramphenicol, streptomycin, or IV gentamycin. Although double intracellular antibiotic therapies help the majority of cases with multiple overlapping bacterial co-infections, many of these infections are "persisters" and require a minimum of three intracellular antibiotics simultaneously in those who are multiply infected. The Horowitz Dapsone protocol, which combines several intracellular antibiotics like doxycycline, rifampin, and Dapsone (a persister drug), with biofilm busters and pulsed cell-wall drugs (like Ceftin) has been helping the majority of those who failed other intracellular therapies, but long-term outcome data is pending.

SIX

Lyme and Other Co-infections: Parasitic, Viral, and Fungal Infections

Parasitic infections, such as Babesia, are frequently found in patients with persistent Lyme disease. Combined with viral and fungal infections, they can intensify and cause chronic symptoms.

Ticks carrying Lyme disease and other bacterial co-infections are also frequently carrying several species of protozoa (single-cell organisms), some of which are parasites. The most common of these protozoal parasites is Babesia, and there are more than one hundred species, which are known collectively as *piroplasms*. However, most Babesia infections transmitted to humans are due to a handful of species: In the United States we often find *Babesia microti* and *Babesia* WA-1 (*Babesia duncani*), with *Babesia microti, Babesia divergens,* and *Babesia venatorum* (EU-1) commonly seen in Europe. Other species are emerging in the United States, like *Babesia odocoilei*, with some species found in animals, such as *Babesia bovis* (which causes Texas cattle fever), occasionally infecting humans. *Theileria parva*, a parasite related to Babesia that causes East Coast fever in cattle, and as-yet unknown organisms similar to tropical Theileria species, are also being discovered in ticks in both the United States and Europe, with *Babesia caballi, Babesia equi* (found in horses), and *Babesia canis* (found in dogs) affecting domestic animals. Co-infection of ticks with multiple bacteria, parasites, and viruses is the rule, not the exception, and in 2016, researchers identified up to eight microorganisms in the same infected tick, including ten Babesia species, two Theileria species, and twenty-four different bacteria.

A study performed in New York State showed that 71 percent of the ticks tested harbored one organism, 30 percent had a polymicrobial infection, with two organisms, and 5 percent were carrying three or more microbes. These included *Borrelia burgdorferi*, *Borrelia miyamotoi*, *Anaplasma phagocytophilum*, Powassan virus, and *Babesia microti*. Other studies are showing evidence of a worldwide epidemic of babesiosis, as it is spreading throughout the United States, Europe, and Asia. For example, although Lyme disease has been rampant in parts of the lower Hudson Valley, New York, where I practice, we have only been able to identify babesiosis there since 1998. In the past ten years, however, the scientific literature has shown that the number of positively diagnosed cases of babesiosis in New York State alone has increased twenty times, and over 40 percent of the ticks in the Hudson Valley are now positive for Lyme and Babesia, with rates of both organisms increasing simultaneously.

Babesiosis is transmitted by the same zoonotic cycle as Lyme disease, involving ticks, deer, and mice. Babesia can also be transmitted from person to person through an infected blood supply, organ transmission, and from mother to unborn fetus. A recent study showed that four out of one thousand blood transfusions are contaminated with Babesia in the United States, and untreated Babesia can cause significant disability, especially in the very young or elderly with impaired immune systems; in some cases, the disease has been fatal.

The Symptoms of Babesiosis

Classic symptoms of Babesia include:

- day sweats
- night sweats (occasionally drenching)
- chills
- flushing
- fever
- cough
- air hunger (unexplained shortness of breath)

These symptoms will not respond to classical antibiotic therapy for Lyme disease alone. This means that if you are diagnosed with Lyme but not tested and treated for other co-infections, such as babesiosis, many of your most aggravating symptoms may not go away, even with long courses of proper Lyme treatment.

Different strains of Babesia may cause different sets of symptoms, yet all can significantly exacerbate a Lyme disease infection. For example, *Babesia microti* and *Babesia duncani* (WA-1) are both found in the United States, and both vary in their presentations from European strains of babesiosis, such as *Babesia divergens*. Most doctors are taught in medical school that Babesia can cause a hemolytic anemia (due to red blood cells breaking down), jaundice, thrombocytopenia (low platelet counts), congestive heart failure, and renal failure. Yet this is not the clinical presentation for all patients who have babesiosis with or without Lyme disease in the United States, and nonspecific symptoms such as fatigue, malaise, and weakness, with an associated fever, shaking chills, and excessive sweating are often mistaken for the signs of a seasonal flu or, in certain regions of the world, another insect-borne parasite: malaria. Although malaria cases are rare in the United States, a 2016 study showed that up to 25 percent of deer in the northeast are infected with malaria parasites (*Plasmodium odocoilei*). Researchers believe the species doesn't pose a threat to humans, but further studies are necessary.

Malaria and Babesia share the same set of symptoms, and the infections may look the same to a laboratory technician viewing parasites under the microscope. Babesia and malaria can both produce ring forms (circular structures) under the microscope, although only Babesia will produce Maltese Cross forms, and these may not always be present on the blood smear for malarial parasites (Giemsa stain) that the laboratory technician is looking at. Doctors therefore may not consider babesiosis as a cause of a patient's symptoms, especially if there is no evidence of an associated hemolytic anemia and thrombocytopenia. It is often only the sickest patients, being admitted to the hospital, who will have both the classic textbook presentations combined with the more common malarial symptoms such as fatigue, malaise, and weakness, with fever, shaking chills, and sweating.

Worse, even if the proper diagnosis is made, some infectious disease doctors are still under the impression that seven to ten days of antimalarial and antibiotic medications, such as Mepron and Zithromax, will cure babesiosis. In my experience, nothing could be further from the truth. Babesiosis occurring in a Lyme-MSIDS patient is one of the most tenacious and dangerous co-infections.

This parasite exacerbates all of the typical Lyme symptoms, causing an increase in fatigue, joint pain, paresthesias, headaches, and cognitive dysfunction, often with the malaria-like symptoms listed above. Psychological problems such as depression, anxiety, and mood swings are also typically worsened with Babesia, which is why it should always be considered in patients presenting with multiple systemic symptoms and severe emotional issues that do not seem proportionate to their present situation or history of trauma.

Other classic symptoms of babesiosis that may suggest its presence in Lyme disease patients are an unexplained cough and/or a shortness of breath with air hunger, without another, more common diagnosis to explain these symptoms (i.e., asthma, allergic rhinitis with a postnasal drip, GERD, COPD/emphysema, interstitial lung disease, or pneumonia). These can occur with or without malaria-like signs or symptoms. The most severe form of shortness of breath is acute respiratory distress syndrome (ARDS), which can occasionally be seen in patients with babesiosis. ARDS can be fatal to those with compromised immune systems.

Other atypical presentations can include severe hemolytic anemia in patients with healthy immune systems and intact spleens, which can also be fatal if not properly treated. This is why we need to be vigilant in trying to avoid prescribing drugs that can suppress the immune system (such as high-dose steroids and other immunosuppressant drugs) for patients with Lyme disease, babesiosis, and associated co-infections. An intact immune system and spleen are needed to properly fight these infections, although rarely even immunocompetent individuals with a spleen can succumb to severe babesiosis, from septic shock.

TESTING FOR BABESIOSIS

Babesiosis is a "persister" parasite, and can go on to develop into a chronic carrier state, like Lyme disease. Early and aggressive treatment is therefore necessary. Testing for Babesia often requires a panel approach to pick up the organism (Giemsa stain, IFA for *Babesia microti* and *duncani*,

Babesia FISH test, and/or PCR), as one negative test does not rule out the disease. An inadequate response to a Lyme regimen, and a positive clinical response to antimalarial therapy with a decrease in day and night sweats, chills, flushing, a cough, and/or air hunger most likely indicates the presence of the organism.

Treating Babesiosis

Babesiosis is much easier to treat successfully if found in the early stages of the illness. If you present with an EM rash and have associated significant day sweats, night sweats, high fevers, and/or shaking chills, then you should clinically suspect an associated co-infection with Babesia, and consider using Mepron or Malarone early in the illness, while testing for Babesia and associated bacterial tick-borne co-infections during the initial evaluation.

Cleocin with quinine remains one of the classical regimens prescribed for babesiosis, but it frequently causes severe ringing in the ears, nausea, vomiting, and rashes. Due to these severe side effects, I will more commonly use rotations for babesiosis, such as Cleocin and a macrolide antibiotic (Zithromax or Biaxin) with (or rarely without) Malarone or Mepron. Mepron can also be used with a macrolide, and adding double-strength Bactrim (a sulfa drug) to a regimen (i.e., Cleocin/Zithromax/Bactrim with Mepron or Malarone) will often significantly increase its efficacy, especially if there is an overlapping Lyme/Bartonella infection. Adding antimalarial herbs, such as *Artemisia*, cryptolepis, and/or neem, to the above regimens, or to other regimens for resistant Babesiosis listed below, may help improve efficacy.

- Doxycycline: Tetracyclines have been used in the past for malarial prophylaxis, and doxycycline covers the majority of intracellular co-infections seen with persistent Lyme disease. We have found that combining doxycycline and Plaquenil (occasionally with Bactrim DS) with other antimalarial drugs, such as Malarone, and antimalarial herbs can be an effective combination.
- Lariam: Although it has good efficacy against malarial organisms, black box warnings and potential neurological side effects restrict its use.
- Coartem: This may be effective in patients with babesiosis whose previous regimens have failed. This is a classical drug regimen

that is used for malaria and is felt to be at least 95 percent effective in eliminating *Plasmodium falciparum* malaria. This is certainly not the case in patients with chronic babesiosis, although it does help to decrease resistant symptomatology. It can be used alone or in combination with other antiparasitic drugs, like Daraprim, but Coartem must be taken away from certain medications (i.e., Elavil, macrolides, quinolones, certain SSRIs, and PPIs) and other antimalarial drugs like Primaquine phosphate (also used for malaria) and Lariam that can affect the QT interval on the electrocardiogram. Due to Lariam's long half-life, it would need to be stopped weeks in advance of taking Coartem. Doing a PDR drug interaction check is advisable, and if some of the medications cannot be stopped, consider checking an EKG.

- Dapsone: My 2016 study in the *Journal of Clinical and Experimental Dermatology Research* showed that Dapsone is an effective treatment not only for Lyme but also for babesiosis. Dapsone helped resistant Babesia symptoms of sweats, chills, and flushing in those failing prior Babesia therapies. Lyme positive, Babesia-positive patients also demonstrated significant improvements in pain, disturbed sleep, and cognitive difficulties, especially when combined with Malarone and antimalarial herbs. The highest dose of Dapsone (100 mg) was oftentimes necessary with Malarone and antimalarial herbs in those patients with severe, resistant babesiosis who previously failed clindamycin, Mepron, Malarone, and other drug/herbal therapies (see Chapter 4 and Appendix A for the full Dapsone protocol). The sickest patients with babesiosis, having high levels of parasites in the blood resulting in the failure of the above regimens, are sometimes given exchange transfusions, in which their blood is taken out of the body and exchanged for healthy, uninfected blood. This can be lifesaving in the right circumstances, but it carries certain risks.

Babesia Is Often Persistent

Conventional wisdom is that Babesia typically resolves spontaneously or after administration of a seven- to ten-day course of treatment. Unfortunately, many highly immunocompromised patients with Lyme-MSIDS who have had babesiosis for years have evidence of persistence, and do not significantly improve after short-term therapy. Babesia can also develop resistance to classical anti-parasitic drugs and herbs, just as malaria has developed multiple drug-resistant strains. Researchers at the University of Oxford discovered genetic mutations that enabled malarial parasites to withstand artemisinin treatment, and Mepron resistance has previously been shown to exist by Dr. Peter Krause. This is particularly important for those who have ongoing chronic symptomatology. Babesia can also persist because it can hide from the immune system, just like Lyme disease.

Several mechanisms could explain Babesia's ability to evade the host immune response:

1. Antigenic variation: changing its outer surface proteins to evade the immune system, like Lyme disease
2. Different gene expressions: how DNA is produced in the organism
3. Cytoadhesion with sequestration: how it binds to cells and hides
4. The ratio of Babesia-infected red blood cells to uninfected cells has also been shown to change the parasites' developmental pathways, enabling swift responses to changing environmental conditions like availability of red blood cells (RBCs) and nutrition, allowing it to persist

Babesia has already been proven to persist in the animal population: It can exist in a carrier state in domestic and wild animals for many years without causing active symptoms. Babesia can similarly suppress the immune system, just like Lyme disease, to a point where our immune system cannot effectively attack other infections and protect the body.

Babesia impairs the elimination of other parasites from the body, such as nematodes (roundworms), Trichuris (whipworms), and trypanosomes, and it may be the case with another parasite, toxoplasmosis, which is genetically similar to Babesia. Toxoplasmosis is often acquired by human contact with cat feces, and it is estimated that between one-third and one-half of the world's population carries a toxoplasmosis infection. We frequently find that patients in our medical practice have been infected with toxoplasmosis, and some do not adequately respond to standard toxoplasmosis therapies. There are also patients who have intestinal parasites that persist despite standard antiparasitic therapies (like Biltricide, Ivermectin, Alinia, PinX, and Albendazole) when they are co-infected with babesiosis. Thus, clearing other parasites from the body may be more difficult when Babesia is present, leading to increased symptoms.

High-dose probiotics (acidophilus) with *Saccharomyces boulardii* two to three times a day should be used in all of the following regimens with broad-spectrum antibiotics, to help prevent diarrhea and yeast infections.

First-Line Treatment Protocols

- Mepron, taken with a high-fat meal, and Zithromax (or Biaxin), Plaquenil, and nystatin tablets. Since there is Mepron resistance in the United States, Malarone may be substituted for Mepron. Clindamycin can be added to this regimen to increase efficacy if the patient's bowels are stable, as can herbal therapies (i.e., *Artemisia* and cryptolepis). IV Cleocin is generally used in patients with severe GI intolerance to oral clindamycin or who have failed oral clindamycin.

- Septra DS may be added if there are resistant or severe symptoms, and if the patient does not have a sulfa allergy. If there is an overlapping Bartonella infection, adding Septra DS may also be useful. Using two or three antibiotics together requires strict sugar-free, yeast-free diets, with high-dose probiotics. Dapsone and Septra should not be combined, due to the increased possibility of adverse side effects (anemia and/or methemoglobinemia).

- Antimalarial herbs such as *Artemisia*, cryptolepis, or neem may also be layered onto this regimen for severe symptoms, and/or if the patient's malarial-type symptoms persist. Other antimalarial herbs that may be effective are Beyond Balance MC Bab-1, 2, 3 and Sida Acuta. Antimalarial herbs are generally used one at a time and may be rotated, depending on the patient's clinical response, but combinations of herbs may be necessary for resistant symptoms.

- Malarone alone, and/or with herbs, is also a good choice for patients with mild babesiosis who can't tolerate stronger protocols due to GI side effects (loose stools, yeast). Malarone is usually dosed at four tablets a day for three days as a loading dose, followed by one tablet two times per day. Some MSIDS patients with severe malarial symptoms require two tablets PO BID to control their symptoms. We have seen clinical and laboratory evidence of persistent and relapsing babesiosis at lower doses and have not seen significant adverse effects in patients using this regimen. Avoid taking CoQ10 as a vitamin supplement while on Malarone or Mepron, as it can interfere with its clinical efficacy. Malarone can be used alone as a single agent, but Mepron should always be used with a macrolide and/or other intracellular medication to prevent drug resistance.

- Patients who previously failed regimens of Mepron or Malarone, or have intolerances to the drugs, should be considered for a Cleocin and Quinine regimen. We do not often use the classically prescribed Babesia therapy of Cleocin and quinine as a first-line therapy (although it may be helpful) because of the severe side effects of quinine. Cleocin and quinine may be reserved for babesiosis in late-stage pregnancy, as it is one of the few regimens that have been proven safe for the fetus. I recently had to treat a woman with Lyme and relapsing babesiosis during her third trimester of pregnancy (twice, during consecutive pregnancies). I used clindamycin, Mepron, and Zithromax (under the supervision of her high-risk OB-GYN), and the babies were completely healthy at birth, with no signs of active babesiosis.

- Many patients who were not treated early relapse once treatment is stopped. They may have positive PCRs (DNA probes) and positive FISH testing (RNA probes), despite months of therapy. In this instance we rotate to other antimalarial regimens such as Coartem, which can be pulsed once a month for several months in resistant relapsing patients if there was initially a positive response without side effects. Coartem can be used alone or with Daraprim for three days in severely ill patients, and/or in combination with doxycycline. We usually follow a course of Coartem with a Lyme-Babesia+/−Bartonella regimen, like Zithromax/Bactrim/Malarone with herbs, or doxycycline/Bactrim/Malarone with herbs, with typical cell-wall, cyst, and biofilm busters added on if the Lyme is active.

- Lariam is an older drug used for malarial prophylaxis, which has clinical efficacy against babesiosis, but we no longer use it due to a black box warning of possible neuropsychiatric side effects, such as seizures, hallucinations, psychosis, increased depression, and paranoia. It also causes vivid dreams with occasional nausea and dizziness (usually at higher doses, not clinically apparent for most patients at a half tablet every three days, or one tablet every five to seven days, which often helps Babesia symptoms). Apart from potential neuropsychiatric side effects, Lariam has an extremely long half-life (three weeks), and can affect QT intervals on the electrocardiogram for up to fifteen weeks post-Lariam in select patients.
- Patients with severe, recalcitrant Lyme and babesiosis who have failed every other drug/herbal regimen should consider a Dapsone protocol, unless they have a significant sulfa allergy. We have been having good success treating resistant Babesia symptoms with this persister drug with antimalarial activity, but it is usually not a first line treatment (at this time) due to potential side effects (which are manageable). We have occasionally seen recalcitrant babesiosis respond well to a combination therapy of Cleocin/Mepron/Zithromax/Dapsone with antimalarial herbs, but long-term follow-ups are lacking to confirm sustained clinical efficacy.

PARASITIC INFECTIONS

Intestinal parasites like giardia, amoeba, pinworm, hookworm, schistosomiasis, and strongyloides are part of the MSIDS map. These infections are found on both serum antibody testing and stool cultures (i.e., local labs, Genova stool CDSA). Although we generally think of parasitic worms as only inhabiting the GI tract, Dr. Alan MacDonald recently found nematode filarial worms in the cerebrospinal fluid of patients with multiple sclerosis and Alzheimer's disease at autopsy. Dr. Eva Sapi has found filarial worms in *Ixodes scapularis* ticks, and Zhang and colleagues found them in lone star ticks, so it is possible that filarial worms are being regurgitated from the gut of the tick into humans after a tick bite. Dr. Steven Fry has found parasites in the bloodstream living in biofilms, called *Pro-*

tomyxoa rheumatica (FL-1953), which are composed of up to eight different genetic types of parasites. Babesia suppresses our ability to clear other parasites, so are multiple parasites partially responsible for chronic illness in Lyme-MSIDS?

Parasites apart from Babesia can play an important role in keeping chronic Lyme patients sick, and antiparasitic regimens are often important. Regimens including Biltricide, ivermectin, pyrantel pamoate (Pin-X), paromomycin, Alinia, and Albenza have been effective in certain patients with not only persistent GI symptoms but also fatigue, headaches, and myalgias resistant to classical tick-borne therapy. Some Morgellons patients report noticing help using antiparasitic drugs in combination with regimens against Lyme and tick-borne co-infections (like Bartonella), and some neuropsychiatric Lyme patients have seen improvement in cognition and behavior with antiparasitic drugs. Make sure you do a comprehensive parasite evaluation if you or your patient is not getting better.

VIRAL INFECTIONS

Vector-borne viral infections can affect those with Lyme-MSIDS. Some of these infections are transmitted by mosquitos, such as dengue fever, Japanese encephalitis, Eastern and Western equine encephalitis, West Nile virus, and the newer Chikungunya and Zika viruses. The Zika virus can also be transmitted by sexual contact. Others are transmitted by ticks, such as tick-borne encephalitis virus (TBEV), Omsk hemorrhagic fever, Kyasanur forest disease (KFD), Congo-Crimean hemorrhagic fever (CCHF), Powassan encephalitis, and the recently discovered Heartland and Bourbon viruses. Researchers have also isolated the Tacaribe virus, which can cause hemorrhagic disease, from 11.2 percent of *Amblyomma americanum* ticks in Florida. It is not known if the tick can transmit the virus to humans.

Chronic viral infections (non-tick borne) may also explain some of the resistant symptomatology that we see among the Lyme-MSIDS population for whom antibiotic therapy fails. Viruses do not respond to antibiotics, and some of these viruses can cause illness in patients with chronic fatigue syndrome and fibromyalgia. I often screen chronic MSIDS patients for associated viral infections, especially if they are presenting with significant fatigue, fibromyalgia, and neurological symptoms. These patients may be carrying viral infections without knowing it, and once they become infected with Lyme disease and other co-infections, it may cause a reactivation of prior viral infections and an exacerbation of their condition.

The most common viral infections that we screen for include:

- Epstein-Barr
- Human herpesvirus 6 (HHV-6)
- Cytomegalovirus (CMV)
- West Nile

We often find elevated levels of HHV-6, which are linked to both chronic fatigue syndrome and fibromyalgia, each of which can cause the same overlapping symptoms that we see with Lyme disease. HHV-6 also causes roseola (Sixth disease) in children, and nearly 100 percent of adults today have been exposed. It can reactivate later in life secondary to immunological and environmental factors and can lead to hepatitis and meningo-encephalitis, as well as being a possible cofactor in ADD, autism spectrum disorder, and multiple sclerosis.

Viruses can also affect autoimmune processes. In 2015, genetic variants of the Epstein-Barr virus were linked to multiple sclerosis, and varicella (Herpes zoster) viral infections were shown to cause an arteritis (inflammation in the arteries). Previously, CMV was shown to increase inflammation in rheumatoid arthritis.

We also will occasionally screen for HHV-8, Coxsackie virus, and parvovirus. Enteroviruses have been linked to neurological disorders with tics; implicating an immune-inflammatory reaction in the patho-etiology of certain brain disorders (like PANS/PANDAS). We may also look for Powassan encephalitis or other types of viral encephalitis if the patient is coming in with a particularly severe neurological presentation. The Powassan virus is now found in increasing numbers of ticks in different areas of the United States (including the Lower Hudson Valley where I practice) and can be transmitted in as little as fifteen minutes of a tick attachment. It can cause fevers, seizures, focal neurological findings, neurological deficits (including loss of consciousness), hemiplegia (paralysis of half of the body), and neurological consequences, including mental status changes, visual deficits, hearing impairments, and chronic motor difficulties.

Nutritional Supplements Help with Viral Infections

Lyme disease patients often report that they feel worse and that their symptoms flare up when they come down with viral infections. It is as if their immune system can only effectively fight so many infections at the same time. Nutritional supplements may help, although most do not see a strong clinical shift in their symptoms.

The following supplements have known scientific efficacy against viruses:

- Colostrum derivatives, such as transfer factors: antibodies that protect against disease and are produced by mammals during lactation.
- Olive leaf extract: Olive leaves and their active component, oleuropein, have been found effective in treating herpes, influenza A, Coxsackie, and other viruses.
- Mushroom derivatives, including 3–6 beta-glucan: The immune-enhancing properties of the yeast beta-glucan have been the subject of more than sixty years of research and more than eight hundred scientific studies. Preclinical research has shown 3–6 beta-glucan to be efficacious against a range of infectious diseases. Beta-glucan's primary effect is to increase natural killer (NK) cells and the phagocytic capacity of immune cells, and to enhance the movement of these cells to the site of a foreign challenge throughout the body via the liver, spleen, and lymph nodes. Clinical research has shown it to have synergistic effects with antibiotics (JH reactions are possible), and 3–6 beta-glucan has been shown to be superior to most other immune supplements. It is therefore useful for those with Lyme-MSIDS fighting bacterial and viral infections with a healthy immune system.

Treating Viral Infections

There is no specific treatment for tick-borne viral encephalopathies like Powassan encephalitis, except supportive treatment, and HIV medications are being studied as a possible option for these patients.

Anyone who does not adequately respond to appropriate antibiotic protocols while addressing the sixteen-point differential on the MSIDS map, and who has high viral titers and/or a positive PCR, may suffer from viral infections that may have been present and/or reactivated, and a trial of antiviral medication is warranted. This could include Valtrex, Famvir, acyclovir, or Valcyte in severe cases. In our experience, classical antiviral drugs such as Valtrex and Famvir do not have a significant clinical effect in the majority of MSIDS patients, except in preventing frequent relapses of herpes viruses. Occasionally Byron White herbal remedies against viruses, such as A-EB/H6, are helpful.

CANDIDA AND FUNGAL INFECTIONS

Candida syndrome with intestinal dysbiosis (a microbial imbalance in the gut) is not an uncommon health problem. It should be suspected in any MSIDS patient who has unexplained fatigue, joint and muscle pain, and neurological symptoms such as brain fog and headaches that are unresponsive or worsen with standard treatment regimens.

I first learned about candida many years ago after one of my patients had developed a strange set of skin rashes that worsened every time she took antibiotics. She also complained of chronic fatigue, headaches, blood sugar swings, trouble concentrating, and digestive problems. In searching for answers I came across William Crook's book, *The Yeast Connection*. In it he described my patient's symptoms perfectly. By placing her on a yeast-free diet and treating the candida with antifungal agents, we were able to reverse all of her symptoms, which had baffled dermatologists and other subspecialists who had been unable to find a cause.

Although we normally have candida organisms present in our gastrointestinal tract in limited amounts, taking antibiotics for bacterial infections will encourage an overgrowth of candida. Antibiotics kill off the good bacteria that keep our normal level of yeast in check. Furthermore, the standard American diet, which is high in sugar and refined carbohydrates, can promote an overgrowth of yeast. Other factors that may contribute to the candida syndrome are:

- Oral contraceptives
- Immune suppression due to stress
- Severe illness or chemotherapy

- Drugs that decrease the acidity of the gastrointestinal tract, such as antacids, H2 blockers (such as Zantac), and proton pump inhibitors (such as Prilosec).

Candida can be confused with antibiotic-resistant Lyme disease. Many patients with adrenal dysfunction and associated hypoglycemia also suffer from candidiasis. These symptoms overlap with those of persistent Lyme disease (except in Lyme there is migratory pain, where symptoms come and go). The most common signs and symptoms of candidiasis include:

- Blood sugar swings with overlapping reactive hypoglycemia and a craving for sweets
- Depression
- Dizziness with poor motor coordination
- Fatigue
- Fungal infections of the nails
- Gas and bloating, which increase with sugar/carbohydrate consumption
- Headaches
- Itching and other skin problems
- Mood swings
- Muscle and joint pain that does not migrate throughout the body
- Poor digestion with nausea
- Poor memory and concentration (brain fog)
- Rashes
- Thrush in the mouth (yeast on the tongue and buccal mucosa, which appears as a white, patchy coating)
- Vaginitis (recurrent vaginal yeast infections)

If you have been tested with both an IgE and IgG food allergy panel and found to be allergic to a multiplicity of foods, suspect overlapping candida and leaky gut syndrome, especially if there is histamine release with associated itching, sneezing, wheezing, and/or nasal congestion after eating certain foods. Pay particular attention to your diet and the acid/alkaline balance of your foods, avoiding allergic foods by following a rotation diet, which we describe in Chapter 16. A comprehensive digestive stool analysis (CSDA) can also be performed through various labs such as Genova Diagnostics to check for bacterial and yeast overgrowth in the stool, while checking yeast sensitivities to antifungal agents.

Treating Candida and Yeast Infections

The most important dietary modifications for dealing with yeast are to eliminate malt, vinegar, simple sugars, and carbohydrates (including fruits early on in the treatment), as well as all yeast-containing foods (most breads and cheeses) and fermented foods (e.g., soy sauce, tempeh, pickles, sauerkraut, and alcoholic beverages such as wine, beer, and cider). Mushrooms should also be avoided (they are fungal, which is a form of yeast), as well as any foods to which you are either sensitive or allergic.

We prescribe nystatin prophylactically if patients need to be on long-term antibiotics, to avoid issues with yeast overgrowth, but often the tablet form of nystatin is insufficient in dealing with severe yeast problems once they have arisen. Powdered nystatin is more effective than tablets, and should be used in cases of severe candida.

Despite explaining the necessity of a strict, sugar-free, yeast-free diet to our patients taking antibiotics, they often have a difficult time adhering to this regimen. Therefore, we sometimes use rotations of antifungal medications such as Diflucan and, rarely, Sporanox. These medications can be very effective, but potential side effects include inflammation of the liver and cardiac symptoms (EKG abnormalities) requiring proper monitoring. If these medications are ineffective or are contraindicated, natural antifungal agents, such as caprylic acid, grapefruit seed extract, garlic, berberine, and oregano oil can be helpful. We also frequently use monolaurin, a biofilm-busting coconut oil extract with antibacterial, antiviral, and antifungal effects, as well as Biocidin with broad spectrum botanicals for intestinal dysbiosis. When combined with good-quality, high-dose probiotics (lactobacillus and/or Bifidobacterium) they can be extremely beneficial in restoring the proper balance of intestinal bacteria and yeast in the colon. We use several strains of high-potency acidophilus and choose brands that are acid resistant and/or coated with sodium alginate to increase the amount of acidophilus that colonizes the small and large intestines.

Not all forms of yeast are detrimental. Apart from prescribing high doses of good-quality probiotics, and occasionally prebiotics containing fructooligosaccharides (FOS) to prevent antibiotic-associated diarrhea, we also give patients *Saccharomyces boulardii*, a type of beneficial yeast that has been shown to decrease the incidence of *Clostridium difficile* diarrhea. *Clostridium difficile* is a bacteria responsible for 95 percent of pseudo-membranous colitis and 30 percent of all antibiotic-associated diarrheas. Saccharomyces is a healthy yeast that acts as a temporary barrier protecting the intestinal mucosa. A 2009 study published in *Infection and Immunity* showed that saccharomyces has a protease that inhibits the effects of *Clostridium difficile* toxins A and B. *Clostridium difficile* has the potential to be life threatening. It is therefore very important to protect against this possibility by using high-dose probiotics and *Saccharomyces boulardii* during antibiotic therapy.

MORGELLONS DISEASE

Morgellons disease, or "fiber" disease, is characterized by unusual skin wounds that appear to have fibers and specks coming out from the lesions, itching or crawling feelings under the skin (peripheral neuropathy), and multisystemic symptoms. This unusual skin syndrome is occasionally seen in Lyme-MSIDS patients like Linda, whom I introduced in Chapter 4.

In 2015, Morgellons was linked to an infectious process with Lyme disease spirochetes. Some believe that parasites are also playing a role (some patient's skin lesions improve with antiparasitic medication) as well as Bartonella and environmental chemicals, and there is even a hypothesis that insects may be involved, since the skin lesions appear to extrude a material that is similar to the chitin found in the hard body of insects. According to the Morgellons Research Foundation, this disease can be characterized by six major signs and symptoms:

1. Skin lesions: both spontaneously appearing and self-generated, with intense itching. The former may initially appear as hives or as "pimple-like" lesions, with or without a white center. The latter appear as linear scratches. Even when not self-generated, the lesions often progress to open wounds that heal slowly and

incompletely. Often patients with Morgellons syndrome are mistakenly accused of self-inflicted skin lesions, because no obvious cause is found.

2. Crawling sensations, both within and on the skin surface: may be described as bugs moving, stinging, or biting intermittently. This can also involve the scalp, nostrils, ear canal, and body hair or hair follicles.

3. Fatigue.

4. Cognitive difficulties.

5. Behavioral problems: Many are diagnosed with psychiatric disorders (obsessive compulsive disorder, attention deficit disorder, attention deficit hyperactivity disorder, or bipolar disorder) and are often labeled as having delusional parasitosis, since well-meaning physicians cannot find an obvious cause for their symptoms.

6. Presence of fibers in and on skin lesions that can be white or black, blue, green, red, and other colors that fluoresce when viewed under ultraviolet light. Patients also report seeing black "specks" or "dots" on or in their skin, and objects described as "granules," similar in size and shape to sand grains, can occasionally be removed from either broken or intact skin.

In addition, many Morgellons patients have been diagnosed with chronic fatigue syndrome and fibromyalgia. Other signs and symptoms include many of the same ones we have been discussing with Lyme-MSIDS: changes in visual acuity; balance problems; ringing in the ears (tinnitus); neurological symptoms, including changes in mood and personality; and painful extremities with arthralgias or arthritis-like symptoms. Obtaining appropriate medical assistance for these patients is challenging, as many physicians do not believe in the diagnosis despite recent scientific evidence.

Treating Morgellons

Although we still do not completely understand this syndrome, I have treated Morgellons patients successfully, starting with using the sixteen-point MSIDS diagnostic map to ferret out underlying health problems and treating them with the same antibiotics used to treat Lyme and associated co-infections. The most effective antibiotics have included intracellular drugs: tetracyclines (doxycycline, minocycline), macrolides (Zithromax, Biaxin), Septra DS, and quinolone drugs (Cipro, Levaquin, Avelox, and Factive), combining at least two intracellular antibiotics for greater efficacy. Often the skin lesions and associated symptoms resolve once antibiotics are used in a comprehensive treatment plan.

SEVEN

Lyme and Immune Dysfunction

utoimmune diseases are caused by an inappropriate immune response in the body; for example, the immune system mistakes some part of the body for a pathogen (foreign invader), and attacks itself. This may be restricted to certain organs or involve a particular tissue, or it may be systemic. More than one hundred diseases are considered to be autoimmune ones, including type 1 diabetes, Hashimoto's thyroiditis, multiple sclerosis, rheumatoid arthritis, Crohn's disease and ulcerative colitis, lupus, psoriasis, Behçet's disease, and scleroderma. More than 50 million Americans are living and coping with autoimmune diseases, and more than 75 percent are women, making them some of the top-ten leading causes of death of women under the age of sixty-five.

It is not uncommon for patients presenting with Lyme-MSIDS to test positively for multiple autoimmune markers on their laboratory blood work. These same patients frequently present with fatigue, joint and musculoskeletal pain with a positive antinuclear antibody (ANA) or rheumatoid factor. Sometimes the lab tests show an elevated C-reactive protein (CRP) or sedimentation rate, which are markers of inflammation. Occasionally patients also test positive for other autoimmune markers. These include: antibodies against double-stranded DNA (dsDNA), which is very specific and sensitive for lupus; Sjögren's antibodies, i.e., anti-Ro (SS-A) and anti-La (SS-B); anti-ribonuclear proteins (anti-RNP), which is seen in several autoimmune syndromes; anti-thyroid antibodies, i.e., anti-thyroglobulin (TG) and anti-thyroid peroxidase (TPO) seen in Hashimoto's thyroiditis; antiganglioside antibodies (anti-GM1, Mag, ASI) seen in autoimmune neuropathies (POTS/dysautonomia, as well as Guillain-Barré syndrome); and are HLA DR 4 positive, which can be associated with increased autoimmune phenomena.

Patients will often come to my medical practice after having been given the diagnosis of lupus, rheumatoid arthritis (RA), or a nonspecific autoimmune disease. Frequently their physicians will have tested them for Lyme disease with a basic ELISA test, and when it comes back negative (as it often does, due to the poor sensitivity of this test), they are told that they do not have Lyme disease but instead have an autoimmune disorder. Then they may be placed on a number of medications for their joint pain, including biologic agents such as methotrexate, Enbrel, Arava, and Cimzia, or immunosuppressive drugs such as Imuran or prednisone. Unfortunately, these drugs do not always help. Worse, these medications can have untoward side effects, including the development of certain cancers, reactivation of underlying infections such as tuberculosis, and exacerbation of active infections such as Lyme disease and associated co-infections. This is because some of these drugs suppress the immune system and allow latent cancers or underlying infections to emerge more powerfully. That was the case with the woman with Lyme, seronegative RA, and Behçet's syndrome (another autoimmune disease, of unknown etiology) that we discussed previously, whose tularemia and Bartonella infections reactivated while on Imuran and prednisone.

The situation becomes even more complicated when there is a true, previously diagnosed autoimmune disease, like rheumatoid arthritis or Behçet's, as well as exposure to Lyme disease and multiple co-infections. For example, a patient may have a positive rheumatoid factor as well as a positive anti-CCP (anticyclic citrullinated peptide) antibody, which is a more specific marker for rheumatoid arthritis. She may also have had a negative ELISA test for Lyme and be told that she has rheumatoid arthritis. However, a more sensitive test for Lyme disease, such as the C6 ELISA and Western blot (done by laboratories like IGeneX in California), may yield different results. What's more, the patient may not have been tested for associated bacterial or parasitic co-infections that can increase fatigue and joint pain; viruses like HHV-6, cytomegalovirus (CMV), or

Epstein-Barr virus (EBV) that increase inflammation, or the newly emerging Chikungunya virus, which mimics rheumatoid arthritis; or tested for heavy metals and other environmental pollutants, which have been associated with autoimmune phenomena. Any of these overlapping medical problems can increase fatigue and musculoskeletal pain.

If you are experiencing these types of symptoms, there are four possibilities that may be occurring:

- You may have an autoimmune disease and not know it.
- You may have an autoimmune disease and know it.
- You may not have an autoimmune disease, but Lyme disease, and/ or co-infections and abnormalities on the MSIDS map are mimicking and exacerbating autoimmune symptoms.
- You have both an autoimmune disease and Lyme disease that, in combination with multiple factors on the MSIDS model, are contributing to making the autoimmune disease symptoms worse.

LYME DISEASE CAN CAUSE AUTOIMMUNE SYMPTOMS

In the medical literature we find that both children and adults who were referred to rheumatologists with presumptive diagnoses of diseases such as juvenile idiopathic arthritis (JIA, previously known as juvenile rheumatoid arthritis), or adult-onset Still's disease (AOSD, a severe form of JIA in adults) were often found to have Lyme disease.

It is interesting that blood tests that indicate rheumatoid arthritis (RA) correlate positively with antibody titers against certain species of borrelia, especially a commonly found borrelia species in Europe, *Borrelia garinii*. In one 1995 study published in *Lupus*, 57 percent of patients with rheumatoid arthritis demonstrated previous exposure to borrelia. Unfortunately, the study's authors dismissed their own findings and assumed these patients had false-positive blood tests. As we have seen, many labs are using insensitive testing for the multiple strains of borrelia and use CDC criteria to make the diagnosis, which will miss many patients with Lyme disease. This suggests that the authors might have dismissed their own evidence, implying a causal link between the two diseases, or at least showing that they may occur together frequently, contributing to the patients' illnesses.

This link has been postulated in the scientific literature and referred to as "Lyme arthritis," a disease caused by a bacterium that can mimic RA. This finding has begged the question of whether infectious agents could be a contributing factor to autoimmune diseases. In animal models, a causal link has been found between borrelia infection and the subsequent development of rheumatoid arthritis. Some of my patients had been diagnosed with "seronegative rheumatoid arthritis" and did not achieve clinical improvement until a diagnosis of Lyme disease with co-infections was made.

Apart from Lyme disease, other infectious diseases may also be driving autoimmune phenomena and joint pain. Let us look at the situation with three commonly found co-infections, Mycoplasma, Bartonella, and Chlamydia. Mycoplasmas have been shown to affect parts of the immune system that can result in promoting autoimmune reactions and rheumatoid symptoms, and they have been found in the joint tissues of patients with rheumatological diseases, suggesting their involvement in the disease process. Bartonella species can also cause polyclonal B-cell activation, commonly found in patients with rheumatologic or chronic inflammatory diseases, and *Chlamydia pneumonia* causes arthritis and joint pain. More than one bacterial organism can be found in the joint fluid of patients with arthritis. These infections are often present in MSIDS patients, and all of them may cause joint pain. These infections are also caused by intracellular bacteria that are sensitive to the antibiotic minocycline, which goes inside the cell to inhibit bacterial growth. This means that when a rheumatologist prescribes Plaquenil and minocycline and believes that their effects on the body for autoimmune diseases are primarily anti-inflammatory as a disease-modifying agent, it may be that the same drugs are also simultaneously treating Lyme disease, Mycoplasma, Bartonella, and chlamydia infections, all of which were undiagnosed.

To complicate matters even further, environmental factors such as heavy metals may also affect whether bacterial organisms cause joint pain. Mercury has been linked in the scientific literature to many autoimmune conditions, and heavy metal exposure reverses genetic resistance to chlamydia-induced arthritis. Other environmental factors such as small particle pollution have also recently been linked to juvenile idiopathic arthritis (JIA) and adult rheumatoid arthritis. Researchers published in *Pediatric Rheumatology* that they found a significant association with high levels of pollution before arthritis onset and linked it to increased production of inflammatory molecules, like IL-6. Environmental toxins and heavy metals drive oxidative stress and inflammation and increase the production of inflammatory cytokines, the specific molecules causing pain, inflammation, and "sickness syndrome" in autoimmune diseases. This may explain the improvement in joint pain in certain patients following detoxification and chelation therapy when heavy metal burdens have been removed from the body.

Other factors in Lyme-MSIDS that may be responsible for autoimmune symptoms are blebs, DNA particles that are shed from *Borrelia burgdorferi*. These blebs can cause an overstimulated immune system to produce antibodies that mimic lupus or RA. Also, our immune system's antibodies go after cells containing blebs, and kill off those host cells, instead of targeting and killing *Borrelia burgdorferi*. The blebs divert the infected host's immunological defenses.

Patients with chronic bacterial and viral infections may have other mechanisms responsible for autoimmune responses, including molecular mimicry (where our immune system cannot differentiate between our own antigens and foreign antigens), as well as intracellular bacteria releasing cell fragments and vesicles with bacterial antigens into the surrounding environment increasing inflammation. Borrelia can also affect the immune system by killing lymphocytes called B-cells (which are essential for our proper immune functioning), and when borrelia exits the lymphocyte it can surround itself with lymphocytic proteins, cloaking itself from the immune system, another mechanism that allows it to persist in the host. This highly evolved defense mechanism helps explain why many patients who have been diagnosed with rheumatoid arthritis, lupus, and multiple sclerosis may not, in fact, have a "true" autoimmune disorder. Instead, they may have an immune system overstimulated by Lyme disease, Mycoplasma and other intracellular co-infections, and exacerbated by exposure to heavy metals and environmental toxins, which further increase inflammation and cytokine production.

Your primary care physician should be able to differentiate between true lupus, true rheumatoid arthritis, and Lyme that is mimicking an autoimmune disease. Have your primary care physician send off blood work that includes a rheumatoid factor (RA), CCP, ANA, and double-stranded DNA (dsDNA), and if either the CCP or the dsDNA return positive, it implies that you may have a true autoimmune disease. The next step would be to find a Lyme-literate rheumatologist.

DO I HAVE LUPUS, RHEUMATOID ARTHRITIS, AND/OR LYME DISEASE?

Lupus is one of the most common autoimmune diseases in the United States, affecting women three times more frequently than men. It is characterized by inflammation in many different organs of the body, including the skin, joints, central nervous system, heart, lungs, and kidneys. Individuals with lupus often present with a constellation of many of the following symptoms: fevers, fatigue, skin rashes with sun sensitivity, hair loss, anemia, arthritis, and inflammation in the heart (pericarditis), lungs (pleurisy), arteries (vasculitis), kidneys (nephritis), and brain (cerebritis).

These symptoms can look remarkably similar to many of those seen in unresolved Lyme disease. Often patients come in with these symptoms and have blood tests that show the presence of a number of antibodies against antigens in the nucleus of the cell, cytoplasm of the cell (the gel-like substance inside the cell membrane containing all of its metabolic structures), and cell membranes.

One way to differentiate between Lyme and lupus, however, is to use the double-stranded DNA test (dsDNA), which is 98 percent specific and sensitive for systemic lupus erythematosus. This is part of the diagnostic criteria established by the American Rheumatological Society.

Rheumatoid arthritis can also look like Lyme disease. Like lupus, it is a chronic systemic inflammatory disease that primarily affects the joints, but it also may involve inflammation in tendons, ligaments, muscle, bone, and various organs in the body. To establish a diagnosis of RA, the joint score (counting and mapping the joints involved at each visit), the presence of synovitis (inflammation in the synovial membrane surrounding the joints), and the physical exam (range of motion, presence of increased fluid in the joints, nodules, and deviations in the joints) are the focus of the criteria. We can get signs of inflammation in both diseases (including positive ANAs and rheumatoid factors), but the presence of positive anti-CCP antibodies differentiates it from Lyme disease and is a more specific marker for true rheumatoid arthritis. Also in RA, there is a symmetric inflammatory polyarthritis (the joint pain is on both sides of the body), whereas in Lyme disease, the joint and muscle pain is often asymmetric and frequently migrates around the body, clinically differentiating it from true RA. Remember that both diseases are possible in the same patient, as no one is immune to getting a tick bite!

Rheumatoid arthritis, lupus, and Lyme disease may all respond to similar treatment regimens. The antirheumatic drug Plaquenil is effective not only in lupus and rheumatoid arthritis but also in Lyme disease, because it modulates an overstimulated immune system, helps increase the effectiveness of intracellular antibiotics, while simultaneously killing cystic forms of borrelia.

DO I HAVE MS OR LYME?

Multiple sclerosis (MS) is a disorder defined by a constellation of symptoms and associated demyelination of nerves—the loss of the myelin sheath surrounding nerves that is essential for proper conduction of electrical impulses—especially of the central nervous system and spinal cord. It can affect the brain, causing white-matter lesions to be visible on an MRI, as well as the optic nerve (leading to varying degrees of visual loss), and it can affect the spinal cord, causing numbness, weakness, and tingling of the extremities as well as urinary difficulties. Other clinical symptoms include difficulty walking, with incoordination, dizziness, hearing loss, difficulties with speech, and pain in varied nerves of the body. It often presents with symptoms that tend to come and go (the remitting/relapsing form of the disease), especially early in its course, and clinically it can be indistinguishable in certain cases from Lyme-MSIDS. In fact, some epidemiological studies suggest an infection may be behind MS (prior scientific studies have shown a link with *Chlamydia pneumonia* and Lyme disease, with newer studies also linking it to Epstein-Barr variants), as new outbreaks have occurred in parts of the world only after Westerners arrived. This was the case when the British troops arrived in the Faroe Islands during World War II, where it was not until years after their arrival that the first cases of MS appeared. Genetic and environmental factors have also been suggested to play a role, as MS is more common farther from the equator. Some have hypothesized that it may be related to a Vitamin D deficiency.

Multiple sclerosis is a clinical diagnosis, as is Lyme disease, and there is no available blood test for it. MS is suspected if there is an MRI of the brain and/or spinal cord with multiple demyelinating lesions, changes in nerve conduction of the eye (as tested by a visual evoked potential, or VEP), and ear (auditory evoked potential, or AEP), with an associated increase in certain markers of the spinal fluid (myelin basic protein, or MBP, and oligoclonal bands). Some of these changes can also be seen in persistent Lyme disease, so it is often a diagnosis of exclusion, when other diseases have been ruled out. Demyelination on a cervical or thoracic MRI, however, is more specific for MS.

Patients with MS often complain of intermittent tingling and numbness in different parts of their bodies, and MRIs of their brains can show varying amounts of white spots. Both of these symptoms and findings are seen in Lyme disease and MS, and since some patients have negative serum Lyme ELISAs, they are often told by neurologists that they have MS and are given an ABC regimen (Avonex, Betaseron, or Copaxone), Rebif, or Rituxan. If these drugs don't help, patients are told that they must have a "relapsing remitting" form of the disease, in which the symptoms come and go, or a chronic, progressive form, and are told to remain on these drugs to stabilize their symptoms. However, just as with the patients diagnosed with lupus or RA, the drugs may not help relieve their symptoms, or even if they do, we may be treating symptoms and not getting to the true, underlying cause(s) of the disease process.

Multiple authors in the medical literature propose that MS is most likely caused by an infection with *Borrelia burgdorferi*, the agent of Lyme disease. There are at least five reasons for the hypothesis that Lyme is the basis for some cases of MS:

1. Spirochetes have been documented in MS pathology specimens.
2. Spirochetal flagellin (the tail of *Borrelia burgdorferi* that allows it to move through the body) is immunologically very similar to human myelin.
3. The demyelination process in MS and Lyme is also similar; they both can cause inflammation in the eye and in the spinal cord, leading to a loss of vision and difficulty walking.
4. If physicians were to do a spinal tap trying to differentiate multiple sclerosis from neurological Lyme disease, they would find

extremely similar results. As with multiple sclerosis, central nervous system infection with *B. burgdorferi* can cause an increased protein synthesis with IgG antibodies, lymphocytic pleocytosis (increased lymphocytes in the spinal fluid), increased protein, increased plasma cells, and oligoclonal bands. Lyme that affects the central nervous system can produce both oligoclonal bands that react with *Borrelia burgdorferi* and ones that do not.

5. We find some of the cystic structures of Lyme disease in the central nervous system of patients with MS. Perhaps certain environmental factors (e.g., low Vitamin D) or co-infections with other organisms, such as chlamydia, are responsible for borrelia coming out of hiding and reactivating cystic forms, driving demyelination and MS-type symptoms. Dr. Alan MacDonald also recently found nematode filarial worms in the spinal fluid of MS patients at autopsy, possibly contributing to demyelination. The significance is unknown, but Ixodes and Amblyomma ticks were recently discovered to contain filarial worms.

The image on the following page is a photo of a larval worm/filarial nematodes found in the cerebral spinal fluid (CSF) of a patient with MS.

The lack of a reliable blood test, and the overlapping of symptoms between the two diseases, would explain the frequent number of patients who have been diagnosed with MS when, in fact, they had Lyme-MSIDS. I have seen many patients with a previous diagnosis of MS who have failed to improve on commonly prescribed MS drugs (the ABC prescription regimen), and Rebif; it was then determined that Lyme-MSIDS was responsible for their demyelination and subsequent fatigue, optic neuritis, tingling, numbness, and difficulty walking.

However, the primary difference between the two diseases seems to be that with MS there were more white-matter lesions on an MRI and higher amounts of myelin basic protein and oligoclonal bands present on the spinal tap. Moreover, Lyme disease did not usually cause demyelinating lesions in the cervical or thoracic spine.

Some patients also have genetic predispositions for autoimmune diseases. For example, the genes expressed as HLA DR 2 and 4, as well as the HLA B 27 chromosomal markers, can predispose certain patients to develop an autoimmune disorder. Dr. Alan Steere has demonstrated that Lyme

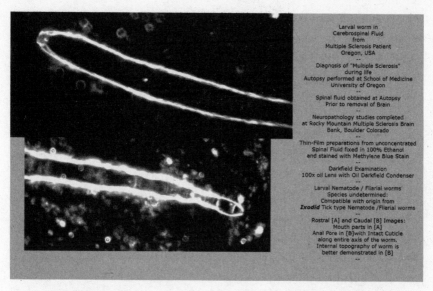

Larval worm in
Cerebrospinal Fluid
from
Multiple Sclerosis Patient
Oregon, USA
--
Diagnosis of "Multiple Sclerosis"
during life
Autopsy performed at School of Medicine
University of Oregon
--
Spinal fluid obtained at Autopsy
Prior to removal of Brain
--
Neuropathology studies completed
at Rocky Mountain Multiple Sclerosis Brain
Bank, Boulder Colorado
--
Thin-Film preparations from unconcentrated
Spinal Fluid fixed in 100% Ethanol
and stained with Methylene Blue Stain
--
Darkfield Examination
100x oil Lens with Oil Darkfield Condenser
--
Larval Nematode / Filarial worms
Species undetermined:
Compatible with origin from
Ixodid Tick type Nematode /Filarial worms
--
Rostral [A] and Caudal [B] Images:
Mouth parts in [A]
Anal Pore in [B]with Intact Cuticle
along entire axis of the worm.
Internal topography of worm is
better demonstrated in [B]
--

LARVAL NEMATODES AND FILARIAL WORMS. *Photo courtesy of Dr. Alan MacDonald, private collection (2016).*

disease patients who test positive for HLA DR4 have more severe autoimmune rheumatological manifestations, and in 2014, researchers identified a specific protein called FSTL-1 (Follistatin-like protein-1), which is an immune modulator induced by an infection with *Borrelia burgdorferi* with an established role in autoimmune arthritis. Infections and autoimmune manifestations are clearly linked in some patients.

As stated earlier, some patients who are genetically predisposed to autoimmune diseases will automatically try to kill off borrelia spirochetes by targeting the flagellar (tail) proteins that are biochemically similar to myelin sheaths. This causes their immune system to attack the myelin sheaths surrounding their nerves as well, leading to demyelination, the process that is the hallmark of MS. Their immune systems are unable to differentiate between the flagellar protein of borrelia and their myelin sheaths. Since up to 70 percent of Lyme patients with unresolved symptoms can have demyelination with associated peripheral neuropathy, it would appear that this process is another common denominator in the two diseases. This is further complicated by other factors on the MSIDS map increasing demyelination and neuropathy, such as other infections (Bartonella), heavy metals (mercury, lead, arsenic), other environmental toxins, vitamin and immune deficiencies, and mitochondrial dysfunction. Searching for multiple overlapping factors driving demyelination is important if we are to get to all of the underlying causes of nerve dysfunction.

Prior scientific studies showed a possible link with bacteria like borrelia, *Chlamydia pneumonia,* and viruses like HHV-6, and recently published research in the journal *Neurology* found that Epstein-Barr virus genetic variants are also associated with multiple sclerosis. We are discovering that multiple infections and environmental factors are responsible for autoimmune manifestations. The scientific literature has recently shown that there are at least six separate etiologies that can independently and together increase autoimmune reactions, including underlying genetic predispositions, bacterial infections, viruses, toxins, hormonal dysregulation (in lupus and RA, estrogen levels can accelerate and androgens, such as DHEA, can inhibit the development of the disease), as well as dysbiosis (an imbalance) of the bacteria within the microbiome of our gut. Two studies released in 2014 link toxins to autoimmune reactions. An endocrine disruptor that affects the mitochondrial function of our cells by disrupting one of the liver's detoxification pathways (BPA) was found in 2014 to provoke autoimmune (AI) reactions, causing molecular mimicry, the same phenomenon seen in infections with borrelia species. Many of us have been exposed to Bisphenol A by drinking out of plastic bottles as well as eating canned goods. Fine-particle pollution, called "nanoparticles," which include cigarette smoke, air pollutants, and asbestos particles, are also being reported to cause autoimmune reactions. These have now been shown to be strong environmental risk factors for RA, JIA, lupus, and scleroderma (an autoimmune skin disease). Their effect may go beyond our generation and be passed onto future generations, as they have also been shown to affect our genetic structure (epigenetic effects).

TREATING GENERAL IMMUNE DYSFUNCTION

Apart from doing our best to address the six factors listed above that affect immune functioning, there are medications and nutritional supplements that may help your immune system to function better. We regularly use drugs like Plaquenil to modulate an overstimulated immune system, except in patients with psoriasis and retinal problems, when it is contraindicated. Low-dose naltrexone (LDN) may also be useful in helping to decrease inflammation. It is published as a useful adjunct in several auto-immune diseases like MS and Crohn's disease, and it has been shown to decrease inflammatory cytokine production, blocking IL-6, IL-12, TNF-alpha, and NFKappa-B. Using natural immune modulators like transfer factors (from colostrum) and 3-6 beta glucan (a potent mushroom de-rivative) may also be helpful in some individuals with low natural-killer cells, T cells, and poor immune function. Since certain bacteria in the GI tract like Prevotella and Clostridium species have also recently been linked to autoimmune diseases like MS and rheumatoid arthritis, it is possible that one day we will be addressing autoimmune diseases by ma-nipulating the microbiome of the gut by introducing anti-inflammatory bacteria, like certain acidophilus and Bifidobacterium, as well as Bac-teroides species.

The study of epigenetics has now demonstrated that nutrients, apart from treating infections, balancing the microbiome, decreasing exposure to environmental chemicals, and increasing our detoxification, have a long-term influence on disease and what genetic characteristics are expressed, and that chronic disease is related to the interaction between our gene-tic inheritance and lifestyle/environmental factors. This allows us the possibility to also use diet, nutrition, and exercise as a means to address chronic illness.

Nutritional substances that have an effect on our epigenetics are compounds found in fruits and vegetables. Many of the colorful com-pounds found in a variety of fruits and vegetables contain important an-tioxidants and phytochemicals. The phytochemicals that have been found to have an epigenetic effect include broccoli compounds such as sulfora-phane (broccoli seed extract, glucoraphanin), the red wine/grape extract resveratrol, curcumin (turmeric), EGCG from green tea, hops, and genis-tein from soy. These nutrients and phytochemicals literally "talk" to our genes and help to affect our epigenetics in a positive way. Infections as well as toxins may both contribute to autoimmune diseases and demye-lination in patients with Lyme disease and co-infections. We need to pay attention to not only addressing the infections, but also detoxifying the chemicals, and using diet, nutrition, and exercise as modulating factors in the disease process.

The inflammatory response caused by these different factors often overlaps, increasing the severity of symptoms, which can be made worse by other factors increasing inflammation, including an improper diet (eating sensitive/allergic foods, gluten), imbalances in the microbiome, lack of sleep (which increases IL-6, an inflammatory cytokine), and mineral deficiencies (like zinc, needed for proper immune function). A comprehensive health plan should address all of these factors on the MSIDS map, which will help you to get well and stay healthy.

BRAD HAD LYME, RHEUMATOID ARTHRITIS, AND "BAGELS DISEASE"

Brad was a thirty-year-old white male from New Jersey with a past medical history significant for eczema and rheumatoid arthritis. He was diagnosed with a torn meniscus on an MRI when he experienced a sudden swelling of his right knee. Afterward, he was fine for two years until a stressful event led to another tear. During the repair his doctors sent off the synovial tissue for examination, which was found to have a significant amount of inflammation, with elevated numbers of lymphocytes. He was sent to a rheumatologist who diagnosed him with rheumatoid arthritis with elevated markers of inflammation (RF+, CCP+, and elevated CRPs and ESRs).

Soon after this diagnosis Brad started taking the classical drugs for RA. The first was methotrexate for several months, but he felt worse. Then they tried anti-inflammatory medication (Meloxicam) with Enbrel for six months, followed by another immunomodulatory medication, Cimzia, for eight months, which didn't help, and then Humira for four months. Nothing helped his severe pain except methylprednisolone at 16 mg twice a day (high doses of steroids that are immunosuppressive), but every time he tried to lower the doses of steroids, he felt worse.

A second doctor diagnosed him clinically with Lyme, started him on doxycycline, and took him off his steroids. The doxycycline didn't help, and one month later his symptoms off steroids were much worse, with increasing fevers, chills, drenching night sweats, and debilitating fatigue, with severe pain in his knees, feet, and calves. He required high doses of oxycodone, OxyContin, and Percocet to even make a dent in the pain, and was placed on Arava with Humira to try and control the pain and inflammation.

When I saw Brad in my medical office, his chief complaints were severe fatigue in the morning (requiring going back on prednisone), drenching night sweats for the past few months, decreased libido, poor sleep even with taking Klonopin (a valium derivative), and diarrhea several times a week. His rheumatoid symptoms included bilateral knee pain and swelling, with migratory pain between the knees and tightness of his calves and feet. He was moody and irritable with some depression and anxiety. He lived in a highly Lyme-endemic area and told me that he had taken hundreds of ticks off his dog, though he denied ever seeing an engorged tick on him or experiencing a bulls-eye rash.

An extensive medical history did not reveal anything beyond the above symptoms. His rheumatological examination showed swollen knees with fluid, with a minimal decrease in range of motion, but without redness (erythema) or heat. The answers to Brad's problems were found, however, in the lab work, which showed multiple abnormalities: severe inflammation with very high C-reactive protein (CRP) values, ranging between 14.2 and 64.8 (normal less than 3); a positive human leukocyte antigen (HLA) DR 4 marker, with negative antinuclear antibodies (ANAs) and rheumatoid factors (RFs); a negative dsDNA and normal complement studies; but an elevated cyclic citrullinated peptide (CCP) that varied between 117 and 229 (normal less than 19), which is a specific marker of RA. He also had an elevated MMP-9 at 1272 (a marker of joint inflammation, normal levels less than 984), abnormal hormones with a low DHEA at 46 (normal between 160 and 449 ug/dl), low testosterone at 6.6 ng/dl (normal between 30 and 85), low salivary cortisol levels on an adrenal test, and low Vitamin D levels. Recent studies show that a low Vitamin D level may also be a marker of inflammation, secondary to intracellular bacteria.

His infectious panel revealed positive exposure to Epstein-Barr virus, positive Mycoplasma and *Chlamydia pneumonia* titers, and Lyme testing with a negative ELISA, but a Western blot showing evidence of reactivity at the 31, 34, and 39 kdA bands (which is specific for exposure to *Borrelia burgdorferi*). Babesia testing was negative, despite the history of drenching night sweats, and other possible etiologies for night sweats (TB, non-Hodgkin's lymphoma, Brucella, hyperthyroidism, and panic disorders) were negative. He was on immunosuppressive drugs for his RA, so a workup to exclude TB or a malignancy was important in his case. A food allergy panel showed multiple allergies and was suggestive of leaky gut.

He was especially allergic to wheat (antigliadin positive, TTG negative), barley, beef, egg whites, and coffee (poor guy, that would be enough to make me moody). Heavy metal testing showed elevated levels of mercury at 85 (normal less than 3), elevated lead at 47 (normal less than 2) with elevated thallium levels. Immunoglobulin levels were normal (IgA, IgM, IgG) with one IgG subclass deficiency (not clinically significant).

Based on the history of living in a Lyme-endemic area with hundreds of ticks on his dog, migratory joint pain, and borrelia-specific bands on a Western blot, I suspected Lyme. Despite a negative Babesia titer, the drenching sweats suggested a malaria-like organism like Babesia was present, as other etiologies had been ruled out. Adrenal suppression due to long-term use of steroids (which would be dangerous for infections with Lyme and Babesia), combined with low testosterone, could be contributing to his fatigue. We sent him for a DEXA scan to be sure there were no early signs of osteoporosis and, fortunately, the test was negative.

We started him on Omnicef, Plaquenil, Zithromax, nystatin, Serrapeptase, and Malarone, to cover cell-wall, cystic, intracellular, and biofilm forms of borrelia, along with a regimen against Babesia, and a low-carb diet with triple probiotics for GI support (over 300 billion live organisms). We added inflammatory and detox support with NAC, alpha-lipoic acid, liposomal glutathione, and high-dose curcumin (greater than 4 grams/day); GI support with his history of occasional diarrhea (Opticleanse GHI, with glutamine and herbs for GI and hepatic support); as well as hormonal support including DHEA, mung bean extract (Testoplex) to increase free testosterone (mung bean helps displace testosterone from sex-hormone-binding globulin [SHBG], where it is tightly bound), and K2D3 for low Vitamin D.

Brad returned the next month. He was feeling a little better. The glutathione helped him with his resistant pain, but he still had a lot of sweats and joint discomfort. We changed his methylprednisolone to hydrocortisone (a bioidentical hormone that is less immunosuppressive), with the aim of eventually tapering him off high-dose steroids, which interfere with Lyme and Babesia treatment. Over several months we managed to slowly taper him off steroids, and his PCP and I worked on dropping down the doses of his narcotics. Due to the severity of his pain and occasional GI symptoms, we changed his Omnicef to Bicillin shots, and added minocycline to the Zithromax for double intracellular coverage (and minocycline/Plaquenil are also part of a disease-modifying antirheumatic drug (DMARD) regimen for RA). This immediately decreased his fatigue and pain, and his stools were better.

The only time the pain significantly increased was on Sundays. Brad liked bagels, and each time he went off his gluten-free diet his knees swelled up to twice their size, with increased pain. It took two days before his knees returned to their baseline size. He also noticed that when he stayed up late and didn't get adequate sleep, all of his symptoms were worse. We added Valerian root and melatonin with small doses of trazadone at bedtime for his insomnia/anxiety, which helped with sleep.

Over time, we tapered him off his Humira and Arava, and got him completely off his prednisone and narcotics. He also was eventually able to taper off hydrocortisone with herbal adaptogenic adrenal support (ginseng, rhodiola, B vitamins, and ashwagandha). His inflammatory markers came down to normal range, and his knees were less than half their size before treatment, but he still had evidence of an active synovitis in his knees and his CCP remained elevated (229). I started him back on methotrexate and sent him back to the rheumatologist, while remaining on Plaquenil and Minocin as a DMARD regimen. His rheumatoid arthritis regimen finally worked once his tick-borne diseases and food sensitivities were properly treated. His synovitis had now resolved (he was almost ready to go for surgery since he couldn't walk on occasion secondary to swollen knees) and he no longer required OxyContin for breakthrough pain once the Lyme and Babesia were adequately treated with detox/inflammatory support. The dietary issues were, however, the last key in his full recovery. The regimen only worked well when he was off sugar as well as gluten. Although he didn't have celiac disease, it was clear he had Bagels Disease.

EIGHT

Lyme and Inflammation

We are seeing a significant number of chronic diseases in the 21st century. These include rising rates of Lyme disease and other tick-borne illnesses, as well as many individuals being diagnosed with cancer, allergies, asthma, ADHD, autism, and neurological diseases like Lou Gehrig's disease (ALS), Parkinson's, and Alzheimer's disease. We usually think of these as being separate illnesses, but there are several common underlying causes and biochemical mechanisms that can explain these varied illnesses. These mechanisms underlie many of the points on the MSIDS model and can be summed up in three connective phrases: free radicals, oxidative stress, and inflammation. Identifying all of the causes of inflammation, and controlling them, is Rule 2 in the MSIDS Action Plan.

Free radicals are atoms and molecules with unpaired electrons. They play an important role in many biochemical reactions in the body, and although they are essential to life, too many can be damaging. We naturally produce free radicals during reactions that take place inside our cells, where oxygen is used to create energy.

Oxidative stress refers to the production of these free radicals. Oxidative stress has been shown to be an important factor in many diseases. In fact, the number one biological mechanism that seems to underlie most chronic disease states is oxidative stress: When there are too many free radicals, oxidative stress occurs, and it leads to inflammation. This process has been shown to be the common denominator underlying premature aging and chronic disease, so if we want to get healthy and stay healthy, we need to control the inflammatory process in our body.

Inflammation is a type of "fire" in the body, and it is characterized by the simultaneous destruction and healing of various tissues and organs. It is identified by five cardinal signs: heat, redness, pain, swelling, and loss of function. Inflammation can occur anywhere in the body—inside or outside. You may have recognized external inflammation that surrounds a cut or a bruise. Internally, inflammation can take many forms, from a headache to nasal congestion to arthritis to heart disease. Any of the disease states that you may have heard of that end in "itis" are forms of inflammation.

Inflammation can be classified as either acute or chronic; with MSIDS we are generally dealing more with the chronic type, except in the case of early Lyme disease and acute exposure to other co-infections. My patients, most of whom have been sick for years, are often suffering from chronic inflammation. The major cells involved in this process are immune cells called "mononuclear cells," which include monocytes that can differentiate into macrophages, lymphocytes, plasma cells, and fibroblasts. These cells produce inflammatory chemicals at the site of injury known as cytokines, such as interferon gamma (IFN-γ), TNF-alpha, interleukin-1 (IL-1), and interleukin-6 (IL-6), as well as various growth factors and enzymes. A subset of cytokines called chemokines are also produced during the inflammatory process, such as the chemokines CXCL9, CXCL10, and CCL19 seen in Lyme disease. These are important signaling molecules that direct the immune cells to the sites of tissue injury. Other inflammatory molecules such as leukotrienes, prostaglandins, and histamine can also be produced once there is cellular activation by sensitized immune cells, such as eosinophils and basophils. This activation further increases inflammation, pain, swelling, and smooth-muscle contraction. Without the proper treatment these cells and their inflammatory products can cause inflammation that lasts for months or years.

When we look at the impacts of free radicals and oxidative stress on multiple organs of the body, we find a broad range of deleterious effects. When free radicals and subsequent inflammation attack the arteries, this can damage the blood vessels and increase atherosclerosis, with oxidized LDL cholesterol eventually leading to heart attacks. Free radicals and subsequent inflammation can also affect the brain and lead to strokes, epilepsy, Parkinson's, or Alzheimer's disease; cataracts and/or macular degeneration; dermatitis, psoriasis, and/or scleroderma of the skin. When it affects the lungs it can worsen asthma or cystic fibrosis, and free radicals and oxidative stress have also been linked to diabetes, aging, and cancer as well as a variety of inflammatory joint diseases, including rheumatoid arthritis.

Persistent inflammation can be due to multiple causes found on the MSIDS map, especially chronic bacterial, viral, parasitic, and fungal infections as well as the type of autoimmune reactions we discussed in the previous chapter. Other important causes include eating allergic or sensitive foods with or without leaky gut, having dysbiosis (i.e., the wrong types of bacteria in our GI tract); having high loads of environmental toxins like heavy metals, mold, and pesticides without the ability to adequately detoxify them; not getting adequate quality sleep; and/or having nutritional deficiencies in minerals like zinc and copper, which are necessary to control free radicals and inflammation. In these circumstances, overlapping multifactorial etiologies increase inflammation and turn on a switch inside the nucleus of cells called NF-KappaB, leading to the production of more inflammatory cytokines. This inflammation and oxidative stress can damage fragile mitochondria, the powerhouse of the cell (causing fatigue and adversely affecting nerve and cardiac function), lead to an imbalance of hormones, and cause a phenomenon known as the "sickness syndrome."

A good example of sickness syndrome is when someone comes down with the flu. The person may complain of fever, fatigue, joint and muscle aches, nausea, mood changes, feeling foggy, and wanting to stay in bed and sleep for long periods. These symptoms are a protective mechanism that is the result of the production of these inflammatory molecules. The same cytokines that are produced during the flu also occur in rheumatoid arthritis, causing joint pain, and they are the causes of muscle aches and pains in fibromyalgia and chronic fatigue syndrome, the brain fog associated with Alzheimer's disease, and the majority of the chronic symptoms we see in Lyme disease. Ordinarily, sickness syndrome forces the individual to stay out of harm's way at a time when the body's resources are needed to fight off the infection. The medical literature contains extensive evidence on the occurrence of sickness syndrome and how it is linked to a variety of disease processes, including major depression, congestive heart failure, anxiety, pain syndromes, and sleep disorders.

If you are complaining of fatigue, muscle and joint pain, an increase in neuropathic pain, headaches, flulike symptoms, difficulty sleeping, mood swings, and cognitive difficulties such as brain fog, you are describing manifestations of a dramatic increase in cytokine production and inflammatory molecules in the body—a kind of inflammation gone wild. The most dramatic example of a severe case of sickness syndrome is a Jarisch-Herxheimer reaction. Killing off borrelia causes a sudden release of these cytokines, leading to a dramatic increase in symptoms. Herxheimer reactions are caused by the release of inflammatory molecules, and we need to find ways to shut down the production of these cytokines that increase inflammation. One way to control inflammation is to activate a molecule found inside of our cells, called Nrf2. When we have oxidative stress and inflammation, Nrf2 goes inside the nucleus of our cells to turn on specialized genes called antioxidant response element (ARE) genes. These enhance detoxification, decrease inflammation, and even help inhibit cancer growth. Eating lots of cruciferous vegetables, as well as brightly colored fruits and vegetables, provides detoxifying phytochemicals that lower inflammation and activate Nrf2. Supplements that are effective in activating Nrf2 include broccoli seed extract (sulforaphane), resveratrol, green tea (EGCG), and the spice turmeric (curcumin).

INFLAMMATION AND THE BRAIN

Inflammation underlies the symptoms in many neurological diseases. In a study published in 2007 in *Lancet Neurology*, researchers reported that the neurological syndromes associated with *Borrelia burgdorferi* are also associated with inflammation in the central nervous system, in particular, amyloid metabolism. Amyloids are proteins that aggregate and change the structure of cells, damaging them. They are found in many diseases, including type 2 diabetes; autoimmune phenomenon, such as rheumatoid arthritis; and neurodegenerative diseases, such as Alzheimer's, Huntington's, and Parkinson's disease. In 2016, researchers at the Drexel University School of Medicine found that biofilms containing borrelia co-localized with the β amyloid plaques in Alzheimer's disease, possibly influencing the destruction of brain tissue.

Amyloid is just one of several neurotoxins: substances that can damage or kill off the brain's neurons that are produced by inflammation and can alter the normal activity of the cells of the central nervous system. Lyme can cause the production of internal neurotoxins like quinolinic acid, and deficiencies in minerals like zinc can cause the production of a chemical called chloral hydrate, also contributing to neurocognitive difficulties. There are also external neurotoxins, the most common being heavy metals and environmental toxins, like mold, pesticides, and volatile organic solvents. In fact, inflammatory processes caused by infections and toxins are involved in many chronic neurological diseases apart from Lyme disease. One of them is the most prevalent and feared neurodegenerative disease of our time, Alzheimer's disease. Neurotoxins and inflammation both can alter the normal activity of the nervous system in such a way as to cause damage to nervous tissue. Neurotoxicity can result from chronic infections; exposure to substances used in chemotherapy, radiation treatment, drug therapies, certain drug abuse, and organ transplants; heavy metals, certain foods and food additives, pesticides, industrial and/or cleaning solvents, and cosmetics; and to some naturally occurring substances. Symptoms may appear immediately after exposure or be delayed. They may include limb weakness or numbness; loss of memory, vision, and/or intellect; uncontrollable obsessive and/or compulsive behaviors; delusions, headache, cognitive and behavioral problems; and sexual dysfunction. Individuals with certain disorders may be especially vulnerable to neurotoxins.

Lyme disease patients, like Alzheimer's patients, often complain of neurocognitive deficits in memory and concentration and difficulties with executive functioning (decision making, for example). Recent studies have reported increased TNF-α levels in the cerebral spinal fluid of AD patients, just as in Lyme disease, and a single genetic change in the TNF-α gene is associated with earlier onset AD. A fascinating study was done on Alzheimer's patients in which the investigators found that inhibiting cytokine production positively affected memory. This may explain why certain patients, who had been previously diagnosed with chronic fatigue syndrome, fibromyalgia, autoimmune diseases, neurological diseases such as Alzheimer's, and psychiatric diseases, find that they feel remarkably better once we have treated their Lyme-MSIDS. By addressing multifactorial causes of inflammation on the MSIDS map, we are treating the underlying biochemical mechanisms causing clinical symptoms.

LYME DISEASE CAUSES INFLAMMATION

Lyme disease can cause significant inflammation in the peripheral and central nervous systems, depending on the specific species of borrelia. For example, *Borrelia burgdorferi* spirochetes express specific lipoproteins— structural complexes of both proteins and fats on the outside of the organism—that can stimulate the immune system and increase inflammation. More than 8 percent of the coding sequence of a common strain of borrelia, strain B31, is devoted to lipoprotein sequences, which attract neutrophils, one of the first immune cells to migrate toward the site of the inflammation. These lipoproteins then stimulate these neutrophils and macrophages (other cells of the immune system that also engulf and digest pathogens and produce inflammatory cytokines). A 1994 study, published in the journal *Infection and Immunity*, reported that borrelia are so powerful that they can cause a much stronger inflammatory response than common bacteria that produce cytokines (like *E. coli*), one that is fifty to five hundred times stronger. This explains in part the extremely strong inflammatory response that some patients can have when exposed to the bacteria that causes Lyme disease. We also now know that there are more virulent strains of the bacteria, which can contribute to more severe symptoms. In the United States we have *B. burgdorferi* infection, which leads to greater inflammatory responses than *B. afzelii* or *B. garinii* infection in Europe, and researchers at Harvard in 2014 identified three *B. burgdorferi* genotypes (substrains of outer surface protein C), called RST-1, RST-2, and RST-3 (accounting for 35, 45, and 20 percent of strains respectively), which lead to different inflammatory responses. This is a genetic variation in the bacteria, which is different from our underlying human leukocyte antigen (HLA) genetic disposition (HLA DR 2 and 4 cause more severe arthritis), influencing the severity of the inflammatory response. Patients who have been infected with the RST-1 strain of borrelia had greater levels of the chemokines CXCL9, CXCL10, and interferon gamma, with an increased severity of arthritis.

Apart from differences in strains, there are also differences in how our immune system responds to the infection. About half of the population in the United States and Europe have a genetic variation, called a SNP (single nucleotide polymorphism), on a receptor on the outside of our T cells that fights infection, which results in higher cytokine and chemo-kine levels with an EM rash. These genetic variations explain in part why some people develop more severe symptoms with antibiotic refractory arthritis.

The effects of proinflammatory cytokines and the symptoms that they produce also depend on whether they act in the central nervous system or peripheral nervous system, as well as on the patient's current health status and genetic predisposition. If cytokines act in the peripheral nervous sys-tem (PNS), they can cause pain and inflammation in the peripheral nerves. A study published in 2005 showed that molecular mimicry can occur in the PNS, with borrelia-specific IgM antibodies reacting against the flagel-lar tail of the organism and cross-reacting with antigens on peripheral nerves, causing neuropathy. This explains the overlap in neurological symp-toms caused by demyelination in both MS and persistent Lyme disease.

Cytokine activity can also take place in the central nervous system, accompanying demyelination (which is seen as "white spots" or "un-identified bright objects" on a brain MRI). It accounts for many of the neurological symptoms we see in Lyme disease, including headaches, sleep disorders, mood swings, memory and concentration problems, and neuralgia/nerve pain. One type of cytokine, known as TNF-alpha, has a principal role in initiating the activation of other cytokines and growth factors in the inflammatory response, causing pain. A 2004 study of the peripheral nervous system found that cytokines induced by TNF-alpha such as interleukin 1-β can cause the secondary production of other in-flammatory molecules, such as nitric oxide, bradykinin, and/or prosta-glandins (chemical messengers that regulate pain, inflammation, and smooth-muscle contraction). When combined together, these inflam-matory cytokines can have a direct effect on the sensory nerves that al-low people to feel pain, pressure, vibration, heat, and cold. Lyme disease patients often complain of symptoms caused by the dysfunction of these sensory nerves: They feel that they are either too hot or too cold, or expe-rience numbness, tingling, or a significant increase in pain usually de-scribed as pinpricks or burning sensations.

Apart from borrelia being able to stimulate proinflammatory cyto-kines, remember that the MSIDS patient usually has multiple overlap-ping infections contributing to the varied symptoms of chronic illness. Mycoplasmal infections increase proinflammatory cytokines and have been found in the joint tissues of those with rheumatoid diseases; Bartonella can cause a host of inflammatory reactions, including arthritis, an encephalopathy and chronic demyelinating peripheral neuropathy (PNP), radiculitis, myelitis, vasculitis, and inflammatory ophthalmologic manifestations. Chlamydia causes reactive inflammatory arthritis. Brucella species have been found in the blood of patients with chronic fatigue syndrome (CFS/SEID), and frequent viruses found in MSIDS, such as Epstein-Barr, cytomegalovirus, and human herpesvirus-6, can cause inflammation. We know that with HHV-6 there is a link to CFS/SEID and fibromyalgia, which are syndromes that overlap with MSIDS.

Other common factors on the MSIDS map can also increase inflammation. I often find that food allergies, and/or sensitivities to foods and chemicals, can cause complex immune reactions in my patients, leading to not only allergic reactions and asthma, but also pain. Even mineral deficiencies can have a profound effect on inflammation. Magnesium is necessary in over three hundred detoxification reactions in the body, and low magnesium levels contribute to increased toxic loads and oxidative stress. You may have copper deficiency, and copper is necessary in superoxide dismutase (SOD), an enzyme essential for controlling free radicals. We also frequently find zinc deficiency in MSIDS patients, and this can lead to increased levels of inflammatory cytokines. In a National Institutes of Health–funded study, elderly patients with zinc deficiencies who were given zinc supplements had decreased incidences of infections, decreased levels of TNF-alpha, and decreased plasma oxidative stress markers. We therefore need to check both serum and red blood cell (RBC) levels of these nutrients, as oftentimes the serum levels are normal but the RBC levels inside the cells are low, indicating a severe deficiency. These are not tests routinely performed in a physician's office, but addressing food allergies/sensitivities, as well as mineral deficiencies, can significantly help control inflammation.

The Relationship Between Sleep and Inflammation

The MSIDS population generally does not sleep well. In fact, they have some of the most resistant and profound insomnia that I have ever witnessed. That is why many patients with Lyme-MSIDS are misdiagnosed with CFS and fibromyalgia, which are also syndromes associated with fatigue and poor sleep.

Sleep deprivation increases inflammation and the production of inflammatory cytokines, causing similar symptoms in these patient populations. Impaired sleep correlates directly with impaired immune functioning, and sleep disorders are commonly associated with chronic inflammatory diseases, such as rheumatoid arthritis, fibromyalgia (FM), and CFS/SEID. Chronic sleep restriction also leads to elevations in IL-6 and pain. Since we already see elevated levels of IL-6 in Lyme disease, sleep deprivation compounds the effects of the elevated level of this inflammatory cytokine.

The Gut and Inflammation

The GI microbiome also plays a role in immune dysregulation and inflammation, and has been linked to diseases as varied as RA, MS, inflammatory bowel disease, diabetes and insulin resistance, cardiovascular and respiratory disease, and even mental illness. One 2013 study found that people with rheumatoid arthritis were much more likely to have the bacteria *Prevotella* in their intestines. We are just discovering the importance of the microbiome in chronic disease.

Heavy Metals and Environmental Toxins Cause Inflammation

We are exposed to hundreds of environmental chemicals every day, and some of those, like plastics, small-particle pollutants, and heavy metals, can increase autoimmune manifestations and inflammation. I am finding mercury exposure in the majority of my patients, using a six-hour urine DMSA challenge. Heavy metals such as mercury increase oxidative stress, and it has been suggested that it causes a multiplicity of autoimmune disorders, including lupus. According to a 2006 article published in *Critical Reviews in Toxicology*, mercury can also cause an increased susceptibility to infections, not a desired effect in MSIDS, where patients often have multiple overlapping co-infections. By detoxifying the patient using chelating agents such as Dimercaptosuccinic acid (DMSA) and Ethylenediaminetetraacetic acid (EDTA), we can remove these metals, and some of our most difficult-to-treat patients find that their fatigue, muscle and joint pain, and cognitive difficulties improve as their heavy-metal burden and inflammation decreases.

HEAVY METALS AND MINERALS WERE AFFECTING STEVE'S HEALTH

Steve came to see me from the Midwest several years ago. He was a young man with a history of severe fatigue, joint pain, headaches, memory and concentration problems, drenching night sweats, and a complete loss of libido. He had seen multiple subspecialists, including eight different rheumatologists, who could not find a cause for his resistant symptoms, which included severe, unremitting joint pain throughout his body. His autoimmune markers were all negative, as was his Lyme ELISA test, even though he reported that he had been bitten by multiple ticks over the years, some of them engorged, remaining on him for days. Because the rheumatologists couldn't find a cause for his resistant pain, he was diagnosed with seronegative rheumatoid arthritis. He had been placed on rotations of high-dose prednisone, methotrexate, Enbrel, Arava, and other antirheumatic drugs over a three-year period. None of them helped his symptoms, and he continued to get worse over time. Eventually he became disabled at twenty-eight years old. He had also been seen by a pain specialist and was on morphine sulphate with oxycodone several times per day for breakthrough pain, yet he still complained of severe, unremitting pain throughout his body. He also had a history of severe kidney stones, and was treated with a high-dose diuretic, chlorthalidone.

My battery of tests painted a different picture. His Lyme Western blot and his Babesia tests were positive. He also tested positive for exposure to mercury and lead, and was severely deficient in testosterone, zinc, iodine, and magnesium. I wasn't surprised by this finding: The diuretics he was taking are known to decrease levels of key minerals in the body.

Once we addressed multiple overlapping factors on the MSIDS map increasing inflammation, and replaced his minerals, lowered his heavy-metal burden, and treated his Lyme, Babesia, and hormone deficiency, Steve felt better and returned to work for the first time in years. What's more, his sex drive increased to age-appropriate levels.

Hormone Production and Inflammation

The hypothalamic-pituitary-adrenal axis (HPA) is the master control center for all hormonal production throughout the body, and it can be affected by inflammation, whether due to Lyme disease or fibromyalgia

(FM). Cytokines can affect hormone levels positively and negatively. Research has shown that cortisol, an anti-inflammatory hormone, is able to shut down the production of cytokines in a healthy individual. However, in someone with Lyme disease and FM, although cortisol production increases, it becomes ineffective due to cortisol resistance, and the result is increased, uncontrolled inflammation. We'll cover hormonal changes in more detail in Chapter 12.

Treating Inflammation

Once we determine that an inflammatory process is present, a multifaceted approach works best, especially for patients with overlapping chronic fatigue syndrome or fibromyalgia who present with severe fatigue, headaches, cognitive dysfunction, neuralgia, myalgias, and arthritis.

- Properly treating Lyme disease and associated co-infections, and lowering the total load of organisms in the body, is essential in order to significantly decrease inflammation and control symptom flares. The antibiotics and herbal regimens discussed in Chapter 3 treat the pain that comes with Lyme disease, and usually the sickest patients will require a combined approach, using pharmaceuticals and nutraceuticals. Classical therapies include immune modulators (Plaquenil, DMARDs), drugs with anti-inflammatory effects (macrolides and tetracyclines), nonsteroidal anti-inflammatory drugs (NSAIDs) and COX-2 inhibitors, and intravenous immunoglobulin therapy (IVIG) for decreased immunoglobulin levels or severe neuropathy, as in small-fiber neuropathy and CIDP (chronic inflammatory demyelinating polyneuropathy).
- To decrease oxidative stress and the production of inflammatory molecules produced along the nitric oxide (NO) pathway (metabolic pathways influencing multiple physiological processes), while increasing the functioning of the biochemical pathways in the liver that help with detoxification, I combine low-dose naltrexone (LDN) with nutraceuticals that decrease inflammation (curcumin, broccoli seed extract [sulforaphane] as well as gluta-

thione and its precursors [NAC], among others). Newer approaches to control and resolve inflammation include using specific derivatives of omega-3 fatty acids, called specialized proresolving mediators (SPMs). We are in the process of evaluating their efficacy for those with severe inflammation who are resistant to standard therapies.

- An alkaline, Mediterranean-style anti-inflammatory diet (low in meat, eggs, dairy, and sugar and high in healthy fruits and vegetables, with olive oil) can be of significant benefit in controlling inflammation, and some individuals need to be on a gluten-free diet, or on a diet without any grains or allergic/sensitive foods, to control inflammation. A 2016 study from the *American Journal of Nutrition* confirmed that Paleo and Mediterranean diets are both associated with lower levels of inflammation and oxidative stress, and should be considered as a baseline/core diet in those with Lyme-MSIDS. Eating the right foods to support better nutrition is part of Rule 6 of the Action Plan.

- As we've discussed, a diet high in antioxidants (multicolored fruits and vegetables) is excellent for assisting detoxification and lowering inflammation. Adding supplements like curcumin, resveratrol, green tea and brocolli seed extracts, CoQ10, B vitamins (especially B_1, B_2, B_6, and methyl B_{12}), α-lipoic acid, minerals such as magnesium and zinc, omega-3 fatty acids, and glutathione precursors such as NAC and glycine, with oral glutathione, can also be beneficial in decreasing the inflammatory response.

If we hope to conquer the chronic degenerative diseases associated with MSIDS, we must put out the fire of inflammation. Comprehensive testing using the sixteen-point differential diagnostic map can help determine which factors may be increasing inflammation, and then, using our multifaceted approach, we can get to the root cause(s) of chronic illnesses.

NINE

Lyme and Environmental Toxins

We are continuously exposed to a variety of environmental toxins, but not everyone feels their effects. The effects on health will depend on several factors: your total load of toxins, nutritional status, immune function, overlapping chronic disease(s) with associated inflammation, and the status of your detoxification pathways. Some people can become ill when the exposure, or load of toxic substances (total body burden), is more than their body can handle.

Heavy-metal burden refers specifically to the exposure to metallic elements, including common heavy metals such as mercury, lead, arsenic, cadmium, nickel, and aluminum. Mercury, lead, and cadmium cannot be fully metabolized and removed from the body through the digestive process and, if accumulated, can interfere with your health in a variety of different ways. These heavy metals are now ubiquitous in the environment, and they accumulate slowly in our bodies over time. That is why many people do not get acutely ill from chronic low-level exposures. However, if you have already been exposed to other chronic illnesses, like Lyme disease, the outcome can be very different.

If you complain of fatigue, muscle pain with fibromyalgia symptoms, joint pain, tingling and numbness of the extremities, and neuropsychiatric abnormalities with memory and concentration problems, and if standard medical testing fails to reveal a cause for your symptoms, many doctors chalk up these experiences as the "aches and pains of daily living," the classic manifestations of getting old, or so-called "normal aging." Unfortunately, the problem is not that simple. Lyme disease, associated co-infections, and heavy metal burdens can overlap in their clinical presentations. Heavy metals might not always be directly responsible for these symptoms but might be a secondary cause, increasing symptomatology through increasing oxidative stress and inflammation.

Every symptom that we find in Lyme disease and co-infections can be mimicked, caused by, or exacerbated by environmental toxins and heavy metals, and no level of heavy metals in the body has been shown to be "safe" and without possible long-term side effects. A small increase in exposure to a toxic metal can lead to a disproportionate increase in the number of individuals who will experience symptoms of toxicity, and additive/synergistic effects among toxic metals may occur.

The most common symptoms/conditions associated with heavy metals include:

- anxiety/irritability
- auditory symptoms (such as ringing in the ears, i.e., tinnitus)
- autoimmunity
- cardiac symptoms (palpitations, chest pain)
- changes in weight (i.e., weight loss)
- cognitive dysfunction
- depression
- fatigue
- fibromyalgia symptoms
- increased susceptibility to infections
- joint pain
- loss of balance and/or incoordination
- paresthesias
- tremors
- urinary symptoms, renal disturbances
- varied abdominal complaints
- visual symptoms

Mercury is considered to be a neurotoxin, affecting brain function. Elevated levels of mercury have been linked to chronic fatigue syndrome, fibromyalgia, joint and muscle pain, tinnitus, memory and concentration problems, tingling and numbness, and a host of autoimmune disorders, and can impair the immune system. Mercury can bind to sulfhydryl groups in the body, increase oxidative stress, which can further drive cytokine production and inflammation, and penetrate into the nerves and bind to acetylcholine receptors in the brain, resulting in neurological dysfunction. Mercury can also affect the central and peripheral nervous systems, causing denervation of nerve fibers similar to the pathology we see in multiple sclerosis, while contributing to peripheral neuropathy. So when a patient presents with an MS-type picture, we need to rule out whether Lyme disease, co-infections (like Bartonella, chlamydia, and Mycoplasma species), Epstein-Barr virus, Vitamin D deficiency, and heavy metals such as mercury are each playing a role in creating similar symptoms with demyelination.

Lead exposure can cause fatigue, encephalopathy with impaired concentration, short-term memory deficits with decreased IQ in children, GI symptoms (i.e. abdominal colic), insomnia, anxiety and depression, irritability, and peripheral nerve dysfunction: Once again we see that these are the same symptoms of Lyme-MSIDS. Lead also can cause anemia and chronic renal failure with elevated blood pressures. Lead is stored in the bones, and may be dumped into the blood as men and women go through hormonal changes and develop osteopenia and osteoporosis. Since lead can raise blood pressure, lead may need to be considered as one of the comorbid conditions causing hypertension, which is now found in over 50 percent of the aging population. As reported in a 2012 *New York Times* article, preliminary results from a New York State Health Department study show that more than half the eggs tested from chickens kept in community gardens in Brooklyn, the Bronx, and Queens had detectable levels of lead. Lead exposure may therefore be more common than most people think. For example, a recent 2013 study by researchers at the University of Alberta in Canada found elevated levels of heavy metals, including arsenic, aluminum, and lead, in over thirty common teas found on supermarket shelves, with seven out of ten teas containing levels unsafe for pregnant women. Certain brands of dark chocolate, cosmetics, and hair dyes have also been found to contain lead in varying amounts, so exposure may be coming from multiple sources.

Arsenic can cause multiple cardiac, vascular, and neurological symptoms including paresthesias and peripheral neuropathy (apart from other effects such as causing aplastic anemia and cancer). Arsenic is found in a wide variety of foods, especially rice, rice products, and apple and grape juice, according to an FDA report in September 2012. Eating one serving of rice at the highest levels found in these studies could expose a person to more arsenic than the EPA allows in drinking water, putting adults at risk for cancer and heart disease, and children at risk for neurological symptoms and poor brain function. Arsenic exposure has also been linked to type 2 diabetes. So regular exposure to arsenic may underlie some of the most common diseases in the twenty-first century, and physicians generally are not checking for exposure to this toxic metal. What's more, there are no federally approved safe levels for arsenic ingestion.

Cadmium, which is also found in trace amounts in some foods, has been linked to chronic fatigue syndrome and toxic brain syndrome as well as hypertension and cardiovascular disease, emphysema, osteopenia, breast cancer, prostate cancer, and renal dysfunction with proteinuria and subsequent loss of amino acids.

Aluminum is a potent neurotoxin and has been associated with increased neurofibrillary tangles and brain degeneration, and it is known to accumulate in the neurons of patients with Lou Gehrig's disease (ALS) and Parkinson's disease. It can cause an encephalopathy with abnormal speech, similar to the encephalopathic symptoms that we see in severe chronic neurological Lyme disease with associated co-infections like Bartonella. It has also been implicated as one of the factors increasing the risk for Alzheimer's disease. We are frequently exposed to aluminum as it is a common food additive in baking, soft drinks, cosmetics, sunscreens, and antiperspirants, as well as being found in some medications such as aspirin or antacids. Although the body naturally excretes aluminum, increased amounts are deposited in the nerves and brain, which may exacerbate underlying degenerative neurological conditions and/or lead to an earlier onset of dementia.

HOW AM I GETTING EXPOSED TO HEAVY METALS?

Whatever toxins have found their way into the external environment will invariably find their way into our bodies. We breathe them in, ingest them from the food and water supply, absorb them through the skin, or they are transferred from mother to infant during pregnancy or breastfeeding. You don't have to live near a landfill to be exposed. For example, a National Wildlife Federation study from 2003 showed that more than 98 percent of rain samples in Texas contained levels of mercury far exceeding what the EPA considered safe for people and wildlife. In New York, the numbers are equally staggering: 84 percent of rain samples exceeded the EPA human health standard.

A 1997 Mercury Study Report to Congress stated that the best estimate of U.S. emissions of mercury from 1994 to 1995 was 158 tons. You read that number correctly. In the mid-1990s we were dumping 158 tons of mercury into the environment every year. Recently, the EPA accidentally spilled 3 million gallons of toxic sludge into the Animas River in Colorado, containing elevated levels of mercury, cadmium, arsenic, and lead. Researchers found levels of mercury 10 times above acceptable levels, cadmium levels 33 times above acceptable levels, arsenic at up to 800 times above acceptable levels, and a sample level of lead in the Animas River was nearly 12,000 times higher than the acceptable level set by the EPA. It can take years or even decades for health problems from metals to develop, but individuals with neurological insults from Lyme and associated co-infections may be more prone to the effects of these heavy metals in the body.

AARON'S ACTING OUT WASN'T ADD

Many years ago, a ten-year-old boy named Aaron came to see me with his mother. They lived in rural Maryland, and Aaron had a history of multiple tick bites. His symptoms started in the second and third grades with reading problems, difficulty retaining information, and temper tantrums. He had a "real attitude problem" according to his mother, who was growing frustrated with his acting out at home and at school.

When I reviewed the physical symptoms that he circled on the questionnaire, I noticed that Aaron suffered from fatigue, muscle pain, joint pain, neck stiffness, headaches, chills with hot and cold feelings, tingling of his extremities, palpitations, and insomnia, along with significant memory and concentration problems. To others, his behavior might seem like he had ADD. But I've seen these symptoms all too often: Aaron was doing an excellent job of "acting out" like an inadequately treated Lyme disease patient with multiple co-infections.

I sat across from Aaron and looked him squarely in the eyes. "What bothers you the most?"

"Doc, I keep losing my wrestling matches. They're kicking my butt. You gotta help me." Not exactly what I expected to hear as the worst symptom, but I wasn't living in his ten-year-old WWF world.

His physical exam was unremarkable, and I sent off his blood to test for Lyme disease and co-infections. His Lyme IFA, his IgG Western blot, and his Lyme dot blot through IGeneX were all positive. He also had a positive Bartonella PCR through MDL Laboratories, as well as a positive Lyme antibody test and a positive Babesia test, which accounted for an increase in the severity of Lyme symptoms, as well as his mood swings and memory and concentration problems.

I started Aaron on a rotation of different antibiotics. Within one month's time the majority of his symptoms had improved, although his energy was inconsistent. His stamina continued to fail him at the gym during wrestling matches. While his energy levels were better, he was still tired in the middle of the day, especially after meals, and around 3:00 P.M. after coming home from school. I suspected reactive hypoglycemia as one of the causes for his fatigue and lack of stamina, but knew that I would have a difficult time convincing him to stay away from pizza, hamburgers, fries, and ice cream, which make up a regular part of the typical ten-year-old's diet. I sent him for a five-hour glucose tolerance test with insulin levels. The test came back positive for significant hypoglycemia. If he could stay on a reasonably strict hypoglycemic diet his energy levels would be stable, and he would be able to get out of a full nelson in his matches.

Over the next six months Aaron was able to return to 98 percent of what he considered to be normal functioning, so later that year we decided to stop the antibiotics. Unfortunately, even with the new diet, Aaron wasn't out of the woods. When he came back two months later, his mother told me that all of his symptoms returned once he stopped taking the antibiotics. His grades were worsening in school. His irritability and temper were worse, and neither he nor his mother was happy.

I wasn't happy with these results, either. Then I remembered a call I recently had with a dentist friend of mine named Randy. He had developed a strong interest in nutritional and functional medicine over the years, and integrated these protocols into his dental practice. Randy had just tested himself for elevated levels of mercury, since he is around mercury vapor all the time in his office. His test results showed that his levels were ten times over the toxic range.

I had occasionally tested patients in the past for mercury and lead, since I was aware that Lyme symptoms overlapped those of an elevated heavy metal burden. Yet these tests always returned negative. Blood serum levels are not highly reliable unless there has been a recent acute exposure. Other tests were more indicative of a high body burden, including a hair analysis, but over the years I've found the best results with DMSA (dimercaptosuccinic acid) urine testing, especially for patients with chronic, resistant, unexplained symptoms including chronic fatigue, fibromyalgia, neuropathy, cognitive difficulties, tinnitus (ringing in the ears), and neuropsychiatric symptoms. Why? Heavy metals can accumulate for years in the body, leave the bloodstream when they are no longer measurable there, and then start compartmentalizing in body tissues. DMSA diffuses into and effectively competes with the tissue-binding sites for the metals, thereby releasing them from sequestered sites in the tissues. They then will redistribute into the blood as a stable complex, and be eliminated in the urine where they can be measured.

After speaking with Randy, I decided to test Aaron for heavy metal burdens. We performed a six-hour urine DMSA challenge and found that his lead level was five times above the normal range, his mercury almost twice the normal range, and his nickel and aluminum were also high. I asked him if he had been playing with thermometers, eating the paint off the wall, swallowing loose change, or eating the siding on his house. Even though the answers to all of these questions were a resounding no (he did not appreciate my sense of humor), he was still carrying a high heavy metal burden.

I started Aaron on oral chelation therapy with DMSA, which addresses elevated levels of mercury, lead, arsenic, cadmium, and other heavy metals. I wanted to use another chelating agent, known as EDTA, which is specific for removal of lead. It is not well absorbed orally, and is more effective by IV or rectal suppository. Do not try and convince a ten-year-old budding wrestler to do EDTA suppositories for elevated levels of lead, although the process of describing it to him and convincing him to do it was quite amusing. Overall we saw a significant improvement in his health over time. How was I sure it was removing the heavy metals that led to his recovery? "I'm kicking their butt in wrestling" was his joyous response when I asked him how he was feeling. He was now Aaron the Invincible.

OTHER TOXINS TO THINK ABOUT

Aside from heavy metals, there are several categories of toxins that may also be present in the Lyme-MSIDS patient. These include industrial compounds and chemical by-products, such as volatile organic solvents, PCBs, plasticizers, pesticides, insecticides, and herbicides, combustion and incineration pollutants, and food and cosmetic additives. Scientific studies have demonstrated that we are exposed to many of these environmental toxins on a daily basis, and cumulatively they can affect our long-term health, contributing to chronic illness.

In 1999 the EPA's Office of Prevention, Pesticides, and Toxic Substances reported that over 4 billion pounds of pesticides are used annually in the United States. This amounts to eight pounds for every individual in the United States each year. If you want to give a laboratory rat Parkinson's disease, immune dysfunction, or cancer, scientific studies have shown that you can do so just by exposing it to one good dose of pesticides.

Pesticides are now accumulating in many genetically modified (GM) grains and soy products, and may be one more chemical contributing to elevated rates of cancer, infertility, and Parkinson's according to research scientists at the Massachusetts Institute of Technology (MIT). In order to educate yourself on the amount of pesticides in foods, the Environmental Working Group (EWG) publishes an annual rating of conventional foods with the most and least pesticides. They have reported that approximately 65 percent of the thousands of produce samples analyzed by the U.S. Department of Agriculture (USDA) test positive for pesticide residues, so reviewing the EWG's top "dirty dozen" and "clean fifteen" fruits and vegetables is one way to help protect you and your family from the effects of pesticides. I also recommend buying organic produce when possible, and thoroughly washing fruits and vegetables.

Other toxins accumulate in the human body. In a 1982 EPA National Human Adipose Tissue Survey, fat biopsies were performed on subjects living in different regions of the United States, from New York to California.

They found that of those individuals tested, 100 percent were positive for different chemicals, including styrene, dichlorobenzene, xylene, ethyl phenol, and TCDD (dioxin). These and other environmental toxins are primarily acting as xenoestrogens (foreign-based estrogens), and have been linked to a variety of cancers, including cancer of the breast, prostate, lung, colon, cervix, and uterus. A follow-up study done by the CDC in 2003 found 116 different pollutants among 2,500 subjects across the United States, and one of those toxins, trichloroethylene (TCE), was responsible for a leukemia outbreak in children in Woburn, Massachusetts.

We especially need to pay attention to these types of chemical exposures in the very young and elderly. Chemicals like TCE, lead, and pesticides can cause learning disabilities, and the American Academy of Pediatrics issued a report in 2012 that warned that children have "unique susceptibilities to [pesticide residues'] potential toxicity," and cited research linking pesticide exposures in early life to "pediatric cancers, decreased cognitive function, and behavioral problems." Based on this prior 2003 CDC study, could TCE, combined with heavy metals such as mercury, which affects memory and concentration, as well as pesticides, be one of the many factors responsible for some of the ADD and learning disability epidemics in children in the United States and worldwide? Could these also be affecting the memory and concentration of my Lyme disease patients when these toxins are combined with the effects of *Borrelia burgdorferi* on the brain, and/or perhaps be an overlapping cofactor increasing dementia rates among Alzheimer's patients? Recent published research says yes! According to a 2014 study in the journal *PLOS ONE*, children exposed to common household chemicals like phthalates saw their IQ scores drop, and a study in *Environmental Health Perspectives* that same year by University of California, Davis, researchers found that pregnant women living near a farm using pesticides had a 60 percent higher risk of having an autistic child. Dr. Philippe Grandjean and Dr. Philip J. Landrigan from Harvard published in the journal *Lancet Neurology* that neurodevelopmental disabilities, including autism, ADHD, dyslexia, and other cognitive impairments, which affect millions of children worldwide, are due to industrial chemicals acting as developmental neurotoxicants, including lead, methylmercury, polychlorinated biphenyls (PCBs), arsenic, and toluene, with six additional developmental neurotoxicants having been documented since 2006, including manganese, fluoride, chlorpyrifos (a widely used pesticide), tetrachloroethylene (TCE), and the polybrominated diphenyl ethers (PBDEs, flame retardants).

Flame retardants like PBDEs or newly discovered ones, like TCEP, have been found in up to 75 percent of Americans tested. These toxins affect developing brains, but they also affect the female reproductive tract, causing pregnancy loss, damaging the nervous and reproductive system, and increasing the risk of autoimmune diseases. Scientists have shown that asbestos and inhaled small-particle environmental pollutants are causing an increase in positive antinuclear antibodies (ANAs), rheumatoid factors, and antibodies to extractable nuclear proteins such as Sm, SSA, and SSB, which are commonly found in patients with systemic lupus erythematosus. Exposure to high levels of ambient particle pollution stimulates inflammatory cytokine production such as IL-6 (also seen in Lyme disease), triggering juvenile idiopathic arthritis (JIA) and adversely impacting other autoimmune illnesses.

Scientists are also reporting toxins as potential risk factors for Alzheimer's disease. Researchers reported in *JAMA Neurology* in 2014 that elevated serum levels of pesticides like DDE were associated with an increased risk for AD, and that both DDT and DDE increase amyloid precursor protein levels, providing a plausible mechanism as to how DDE exposure may cause AD. Although those who are genetic carriers of the ApoE4 allele may be more susceptible to the effects of DDE, it is becoming clear that the higher our infectious burden, and the higher our load of environmental toxins, the greater our risk of neurodegenerative disease.

NATURAL-BORN TOXINS

Some toxins are externally produced, like molds, or are internally produced in the body, significantly impacting both physical and neurological symptoms. Dr. Joseph Brewer published in the journal *Toxins* in 2013 that many patients with chronic fatigue syndrome test positive for mold toxins. We have similarly found that a significant number of our resistant Lyme patients test positive for multiple mold toxins (aflatoxin, ochratoxin, trichothecene) on a urine mold assay through RealTime Labs in Texas. We recently discovered a new class of mold toxins called gliotoxins in our patients, which has immunosuppressive effects that could be impacting the immune system's ability to combat Lyme and multiple co-infections.

We are also exposed to multiple internal toxins. These include molecules like chloral hydrate, which can be produced when the liver doesn't have enough zinc to convert aldehydes to alcohols; alcohol molecules produced in some with Candida overgrowth in the GI tract; or quinolinic acid, which is a neurotoxic metabolite of certain biochemical pathways in the brain used to make neurotransmitters (such as the L-tryptophan pathway), which when produced in the brain by activated microglia and macrophages is involved in neurodegenerative diseases such as Parkinson's disease, Lou Gehrig's disease (ALS), Huntington's disease, MS, and Alzheimer's disease. Lyme disease patients have also been shown to have increased levels of quinolinic acid. This toxin may be playing a key role in the cognitive processing issues and mood disorders that Lyme patients frequently complain of after having been exposed to borrelia and associated co-infections. It could explain in part why certain patients continue with ongoing symptoms despite seemingly adequate antibiotic therapy. The scientific literature has shown that once you suppress the production of quinolinic acid, using antioxidants such as curcumin, or the ones found in green tea (epigallocatechin), or protect against the effects of quinolinic acid using COX-2 inhibitors (like the medication Celebrex), some patients will clinically improve.

Treatments for Removing Environmental Toxins

Detoxifying external toxins like mold and heavy metal burdens, or internally produced chemical compounds like quinolinic acid, can make us feel better. That's why detoxification is Rule #3 in our Action Plan. We recommend a three-step process: detoxification, chelation, and nutritional supplementation.

Step 1: Detoxification

There are four main organs involved: the skin, from which we sweat out toxins; the liver, which transforms toxins into less toxic substances; and the colon and the kidneys, which remove toxins via excretion.

Far infrared saunas, a specific type of sauna therapy, are extremely effective for removing chemicals by sweating them out through the skin. Individuals with chemical sensitivity/environmental illness (EI), and/or high levels of biotoxins such as quinolinic acid or mold neurotoxins may benefit from infrared saunas, especially when combined with binding agents (bentonite clay, charcoal, zeolite, cholestyramine, or WelChol), with high-dose oral or IV liposomal glutathione (GSH), and phosphatidylcholine (PC) with N-butyrate. Nutritional supplementation that supports the detoxification pathways (magnesium, NAC, glycine, α-lipoic acid, DIM, sulforaphane glucosinolate, and methylation cofactors) is also important so that the liver can effectively remove toxins.

The liver helps transform chemicals, drugs, hormones, and toxic compounds into nontoxic substances. This takes place through two essential phases, known as phase I (oxidation) and phase II (conjugation). In phase I, an electron is added to a molecule (oxidizing it) by a series of enzymes in the liver called the cytochrome P 450 system, which prepares it for phase II. Then biotransformation of the chemical compound takes place: It shuttles through one of six different detoxification pathways, where a series of molecules are added (conjugation) to help make it more water soluble, increasing its ability to be excreted out of the body through the kidneys. We recommend using high-quality protein with essential amino acids, combined with specific vitamins, minerals, herbs, and nutritional supplements, to support phase I and phase II liver pathways and help to convert toxic substances from fat-soluble toxins that are stuck in body fat to water-soluble substances that can be more easily eliminated.

A second useful approach to removing toxins from the body via the liver in phase II involves glutathione (GSH). Glutathione is made by the liver to help the body detoxify foreign chemicals, as well as to help remove hormones and medications that we may be taking. Glutathione takes fat-soluble toxins stored in our tissues that are not easily eliminated and helps make them water soluble, so they can be removed from the body. It also helps with many other important metabolic functions, such as making enzymes, hormones, and new genetic material. It has even been found to be helpful in treating neuropsychiatric disorders and cognitive problems, as it helps supply neural glutamate, the principal excitatory neurotransmitter in the brain, important in learning and memory.

We make glutathione all the time, but if you have inadequate stores of it because of increased exposure to internal and external toxins, the glutathione levels in the body will be depleted. Hence, less glutathione would mean a possible increase in toxic chemicals from the environment, or in the case of a Lyme-MSIDS patient, an inability to properly deal with a sudden release of cytokines during a Jarisch-Herxheimer flare, making the patient sicker.

One way to assist the body in making its own glutathione is by supplementing with N-Acetylcysteine (NAC), and alpha-lipoic acid (ALA), which can facilitate the regeneration of glutathione. Alpha-lipoic acid has other beneficial effects, such as mildly chelating heavy metals and providing antioxidant support against free radicals and lowering inflammation; decreasing insulin resistance and lowering blood sugars (those with significant hypoglycemia may need to use lower doses), and high doses can even be helpful for diabetic neuropathy.

Glutathione has been shown to be a safe treatment in our clinical trials. Improvements from a single dose of IV GSH lasted from several hours to two to three days in some patients before they experienced a relapse in symptoms. There were generally no significant adverse effects. An occasional patient complained of temporary nausea, rare, fleeting pressure in the head, and a temporary increase in tingling in the extremities. These symptoms all disappeared within several minutes of the injection. There are, however, rare patients with a sulfa sensitivity or environmental sensitivities who do not tolerate IV GSH and may get adverse effects (a rash/allergic reaction, or increased symptoms as their detoxification pathways are severely impacted), so asking about allergies, prior use of sulfa drugs, and sensitivity to removing toxins is important.

We use both a liposomal form of oral glutathione and IV glutathione with resistant Lyme-MSIDS patients on a regular basis. Overwhelmingly, I have found that for most treatment-resistant patients with symptoms unresponsive to antibiotics and other interventions, we see marked clinical improvements when we enhance their detoxification pathways using glutathione.

In terms of detoxifying through the colon, we use nutritional fiber, probiotic supplementation (i.e., Acidophilus, Bifidobacteria, and other healthy bacterial flora), and occasional colon cleanses. Probiotic enemas have also been helpful in replacing healthy bacteria in the microbiome.

For detoxification through the kidneys, drinking two to three liters of water per day will help flush toxins. This is safe unless there is a medical contraindication (certain forms of heart, liver, or kidney disease).

Step 2: Chelation

Chelation is the process by which we remove heavy metals from the body. It can be done at a doctor's office by an IV preparation, or by taking medication orally. Treatments are individualized and based on the patient's levels of heavy metals, possible drug allergies, and side effects (although these are few and far between, except in patients with extremely poor detoxification abilities).

Common oral chelation regimens include DMSA (for removing lead, mercury, arsenic, and other heavy metals), as well as 2, 3-Dimercapto-1-propanesulfonic acid (DMPS), which is more specific for mercury. For those who cannot tolerate the above two sulfa drugs, another option is D-penicillamine (Cuprimine), but it is more labor-intensive to use and may have more side effects. Transdermal chelation (DMSA) can be used for children who cannot swallow pills.

DMSA should initially be started in low doses to test for tolerance, as some patients may get Jarisch-Herxheimer reactions with chelation if their detoxification pathways are not functioning properly. We generally use low-dose oral DMSA at bedtime every several days or pulsed DMSA two days in a row on the weekends, and higher dose DMSA (5 to 10 mg/kg TID), one hour before meals, three days on, eleven days off (standard chelation protocols) can be used in patients with very high levels of heavy metals, usually once they are off antibiotics, if their detoxification pathways are functioning properly. I have never seen any long-term adverse effects of using DMSA, although an occasional patient may become chemically sensitive to DMSA over time if he or she is sulfa sensitive (and develop a rash). However, there are patients who are sensitive to sulfa (i.e., cannot take drugs like Bactrim or Septra double-strength) and are able to tolerate DMSA without a problem. If chelation is absolutely necessary, and DMSA must be used, and there is any possibility of an associated sulfa sensitivity (history of a rash or itching), an H1 blocker (i.e., over-the-counter Allegra, Zyrtec, or Claritin) and an H2 blocker (over-the-counter Zantac or Pepcid) can be used simultaneously to help prevent allergic reactions by blocking H1 and H2 histamine receptors. This seems to prevent any significant reactions in patients who have questions about sulfa sensitivity, and can be used for the initial DMSA challenge. Discuss this option with your physician. If there is a history of a severe sulfa sensitivity such as wheezing, shortness of breath, or severe skin reactions, then another chelating agent is advisable.

Intravenous chelation therapy is available for both DMPS and Disodium EDTA, which are primarily used for mercury and lead toxicity respectively. Intravenous EDTA has also been used to treat atherosclerosis and was recently found to modestly reduce the risk of adverse cardiovascular outcomes. Rectal suppositories with EDTA (Detoxamine) can be used in a comprehensive chelation protocol when high levels of lead are present and IV treatments are not available or convenient. The rectal suppositories can be combined with oral chelation therapies.

There are many misconceptions about chelation and its safety. We have never seen a life-threatening reaction, nor any long-term problems in chelating several thousands of patients using the protocols that I am describing, and many have experienced the clinical benefit. Approximately 20 percent of my resistant Lyme-MSIDS patients had improved fatigue, decreased muscle and joint pain, and improved neurocognitive functioning following chelation therapy. This included a reversal of memory loss and improved concentration, with fewer mood swings. This improvement was independent of any antibiotic protocols used to treat these same patients.

Chelation first requires an evaluation that determines if there are heavy metals in the body. This can be done through blood work, although it will only pick up a recent, acute exposure. Some healthcare providers will perform a hair analysis to evaluate the burden of heavy metals, but this is not as specific as performing a six-hour urine DMSA challenge, which pulls heavy metals from the body's tissues into the urine, where it can be measured.

We also frequently use NAC and oral liposomal glutathione in combination with these medicines, to both help chelate heavy metals and protect against side effects and associated increased oxidative stress.

I do not use IV chelation, and have found that combining oral DMSA with EDTA suppositories works well without significant side effects for the vast majority of patients if high levels of mercury, lead, and other heavy metals are present.

Avoid taking mineral supplements on the days of chelation—such as antacids, including Tums, multivitamins with minerals, or calcium supplements with magnesium—since minerals may bind to the chelating agents, making them ineffective. These supplements, especially a broad multimineral supplement with magnesium, should be taken on the days not chelating, because they are essential in helping to prevent any side effects, such as increased oxidative stress and muscle spasms, as chelation can pull magnesium and other minerals out of the body.

If high levels of aluminum are present, we will also add malic acid (a natural substance found in fruits) to our chelation regimen. Malic acid is naturally found in apples and grapes and also can be taken as a nutritional supplement.

Some patients doing a chelation regimen will only notice mild improvements, but for others it may be much more dramatic. But even for those patients who do not notice a clinical shift in symptoms, it is still wise to chelate these heavy metals. Remember, heavy metals and other environmental toxins have been linked to autoimmune diseases and may be responsible, with borrelia infections, for some of the autoimmune manifestations we see contributing to chronic illness. This includes mercury's effect on nerves, causing neuropathy, a common symptom. Second, heavy metals, such as mercury, can increase oxidative stress and increase inflammation, which we have shown to be a common denominator in causing symptoms of Lyme-MSIDS as well as those of many other chronic illnesses. Finally, mercury has been shown to increase susceptibility to chronic infections, which is a problem for anyone who has an impaired immune system that is overwhelmed by multiple co-infections.

Step 3: Nutritional Supplementation

We also need to remove toxins because a high load of environmental chemicals may worsen mineral deficiencies, as these can be used up in detoxification reactions. Up to 25 percent of our chronic MSIDS patients with heavy metals are deficient in one or more minerals, such as iodine, magnesium, copper, and zinc. It is important to check both serum and red blood cell (RBC) levels of all these minerals, because many, such as magnesium, are primarily intracellular and cannot be adequately tested by serum levels alone.

Proper levels of trace minerals (micronutrients) are essential for optimal biochemical functioning at the cellular level. Minerals are also essential components in complex biochemical detoxification reactions. For example, magnesium is necessary in approximately three hundred detoxification enzymes in the body. A magnesium deficiency can result in muscle spasms, tremors, anxiety, Raynaud's phenomenon, and cardiac arrhythmias. Copper is involved in the production of superoxide dismutase (SOD), which is an essential enzyme in dealing with free radicals and oxidative stress. Copper is also found in other enzymes: polyphenol oxidase, which is necessary to detoxify chemicals, tyrosinase and dopamine oxidase (essential for neurotransmitters), and cytochrome c oxidase (essential for energy production). Zinc is necessary in over ninety enzymes, including alcohol dehydrogenase, which is one part of the liver's detoxification pathways, when it converts alcohols to aldehydes. Many of our Lyme-MSIDS patients are zinc deficient.

For mineral replacement, I generally prescribe calcium, magnesium, and zinc, with a high-potency multimineral supplement containing trace minerals like copper, on the days that the patient is not chelating. I will test the patient's mineral levels intermittently (serum and RBC magnesium, serum and RBC zinc, serum and RBC copper, and iodine) and get a complete blood count (CBC) and biochemistry profile every few months to check liver and kidney functions. If on Lyme treatment, these mineral supplements should be taken at least several hours away from the antibiotics to avoid interfering with absorption.

Nutritional supplements used during chelation with DMSA and/or EDTA usually include Chlorella with NAC, alpha-lipoic acid, liposomal glutathione, and occasionally Med Caps DPO (Xymogen) if phase I and phase II liver detoxification pathways are not functioning efficiently. Using this protocol, and properly supporting the detoxification pathways, we have seen heavy metal burdens decrease (although different metals may come out in stages as more are found during chelation).

These three important steps are detoxification, chelation, and nutritional supplementation and are necessary for removing toxins from the body and promoting healing. Once these toxins are removed, the majority of our patients feel better. Remember, both infections and toxins drive inflammation, and both have to be treated in order for you to get better.

TEN

Lyme, Functional Medicine, and Nutritional Therapies

Functional medicine offers a different perspective from the way medicine is commonly practiced, which is primarily concerned with naming a disease and then finding drugs to treat it. According to the Institute for Functional Medicine, "Functional medicine is a science-based healthcare approach that assesses and treats underlying causes of illness through individually tailored therapies to restore health and improve function."

One of the ways we do this is by looking at nutritional and metabolic profiles that address the various organ systems of the body. These specialized tests must be ordered by a healthcare practitioner. They are performed at functional medicine laboratories such as Genova Diagnostics and Doctor's Data. These tests monitor gastrointestinal function, immunity, toxicity, nutrient and toxic elements, amino acids and fatty acids, vitamins, oxidative stress, and endocrine profiles, and they are not typically performed in standard laboratories. These allow us to look at the body through the eyes of a nutritional biochemist, evaluating illness at the deepest cellular and biological levels.

These profiles are extremely important for the typical MSIDS patient. Remember, standard laboratories do not adequately screen for environmental toxins and for specific detoxification problems, whereas testing through a functional medicine laboratory such as Genova Diagnostics can give a more comprehensive biochemical picture of your health.

Other examples of how we might use functional medicine testing include evaluating for *Candida* (intestinal fungal overgrowth), leaky gut (increased intestinal permeability), and food allergies and sensitivities in those with resistant fatigue, aches and pains, headaches, and gastrointestinal complaints. Standard allergy testing may only look at IgE antibodies (antibodies involved in immediate reactions to allergens), but functional medicine laboratories also do extensive IgG food antibody panels (antibodies involved in delayed immune reactions against foods) and can therefore pick up food sensitivities and allergies missed by other labs. Similarly, standard stool cultures do not give us the detailed analysis necessary to rebalance the microflora in the intestine and see if digestive enzymes may be necessary. By ordering a Comprehensive Digestive Stool Analysis (CDSA), which looks at digestive and pancreatic functions as well as levels of bacteria, yeast, and parasites in the intestine, we can get a much better look at the gut. These types of tests are critical because nutrition and enzyme deficiencies that cause digestive disorders are commonly seen with chronic fatigue syndrome (CFS), fibromyalgia, and those suffering from chemical sensitivity. These enzyme deficiencies lead to poor digestion, thereby causing a deficiency of vital nutrients necessary for proper cellular function.

There are six basic functional medicine principles that need to be a part of every good health plan. They allow us to properly "detoxify," which is Rule 3, "repair the damage," which is Rule 4, and "provide internal balance," which is Rule 5 of the Action Plan:

- Minimize toxic exposure
- Ensure hydration
- Optimize bowel health
- Increase antioxidant reserves
- Optimize mitochondrial function
- Assist and balance liver biotransformation

How Can I Minimize Toxic Exposure?

- Do not use pesticides in your home or close to the home
- Try to avoid using chemical products indoors

- Use natural cleaning products when possible
- Use water and air purifiers when possible
- Check your home for radon and mold
- Reduce cell phone radiation by avoiding close contact with your body

How Do I Know I'm Drinking Enough Water?

As Dr. Sherry Rogers says, "Dilution is the solution to pollution." Drink at least two to three liters of fluid per day (unless you have a medical condition that requires fluid restriction, such as congestive heart or kidney failure). Staying well hydrated helps flush toxins from the bloodstream and out through the kidneys. Fluids also help us maintain proper bowel health, preventing constipation and moving toxins more quickly through the GI tract.

The water you drink should be pH neutral and preferably alkaline to enhance cellular function. A neutral pH for water is around 7.0 to 7.4, and acidic water has a pH below 7.0, while alkaline water has a pH of 7.5 or higher. You can determine the pH of your water using test strips purchased at a local pharmacy or through a company that specializes in water testing (i.e., Culligan or swimming pool and hot tub suppliers). Reverse osmosis systems take minerals out of the water, making it more acidic, and alkalizing water purifiers are commercially available to correct this problem.

Drinking regular purified water (not distilled water, which has no minerals, and not club soda or other carbonated beverages, as they are acidic in the body) is the easiest way to achieve your daily intake. Neither caffeinated coffee or tea counts in your total fluid intake, as the caffeine can cause additional excretion of fluids and can lead to a negative fluid balance, with dehydration. Fresh vegetable juices (organic, with lots of greens) are also an excellent option, as these are high in vitamins and minerals and are alkaline in pH.

One easy way to tell if you are adequately hydrated is by observing the color and smell of your urine. A dark, strong-smelling urine usually means that you are not drinking enough water.

How Can I Optimize Bowel Health?

The GI tract is one of the first lines of defense for protecting us from certain pathogenic bacteria and viruses. We also need a healthy GI tract to properly absorb all of our essential vitamins and nutrients, and the bowels play an important role in detoxifying chemicals and toxins that may enter the body through the foods we eat or the fluids we drink.

Many Lyme patients have overlapping food allergies and sensitivities, usually secondary to an associated problem with Candida and a leaky gut. Increased intestinal permeability has also been associated with elevated levels of mercury, increasing oxidative stress, and adversely affecting the tight junctions in between cells. Classical treatment includes avoidance of allergens, rotation diets, and occasional immunizations against offending allergens. Integrative treatment includes treating an underlying Candida syndrome or leaky gut with dysbiosis if present, using enzyme therapy if the patient is deficient, and using antioxidants and chelators to lower heavy metal burdens. Some patients have reported benefits from using techniques such as Nambudripad's Allergy Elimination Techniques (NAET) to clear resistant food allergies, but we have not had enough experience with the technique to validate its effectiveness in our patient population. Herbal therapies to treat Candida include garlic (allicin), berberine, olive leaf extract, grapefruit seed extract, monolaurin (Lauricidin), Pau D'Arco, and Biocidin, with classical treatments including nystatin (tablet, compounded), Diflucan, Sporanox, Voriconazole, and Amphotericin B. We usually find combining herbal therapies with classical therapies works best for resistant cases of Candida (with a very strict diet).

We can maintain proper bowel health by drinking adequate amounts of fluids and by taking in high amounts of fiber, which helps prevent constipation and diverticulosis, a potentially painful condition which can lead to inflammation in parts of the colon. Occasionally colon cleansing may also be necessary in certain individuals who are chronically constipated, as toxins that are not properly removed from the colon may find their way back into the body through the enterohepatic (intestinal-liver) circulation. Nutrition that supports the enterocytes (cells that line the intestines), using products like glutamine, and by using high-quality probiotics, are other ways to ensure optimal bowel health.

Probiotics produce substances that prevent harmful bacteria and yeast from establishing themselves in the colon. These include lactic acid, bacteriocins, and hydrogen peroxide (H_2O_2). They also inhibit dangerous bacteria, such as *Salmonella,* from attaching to the intestines. Other important functions of probiotics include specific metabolic activities, such as the breakdown of microbial toxins and the modulation of the immune system, the latter by helping to regulate certain proteins and signaling molecules, such as interleukins and cytokines, the molecules that cause inflammatory and autoimmune reactions in the body. Certain probiotics that are Bifidobacterium strains can also help with constipation by speeding up transit time, reducing bloating and discomfort in people with functional bowel disorders, enhancing immunity, and decreasing allergic reactions.

We routinely use a variety of high-potency probiotics for those who are on long-term antibiotics, because antibiotics can adversely impact intestinal flora. The probiotic *Lactobacillus rhamnosus* has been shown to help prevent antibiotic-associated diarrhea, as well as preventing *E. coli, Salmonella,* and *Shigella,* which are pathogenic organisms that cause diarrhea, from adhering well to the intestinal lining. *Lactobacillus rhamnosus* accomplishes this by lowering the intestinal pH where the lactic acid produced inhibits the growth of the harmful bacteria responsible for outbreaks of gastroenteritis and diarrhea.

Another organism that is frequently associated with diarrhea is *Clostridium difficile,* which is normally present in the colon, but antibiotic use increases its production, leading to inflammation in the colon. It is the bacteria responsible for 95 percent of pseudomembranous colitis (a serious and potentially life-threatening inflammation of the colon). Based on a 1999 study published in *Infection and Immunity,* we've long since known that by using a different type of probiotic, *Saccharomyces boulardii,* which is a healthy yeast, we can create a temporary barrier in the colon protecting the healthy intestinal bacteria.

We can also improve intestinal health by adding fiber to the diet, which cleanses the bowel of toxins by increasing bowel movement frequency. Food sources of dietary fiber include the indigestible portion of plants, which contain two main components, soluble and insoluble fiber. Soluble fiber is readily fermented in the colon into gases and active byproducts, and insoluble fiber may be metabolically inert, and it facilitates the bulking of the stools. Insoluble fibers can absorb water as they move through the digestive system, making it easier to have a bowel movement. However, some forms of insoluble fiber, such as wheat bran, may actually decrease bowel frequency, so choosing the right type of fiber is important.

Flaxseeds contain an insoluble fiber that can increase bowel frequency, and it also has high amounts of lignans, a type of fiber that modulates hormone levels and may be useful in treating hormonal imbalances for adult men and women. Current recommendations from the United States National Academy of Sciences' Institute of Medicine suggest that adults consume 20 gms to 35 gms of dietary fiber per day and 1 tbsp to 2 tbsps per day of milled flax. One hundred grams of ground flaxseed supplies 28 gms of fiber and 20 gms of protein.

If you experience other inflammatory conditions in the gut (e.g., inflammatory bowel diseases such as Crohn's disease and ulcerative colitis), which produce symptoms of abdominal pain, cramping, frequent bowel movements, and/or bloody diarrhea, you may benefit from using certain lactobacillus (*L. gasseri*) and bifidobacteria (*B. longum*), which lower inflammatory cytokines; getting off gluten, grains, and allergic foods that may increase inflammation; as well as other strategies that support colon health, like using low-dose naltrexone (LDN), which has been published to decrease inflammation in Crohn's disease. The functional medicine approach suggests that we evaluate and balance the microbiome in our GI tract; treat enzyme deficiencies, bacterial dysbiosis, Candida, and parasites (if present); heal leaky gut and food allergies/sensitivities; decrease inflammation, and reduce the burden of toxic substances in the body by increasing transit through the GI tract while supporting detoxification pathways in the liver.

This approach recommends nutritional support for gastrointestinal and liver functions, including glutamine, which can come from either foods or dietary supplements, a naturally occurring amino acid essential for recovering from illness or injury. Glutamine provides essential fuel for colon cells, enabling them to act as a functional barrier to dangerous microorganisms that can cause inflammation. Intestinal inflammation can cause leaky gut syndrome, in which large molecules of food pass across the intestinal barrier, creating increased food sensitivities, food allergies, increased histamine release, autoimmune reactions, and further inflammation. Leaky-gut syndrome has been identified in the medical literature in such diverse conditions as ankylosing spondylitis (a chronic, inflammatory arthritis in which immune mechanisms affect joints in the spine and the sacroiliac joint, leading to eventual fusion of the spine), rheumatoid arthritis, asthma, eczema, and inflammatory bowel disease (IBD).

Dietary sources of L-glutamine include:

- Beef
- Beets
- Cabbage
- Chicken
- Dairy products
- Eggs
- Fish
- Parsley
- Spinach
- Vegetable juices
- Wheat

Other ways to support gastrointestinal function include *larch arabi-nogalactan*, an immune-enhancing polysaccharide, as well as immuno-globulins. Polysaccharides are components of soluble dietary fiber that can bind to bile acids in the small intestine, making them less likely to enter the body. This helps lower cholesterol and sugar levels (decreasing the risk of diabetes), while also lowering the levels of toxins, as some are bound to bile acids.

Supplementing with immunoglobulins can support the immune system and control inflammation in the gastrointestinal tract. Immunoglobulins are proteins made by the immune system to identify and control bacte-rial and viral infections. You can also supplement the body's production by taking whey protein capsules or adding whey protein powders to shakes. Increasing your intake of immunoglobulins can help neutralize endotoxins and prevent and treat infections caused by pathogenic bacte-ria, viruses, parasites, and yeast, and they are an important addition to antimicrobial prescription medications.

Immunoglobulins have been looked at as a treatment for inflamma-tory bowel disease. Immunoglobulins may also neutralize endotoxins, the molecules found on the outer cell membranes of dangerous bacteria, which are made up of lipids and sugars (lipopolysaccharides, i.e., LPS). LPS appears to increase inflammation in our cartilage and contribute to arthritis by turning on NFKappa-B and increasing inflammatory cyto-kines, so it may be helpful to neutralize LPS in Lyme and autoimmune arthritis. If large amounts of endotoxins are released when certain toxic bacteria in the gut are killed or destroyed, then these endotoxins can go on to produce fever and lower blood pressure (causing hypotension) and further activate inflammatory and coagulation pathways in the body, leading to severe illness.

In the table that follows you can see the relationship between the gastrointestinal system and the liver, and the overlapping syndromes found in Lyme-MSIDS. The diseases shown are ones that we would not normally consider to be related to problems in the gastrointestinal tract, but may appear as a result of inflammatory cytokine production, as is the case with chronic fatigue syndrome and Lyme disease. Helping to establish a healthy GI environment and microbiome, while lowering inflammatory cytokines by decreasing the absorption of endotoxins and preventing leaky gut, can positively influence these varied disease processes. What's more, lowering the toxic burden in both the GI tract and the liver while providing the nutrients essential to their proper functioning also contributes to the treatment of these diseases.

How Can I Increase Antioxidant Reserves?

Oxidative stress increases cytokine production and inflammation. It is therefore essential to have adequate amounts of antioxidants to decrease free radical damage and to prevent the turning on of NFKappaB—the switch inside the cell's nucleus that increases the production of the cytokines IL-1, IL-6, and TNF-α—which increases inflammation.

Glutathione is one of the most important antioxidant systems that we have in the body, along with superoxide dismutase (SOD). Whey-based proteins and nutritional supplements such as N-Acetylcysteine (NAC) and glycine will help in the production of glutathione, because they contain amino acids that are essential parts of the glutathione molecule. Other nutrients and antioxidants can modify detoxification reactions and promote enzymes that make glutathione, including glutathione reductase, glutathione S transferase, and glutathione peroxidase.

Alpha-lipoic acid is another excellent nutritional supplement that can decrease free radicals and increase the production of other antioxidants, such as Vitamins C and E and glutathione. A 2002 study published in *Alternative Medicine Review* showed that alpha-lipoic acid has the ability to chelate heavy metals, and that it plays an important role in the treatment

Table 9.1: GI Dysfunction and Other Medical Conditions	
Inflammatory Bowel Disease	• Glutamine is a primary fuel for the formation of healthy intestinal cells. • Fiber/probiotics promote the formation of short-chain fatty acids (SCFA), helping decrease inflammation. • Essential oils promote healthy GI function.
Chronic Fatigue Syndrome	• Bowel permeability results in systemic translocation of toxins, which may uncouple adenosine triphosphate (ATP), causing fatigue.
Fibromyalgia	• O_2 deprivation (Krebs cycle) results in cell death and tissue damage, leading to tender muscles.
Chronic Inflammation (Arthritis)	• Bowel permeability results in the uptake of antigenic protein, which may be deposited in joints.
Food Allergies	• The translocation of antigenic proteins results in allergic reactions or sensitivities with subsequent inflammation.
Hormone Imbalance (PMS, Menopause)	• Enterolactone (good estrogen) is formed in the bowel by the bacterial fermentation of fiber (i.e., flaxseed, lignans). • Impaired liver function (phases I and II) results in excessive circulating estrogens.
Cognitive/Neurological Dysfunction	• Impaired liver function facilitates free radicals attacking the CNS (myelin sheath). • Heavy metal deposits in neurons result in neurological disorders (e.g., aluminum and Alzheimer's).

218 • RICHARD I. HOROWITZ, MD

of toxicity of mercury and other toxic metals, such as arsenic and cadmium. It is also useful for treating metabolic syndrome with insulin resistance, polycystic ovarian syndrome (PCOS), and diabetes, as it helps lower blood sugar and reduces one of the primary neurological conditions in diabetes, diabetic neuropathy.

Dietary protein is essential for the synthesis of glutathione. Amino acids such as glycine, glutamine, cysteine, and taurine (which are found in most proteins, dairy products, grains, and vegetables; each can also be taken as a nutritional supplement) are also involved in the conjugation of drugs and their metabolites as well as aiding in detoxifying environmental chemicals. Conjugation reactions are one of the six essential phase II detoxification reactions that take place in the liver. These phase II reactions help to make fat-soluble substances (such as toxins) that cannot be excreted from the body into water-soluble molecules, which can then be eliminated through the kidneys.

Certain phytochemicals such as resveratrol (derived from grapes and dark berries) curcurmin (i.e., turmeric, a common Indian spice), green tea extract, and broccoli seed extract (sulforaphane glucosinolate) are all important antioxidants that can be obtained through foods or taken as nutritional supplements, which have a positive effect on our genes (epigenetic effects) while also helping to decrease inflammation. All four substances in the presence of oxidative stress help translocate Nrf2, located in the cytoplasm of our cells, into the nucleus, where it turns on antioxidant response element (ARE) genes. These DNA-binding sites primarily activate phase II enzymes in the liver (with a minor effect on phase I) plus numerous other cytoprotective enzymes, enhancing detoxification, decreasing inflammation, and inhibiting cancer growth. Nrf2 also interacts with important cell regulators such as tumor suppressor protein 53 (p53) and nuclear factor-kappa beta (NF-κB), helping to protect against many age-related diseases including cancer and neurodegeneration. In a recent placebo-controlled, randomized, double-blind clinical trial, daily oral administration for eighteen weeks of the phytochemical sulforaphane, derived from broccoli sprouts, given to twenty-nine young men with autism spectrum disorder (ASD), substantially (and reversibly) improved behavior compared to that of fifteen placebo recipients. I regularly advise using sulforaphane, curcumin, green tea extract, and resveratrol to upregulate genes that protect aerobic cells against oxidative stress, inflammation, and DNA damage, while supporting detoxification.

Other nutritional substances high in antioxidant compounds are fruits and vegetables. The American Cancer Society suggests that we consume as many as five to eight cups of fruits and vegetables every day to maintain health. Many of the colorful compounds found in a variety of fruits and vegetables contain important antioxidants and phytochemicals.

Lastly, replace vitamins, minerals, amino acids, essential fatty acids, and enzymes as per test results from both functional medicine laboratories and standard laboratories.

How Can I Optimize Mitochondrial Function?

The mitochondria are the energy powerhouses of the cell. If they are damaged by free radicals and toxic chemicals, they are unable to work correctly. We can optimize mitochondrial function by taking the vitamins, minerals, complex carbohydrates, and phospholipids necessary for proper energy metabolism, such as CoQ10, acetyl L-carnitine, D-ribose, Nicotinamide adenine dinucleotide (NADH), and glycosylated phospholipids (NT factors). These all help to ensure more efficient adenosine triphosphate (ATP)/energy production. This will be discussed in more detail in Chapter 11, "Lyme and Mitochondrial Dysfunction."

How Can I Enhance My Liver Function?

The liver is one of the primary organs that help transform chemicals, drugs, hormones, and toxic compounds into nontoxic substances that are water-soluble, allowing the body to excrete them through the urine.

Good quality proteins—such as lean red meats, chicken, turkey, cottage cheese, Greek-style yogurt, and nut butters—are especially important for maintaining liver health. Broccoli and other cruciferous vegetables contain active compounds that convert toxins acting as xenoestrogens (foreign chemicals with estrogenic effects) into healthier compounds. Lastly, other food and dietary compounds known as "bifunctional modulators" are also important to include in the diet. Substances that help to modulate phase I (and some phase II) metabolic reactions in the liver include:

- Ellagic acid (found in pomegranates, raspberries)
- Green tea

- Watercress
- Silymarin (milk thistle)
- Minerals (like zinc)

Substances that help to upregulate and support phase II metabolic pathways include:

- Amino acids (cysteine, glycine)
- Artichoke leaf
- B vitamins (B_6, B_{12}, pantothenic acid, folic acid)
- Glutathione and substances supporting sulfation (i.e., alpha-lipoic acid, sodium sulfate, MSM)
- Minerals (like magnesium)
- Methylation cofactors, i.e., SAMe and 5-methyltetrahydrofolate (5-MTHF)

Methylation is important in removing heavy metals and controlling gene expression, like the p53 cancer gene, and NFKappaB, involved in inflammation. We discussed in the last chapter the important effect that zinc has on immune function, inflammation, and cytokine production, and in supporting phase I detoxification in the liver. Combining zinc, SAMe, and 5-MTHF has improved many of our patients' overall functioning.

IMPORTANT HERBAL PROTOCOLS FOR LYME NUTRITIONAL THERAPIES

I started using herbal protocols for treating Lyme disease back in 2002. The majority of my patients were relapsing once they were taken off antibiotics, especially the ones who had been ill for many years before receiving a proper diagnosis. However, I knew that I couldn't leave my patients on antibiotics forever.

There are a few different regimens that I have found effective. The first is based on traditional Chinese herbs that had been studied in China for bacteria and parasitic infections that are similar to borrelia, such as syphilis and malaria. The one that I frequently use is called the Zhang protocol, after the doctor who introduced it to me. There are published references in the Chinese medical literature on their use and safety. The Zhang protocol consists of using several herbs in varied combinations. Many feature the herbs called HH and HH2 (different strengths of Houtiyana) and Circulation P (which helps get the herbs deeper into the tissues). We often end up rotating combinations, such as 2 *Coptis* TID, one HH TID, and one Circulation P TID, or 2 R-5081 TID, with HH (or HH2) and Circulation P. We also add the herbs *Cordyceps* (2, TID) when there is significant fatigue and lack of stamina; Puerarin (2, TID) if there are memory and concentration problems; Artemisia if there are ongoing sweats and chills (history of babesiosis); and, finally, the herbal product AI#3 (autoimmune III), when there is evidence of an overstimulated immune system with inflammation. AI#3 should only be used for two to three months consecutively, 3–5 capsules a day, and then stopped, although it can be used again months later if necessary for those with resistant inflammation.

A second herbal combination is called the Cowden protocol after Dr. William Cowden, an internist and cardiologist who specializes in integrative medicine. He was getting good results helping people with Lyme disease. These herbs are supplied by a company called NutraMedix, and include Samento, Banderol, Cumunda, and *Quina* (all up to 30 drops BID before meals), parsley and Burbur (10 drops BID), Serrapeptase, and Stevia. Dr. Cowden told me that his protocol was highly effective in helping to relieve the symptoms of Lyme disease, and that his herbs had also been studied in the laboratory for efficacy and safety. I did my own study and confirmed their efficacy. Samento, Banderol, Cumunda, and *Quina* target *Borrelia burgdorferi* and may affect different co-infections by their antibacterial, antiviral, antiparasitic, and antifungal effects. Dr. Eva Sapi took Samento and Banderol into the laboratory and proved that they were in fact killing borrelia, and that Stevia was breaking up biofilms. Burbur and parsley are used to help support detoxification during treatment, especially during Jarisch-Herxheimer reactions, where they can be used more frequently (up to 6 to 8 times per day if necessary). I have found significant improvements with fatigue, muscle and joint pains, neurological symptoms (light sensitivity, dizziness, headaches, and cognitive problems), as well as with sleep and moods.

I refer to a third combination as the Buhner protocol, named after Stephen Buhner, the author of *Healing Lyme*. He suggests using Samento in combination with other herbs, such as *Andrographis, Polygonum* (Japanese knotweed/resveratrol), *Stephania* root, and *Smilax* in patients with Lyme disease. I liked that these herbs had been studied extensively, and that the results were published in the scientific literature. These are the primary actions for these herbs:

1. ***Andrographis paniculata***: antibacterial, antiviral, anti-spirochetal, antifilarial, antimalarial, anti-inflammatory, and analgesic. It crosses the blood-brain barrier and helps decrease inflammation in the central nervous system, as well as helping modulate autoimmune reactions.

2. ***Polygonum cuspidatum* (Japanese knotweed/resveratrol):** antibacterial, antiviral, anti-spirochetal, antifungal, immunomodulatory (affects autoimmune reactions), anti-inflammatory, and has antioxidant properties.

3. ***Smilax* (sarsaparilla):** anti-spirochetal, antiparasitic, immunomodulatory, lessens Jarisch-Herxheimer reactions, binds endotoxins, anti-inflammatory, neuroprotective (crosses the blood-brain barrier), enhances cognitive function, protects the liver, and normalizes liver functions.

4. ***Stephania* root:** antiparasitic, anti-inflammatory, antioxidant, decreases cytokines (IL1-Beta, TNF-α, IL-6).

We find that we are able to use these herbs alone or in combination, with patients both on and off antibiotics, to help improve resistant symptomatology. For example, some with severe Jarisch-Herxheimer reactions have taken *Smilax* in combination with other herbs, such as redroot, boneset, and/or Teasel root (Researched Nutritional's BLT formula, or Greenwood Herbal's Herxheimer formula) and found it to be effective, especially when alkalizing and using oral glutathione have inadequately controlled their symptoms. Green Dragon Botanicals in Vermont is another well-known source for these herbs. We have found them to be safe, but just as with classic medications, they are contraindicated under certain conditions (pregnancy, active gallbladder disease) and can have side effects, such as gastrointestinal upset, allergic reactions, or changing drug levels in the body. The use of these herbal compounds should therefore be monitored carefully by a healthcare practitioner, and the suggested dosages can be found on the manufacturers' Web sites.

The last herbal regimen that we often use is the Byron White protocol. This is another Chinese-based regimen with multiple herbs in combination formulas (i.e., A-L has allicin and *Coptis* to treat Lyme disease and includes antiparasitic herbs, such as clove, black walnut, and wormwood). There are many formulas for co-infections (i.e., A-Bart for Bartonella, A-Myco for Mycoplasma, A-Bio for a broad range of bacteria), and include antiviral (i.e., A-EB/H6, A-V, A-CM), antifungal (A-FNG), antiparasitic (A-P), detoxification (NT detox, BT detox, Detox I and II), as well as anti-inflammatory formulas (like A-Inflam). We find them to be very promising for resistant patients who fail antibiotics, other herbal protocols, or continue to relapse when they are off antibiotics. They also can cause severe Jarisch-Herxheimer reactions if not used properly (requiring decreased dosages, as per individual sensitivity), as is the case with the other herbal protocols described above, and they should only be used under the guidance of a healthcare practitioner. Oftentimes patients only require small doses of several of these formulas (like A-L and A-Bart several drops twice a day) to be effective.

Other herbal protocols exist for the treatment of Lyme and co-infections like the Beyond Balance formulas (i.e., BB-1, BB-2, MC-Bab-1, MC-Bab-2, MC-Bab-3, Bar-1) as well as the Researched Nutritional formulas, BLT and Cryptoplus, which can all be helpful. We have also used the Biocidin protocol, which contains essential oils, to treat dysbiosis of the gut (Candida, parasites). Some patients report overall feeling better, and recent scientific studies have shown it may also be effective in some suffering from tick-borne disease. We have not personally studied other herbal protocols on the market for safety and efficacy. However, the ones we use on a regular basis assist with many of the frequent symptoms we see in Lyme-MSIDS, including fatigue, memory problems, muscle and joint pains, sleep problems, and mood disorders. They also can help support the detoxification pathways and relieve Herxheimer reactions, improving quality of life.

OTHER INTEGRATIVE THERAPIES FOR LYME AND ASSOCIATED CO-INFECTIONS

Other therapies being used to treat resistant Lyme and co-infections, unfortunately, have not all been well studied scientifically for either side effects or long-term efficacy. While I don't generally perform the following treatments, I have heard anecdotal results from both patients and practitioners that some of these therapies have been effective. These include:

1. Oxidative therapies (ozone, H2O2, UV light therapy)
2. Homeopathy: i.e., Ledum, syphilitic and malarial nosodes, and others
3. Salt and Vitamin C protocol
4. Rife machines, Coil machines, Bionic 880, other frequency generators
5. Heat therapies, including hyperthermia (clinics in Germany)
6. Magnet therapy
7. Essential oils (such as Young's living oils and Rainbow therapy)
8. CBD oil (Cannabidiol, for seizures, pain; federal and many state laws restrict use)
9. Liposomal Vitamin C (oral, IV Vitamin C)
10. Silver, oral or IV (Argentyn 23, other Nano or colloidal preparations)
11. Fecal transplant therapy (for inflammation, not C. difficile)
12. Master Miracle Solution (MMS): sodium hypochlorite
13. Stem cell therapies or other live cell injections
14. Hormonal therapies (i.e., human growth hormone)
15. Hyperbaric treatments (standard [-2.4 ATM] and lower O_2 therapy)
16. IV Mold toxin therapy (such as the Kane protocol)
17. IV chelation for heavy metals (IV EDTA, IV DMPS)
18. IV detoxification therapies (i.e., Meyers Cocktails, others)
19. Low-dose immunotherapy

As integrative medicine/functional medicine is adopted in major universities, clinics (e.g., Cleveland Clinic), and hospitals across the United States (including Harvard), it would be beneficial for these institutions to establish a partnership with integrative practitioners and/or the office of alternative medicine (OAM) at the National Institutes of Health to properly study these therapies, in order to best serve the rapidly expanding number of individuals suffering from Lyme and associated co-infections.

ELEVEN

Lyme and Mitochondrial Dysfunction

Constant fatigue is one of the most common complaints of individuals with Lyme-MSIDS. Even when we are relatively healthy, many of us feel that we don't have the energy we should have to get through our busy lives. But where does our energy really come from?

The energy that keeps us going is made through a complex series of biochemical reactions known as the Krebs cycle, which takes place in the powerhouse of every cell known as the mitochondria. Adenosine triphosphate (ATP), the most important energy molecule in the body, is produced by the mitochondria. Adenosine triphosphate transports chemical energy to help power our metabolism; however, when the mitochondria are not working properly they cannot make enough ATP, and we experience fatigue.

The energy made in the mitochondria is determined by our diet. If we do not have an adequate supply of healthy fats (the preferred energy source for mitochondria), carbohydrates, and proteins to feed into stage 1 of the Krebs cycle, we will experience fatigue. This is seen in chronic fatigue syndrome, when nutritional and enzyme deficiencies lead to poor digestion. And if our diet is deficient in the amino acids found in protein-rich foods, we will not be able to keep up with the energy requirements of our cells.

If we are exposed to a large load of environmental chemicals that need to be detoxified, we may use up nutrients like B vitamins and magnesium, which are essential for mitochondrial energy production. These environmental chemicals also stimulate free radical production, which damages fragile mitochondrial membranes. Again, the result is fatigue, which is seen in diseases such as chemical sensitivity and environmental illness (EI).

THE CAUSES OF MITOCHONDRIAL DAMAGE

Mitochondrial dysfunction is one of the common pathways to many chronic diseases. Each mitochondrion has four main compartments: the outer membrane, the inner membrane, the matrix, and the intermembranous space. Any abnormal functioning in these areas will directly impact the mitochondria. Mitochondrial damage also occurs when free radicals are released during the process of creating ATP, when you eat a high-sugar diet, or when there is oxidative stress from environmental chemicals. Many infections and even medications can damage mitochondrial structures, thereby complicating the diagnosis, since both the diseases and their drug treatments can cause similar symptoms, primarily fatigue. These medications include:

- Analgesics (aspirin, acetaminophen, and other anti-inflammatory drugs such as NSAIDs)
- Angina medications and antiarrhythmics (Cordarone/amiodarone)
- Antianxiety medications, such as Xanax (alprazolam)
- Antibiotics (tetracyclines)
- Antidepressants, such as amitriptyline (Elavil) and SSRIs, such as Prozac (fluoxetine)
- Antipsychotics (haloperidol, risperidone)
- Bile acid sequesters (cholestyramine/Questran, colesevelam/WelChol)
- Cancer drugs
- Cholesterol medications, including the statins (atorvastatin/Lipitor, fluvastatin/Lescol, lovastatin/Mevacor, pravastatin/Pravachol, rosuvastatin/Crestor)
- Diabetes medications (Glucophage/metformin, troglitazone, rosiglitazone)
- Epilepsy medications (valproic acid/Depakote)

- Mood stabilizers (lithium)
- Parkinson's disease medications (tolcapone/Tasmar, entacapone/Comtan)
- Treatments for alcoholism (Antabuse/disulfiram)

However, many people need these drugs to treat chronic diseases (like tetracyclines for Lyme disease) and at the same time, feel better with more energy, not worse. Understanding the above drugs' potential effects on the mitochondria suggests, however, that mitochondrial support during and after treatments with the above medications may be useful. Researchers at the University of Manchester in 2015, working with the Kimmel Cancer Center in Philadelphia, identified a novel way to use the side effects of antibiotics on mitochondria: to kill cancer stem cells. The team used five types of antibiotics, including doxycycline, on cell lines of eight different types of tumors, and found that four of them eradicated the cancer stem cells for glioblastoma (a very aggressive type of brain tumor recently linked to excessive cell phone radiation), as well as ovarian, breast, prostate, lung, pancreatic, and skin cancer. This research opens up potentially new avenues in cancer treatment, because mitochondria are the source of energy for not only our cells but also cancer stem cells as they mutate and divide to form tumors.

A list of medications that should be avoided (as well as ones for treatment) is available in a 2009 published paper, "The Modern Treatment of Mitochondrial Disease," and it can be found on the Web site of the Mitochondrial Medicine Society (www.mitosoc.org). Many common infections, like herpes virus infections (herpes virus I, cytomegalovirus, Epstein-Barr), can be found as latent infections in neurons, and they are also known to cause mitochondrial DNA (mtDNA) damage, leading to neurodegenerative diseases like Alzheimer's. If we are to address the multifactorial overlapping causes of chronic fatiguing, musculoskeletal illnesses, and neurodegenerative diseases, we must find a way to decrease mitochondrial damage and repair these essential organelles inside our cells.

How Do I Know If I Have Mitochondrial Damage?

We can indirectly determine if there is damage to the mitochondria by measuring markers of free radical/oxidative stress on membrane lipids (lipid peroxides), proteins (protein carbonyls), and DNA

(8-oxo-dG), as well as measuring levels of nutrients essential for proper mitochondrial function, like CoQ10, and acetyl-L-carnitine (which shuttles fatty acids as a fuel source into the mitochondria). In a study of those suffering from chronic fatigue syndrome and fibromyalgia, CFS/FM patients had significantly increased levels of lipid peroxidation, respectively ($p<0.001$ for both CFS and FM patients with regard to controls) that were indicative of oxidative stress-induced mitochondrial damage. Great Plains Laboratories also recently created a Toxic Organic Chemical Exposure Profile (GPL-Tox), which measures 168 different toxic chemicals including organophosphate pesticides, phthalates, benzene, xylene, vinyl chloride, pyrethrin insecticides, and Tiglyglycine (TG), a marker for mitochondrial disorders resulting from mutations of mitochondrial DNA. These mutations can be caused by exposure to environmental chemicals, infections, inflammation, and nutritional deficiencies. By measuring oxidative stress, mitochondrial nutrients, environmental chemicals, and TG, we can get a picture of the health of our mitochondria.

We can also check for inherited genetic conditions associated with mitochondrial dysfunction by doing muscle biopsies and looking at histopathological findings and Krebs respiratory chain enzymes, checking for high levels of lactic acid in the blood, doing exercise testing and electromyography (EMGs) to check for peripheral neuropathy, as well as testing mitochondrial genes and/or nuclear genes. Since the brain and CNS is involved in up to 60 percent of those with mitochondrial disorders, brain magnetic resonance imaging (MRI) and magnetic resonance spectroscopy (MRS) are other diagnostic tools that can respectively identify relatively specific abnormalities (such as basal ganglia calcification) and nonspecific abnormalities (such as white-matter changes) as well as intracerebral lactate elevations. Inherited disorders of mitochondrial dysfunction can cause some of the same symptoms we see in persistent Lyme disease (i.e., neurological symptoms, including cognitive impairment, neuropathy, encephalopathy, and musculoskeletal symptoms), and they may be among the underlying causes driving resistant symptomatology for those with MSIDS.

Diseases Related to Mitochondrial Dysfunction

Apart from fatigue, there is a link between mitochondrial dysfunction and many other diseases. Mitochondria are found in all of the cells of our bodies (except red blood cells), but they are particularly abundant in those organs that are needing active and abundant sources of energy, such as the skeletal muscles, heart muscle, liver, kidneys, and brain. If mitochondrial dysfunction were to happen in the heart, it could lead to various cardiac conditions, including conduction defects, cardiovascular disease, cardiomyopathy (an enlargement of the heart that leads to poor cardiac output and congestive heart failure), and atherosclerosis. Mitochondrial dysfunction in skeletal muscles leads to weakness, low muscle tone (hypotonia), exercise intolerance, and myofascial pain. If it were to affect the liver, it could cause hypoglycemia, with low blood sugars secondary to defects in glucose production (gluconeogenesis), nonalcoholic fatty liver disease (steatohepatitis), cancer, and hepatitis C–associated hepatocellular carcinoma. In the kidneys, it can result in proximal tubular dysfunction (Fanconi's syndrome) and cause a loss of essential amino acids, electrolytes, and minerals such as magnesium.

When mitochondrial dysfunction affects the brain, it sets the stage for a host of neurological diseases, including ADHD, autism, Alzheimer's disease, Huntington's and Parkinson's disease; psychiatric disorders, such as schizophrenia, bipolar disorder, depression, and anxiety disorders; or as various dysfunctions of the central and peripheral nervous system. When the optic nerve and visual systems are affected, we can experience optic neuritis and visual loss. When the eighth cranial nerve, which sends signals from the inner ear to the brain, is affected, we can experience hearing loss. When the peripheral nerves are affected, we can experience neuropathic pain, chronic inflammatory demyelinating polyneuropathy (CIDP), and problems with the autonomic nervous system, such as postural orthostatic tachycardia syndrome (POTS), which can result in low blood pressure, palpitations and fainting, absent or excessive sweating, and problems with temperature regulation. It can even contribute to autoimmune disorders, type 2 diabetes, premature aging, and cancer.

These different diseases, all caused by mitochondrial dysfunction, may also be worsened with oxidative stress, and exposure to multiple environmental chemicals including heavy metals—mercury, lead, arsenic, cadmium, and aluminum—can increase oxidative stress. The resulting increase of free radicals adversely affects many different neurological conditions, including Alzheimer's and Parkinson's disease, and a wide variety of central nervous system disorders, including Lyme-MSIDS. Free radicals are produced in Lyme disease patients infected with *Borrelia burgdorferi*, and these not only damage mitochondrial cell membranes but also activate microglia in the brain, the cells that act as the main form of active immune defense in the central nervous system. This stimulates the production of proinflammatory cytokines, which cause symptoms of fatigue, muscle and joint pain, neuropathy, headaches, mood disorders, and cognitive difficulties.

Some of my Lyme-MSIDS patients experience episodes of optic neuritis and visual and hearing loss. Many have neuropathy (present in up to 70 percent of persistent Lyme disease patients), and CIDP (chronic inflammatory demyelinating polyneuropathy), as well as POTS and autonomic nervous system dysfunction. Neuropathy is common in all of these diseases, in which there is a loss of myelin sheathing that protects nerve fibers. This may be the result of multiple infections, immune damage, environmental toxins, or problems with proper detoxification, all of which can produce free radicals and damage the fragile mitochondrial membranes. The first human mitochondrial DNA (mtDNA) diseases causing neuropathy and myopathy were reported in 1988, such as Leber hereditary optic neuropathy (LHON). Many genetic variants have been identified since that time.

MITOCHONDRIAL DYSFUNCTION AND METABOLIC SYNDROME

Metabolic syndrome is defined as a cluster of at least three of the following five metabolic conditions: hypertension, truncal obesity (abdominal belly fat), abnormal glucose tolerance, elevated triglyceride levels, and low HDL cholesterol. Several scientific studies have now shown that one of the defects in metabolic syndrome and its associated diseases is excess cellular oxidative stress, with associated damage to the mitochondria.

Mitochondrial damage can also be a by-product of metabolic syndrome and insulin resistance. In metabolic syndrome, higher than normal levels of insulin are required to regulate blood sugar levels. One of insulin's primary effects in the body is to take sugar and convert it into fat, which is stored as a source of energy. When fat is being stored abnormally in muscle and liver cells, it causes a breakdown of the cells' normal functioning, which subsequently affects the mitochondria. Researchers have also determined that vascular endothelial growth factor B (VEGFB), which is produced by skeletal muscle, heart muscle, and brown adipose tissue, also promotes the movement of fat from the bloodstream across vascular endothelial cells and into the target organs. Researchers have seen a strong positive correlation between VEGFB and mitochondrial function.

We see metabolic syndrome frequently among our MSIDS patients. Although clinicians often rely on weight gain and abnormal lipid levels as warnings of disease risk in metabolic disorders such as type 2 diabetes and associated heart disease, we now know that fat accumulation in the metabolic organs (i.e., skeletal muscle, liver, and heart) is an even stronger predictor of morbidity and mortality. What's more, a diet high in sugar often causes reactive hypoglycemia (blood sugar swings) and fatigue, increases the risk of fungal and Candida overgrowth, causes weight gain with increased abdominal obesity (which increases production of cytokines), and adversely affects mitochondrial function. Therefore, try and avoid simple carbohydrates as much as possible, especially since certain sugars, such as fructose and lactose (found in milk products), have approximately ten times the glycation activity of glucose, the primary body fuel. Glycation is when a sugar molecule attaches to the proteins or lipids of our body without an enzyme, causing new types of sugar molecules to form; these are known as advanced glycation end products (AGEs). These bind to receptors for advanced glycation end products (RAGEs), and the result is increased inflammation driving cytokine production. Diseases linked to RAGEs include: diabetes, with eye, kidney, and nerve complications (retinopathy, nephropathy, and neuropathy); atherosclerotic heart disease; peripheral vascular disease; and neurological diseases, such as Alzheimer's. Strictly avoiding simple sugars, keeping down the total carbohydrate load to less than 60 grams of sugar per day, and eating a Paleo type diet that is higher in healthy fats forces the body into a ketogenic state, which can be very helpful to increase our energy stores, lower inflammation, and support mitochondrial function.

What exactly are healthy fats? Eating too much saturated fat (animal fat) and trans fats (like margarines) is unhealthy, but increasing healthy dietary fat like olive oil and avocados in a low carbohydrate Mediterranean diet, is helpful for sustained weight loss and health. Also, ketones are formed when we break down fats, and they are a healthier form of energy than sugars (except in poorly controlled type I diabetics). Mitochondria are primarily designed to use fat, not sugars, to make energy, and high-fat, ketogenic diets have been used in medicine for conditions as diverse as resistant epilepsy, autism, ADHD, Alzheimer's disease, ALS, Parkinson's disease, migraines, obesity, cardiovascular disease, and type 2 diabetes.

Mitochondria are significant players in many complex diseases and contribute to the process of inflammation through the assemblage of a large molecular complex called the "inflammasome." This is created when mitochondrial membrane damage occurs, and the inflammasome further stimulates the production of inflammatory cytokines, leading to a vicious cycle of fatigue and inflammation, contributing to diseases like CFS/FM, autoimmunity, as well as a broad range of cardiovascular, GI, and neurological conditions.

HOW CAN I INCREASE MITOCHONDRIAL PRODUCTION?

The benefits of increasing the production of mitochondria can include an increased energy level, better exercise performance, increased metabolic functions in major organs, a subsequent loss of body fat and increased lean muscle mass, less oxidative stress, and the possible reversal of metabolic syndrome. In order to do this, we need to turn on a switch inside the mitochondria, called PGC-1α, which is one of the master regulators of mitochondrial development and metabolism. If the PGC-1α switch is turned off, whether through inactivity or obesity, we don't produce as many new mitochondria, or the existing mitochondria do not function as efficiently, which can lead to decreased energy production, decreased oxidation of fats, and the accumulation of lipids in skeletal muscle. Cutting back on our food intake and decreasing the number of calories and sugar (i.e., a ketogenic diet) while increasing our exercise is one way to turn on this PGC-1α switch and increase mitochondrial biogenesis, which is also important for preventing chronic disease.

There are three different types of nutritional supplements that can also positively affect PGC-1α and turn on the switch:

- L-arginine is an essential amino acid that works on increasing mitochondrial function through its effects on the nitric oxide pathway.

- Alpha-lipoic acid, through food or supplements, can turn on an enzyme called 5' adenosine monophosphate-activated protein kinase, or AMPK (AMP-activated protein kinase). AMPK acts as a metabolic master switch; it regulates several intracellular systems, including the cellular uptake of glucose for energy production and the formation of new mitochondria. When ATP levels go down with exercise, AMPK is stimulated, helping replenish it.

- Resveratrol, either through foods or supplements, activates the sirtuin genes (SIRT1) in the body, stimulating PGC-1α. The sirtuin genes appear to be responsible for preserving the lives of cells, and they influence age-related diseases such as cancer, heart disease, osteoporosis, diabetes, and neurodegeneration. Resveratrol from grapes and berries, and quercetin found in fruits, vegetables, and tea, both exhibit chemical properties that allow them to activate SIRT1 and the sirtuin genes of longevity. Resveratrol can also increase mitochondrial production and enhance exercise tolerance, as well as inhibiting AMPK in the hypothalamus and activating AMPK in the peripheral tissues. To date, it is the only supplement known to do this.

Combining alpha-lipoic acid and resveratrol (occasionally with L-arginine) to stimulate mitochondrial production may therefore be useful in certain chronically fatigued individuals with mitochondrial dysfunction. Using L-arginine may be contraindicated in certain patients with Lyme-MSIDS, who experience sickness syndrome, or certain diseases, such as migraines and inflammatory bowel disease, as it can exacerbate all of these conditions. Antioxidants that protect fragile mitochondrial membranes may also be helpful (Vitamins C and E), especially those that also act as epigenetic modifiers (like broccoli seed extract [sulforaphane], curcumin, and green tea extract), as well as B vitamins, minerals like magnesium, and interventions (dietary, meditation) that positively affect telomeres, the ends/caps of our DNA strands. Long telomeres equate with increased longevity, and when there is a shortening of telomeres, it disturbs mitochondria function and decreases energy production, increases oxidative stress/free radicals, and leads to the cell's self-destruction.

Two newer methods that may improve mitochondrial function and increase energy are high intensity interval training (HIIT) and intermittent fasting. Exercising with HIIT techniques for one minute (i.e., three twenty-second intervals) has been shown to be equivalent to exercising for forty minutes. You may need to gradually increase your exercise before attempting HIIT, which should be done under the supervision of an exercise physiologist/physical therapist.

Intermittent fasting is known to increase metabolism, mental clarity, mitochondrial function, and energy, while decreasing blood pressure, glucose and LDL cholesterol, weight and visceral fat (improving metabolic efficiency), as well as inflammation/CRP. It can reproduce some of the cardiovascular benefits associated with physical exercise.

REPAIR THE DAMAGE: LIPID REPLACEMENT THERAPY

Lipid replacement therapy (LRT) is part of Rule #4 of the Action Plan. It involves replacing unhealthy fats in the body with healthy ones at the cellular membrane level. Lipid replacement therapy is different from just the substitution of certain dietary fats with others for proposed health benefits. We are specifically referring to phospholipids, such as phosphatidylcholine (PC), which are major components of our cell membranes. They can be obtained from a variety of readily available sources, such as egg yolk or soybeans, and are also found in supplements and foods containing lecithin. As we age and accumulate toxins in our bodies, like mold, the PC layer of our cell membranes may be damaged. Lipid replacement therapy assists in exchanging damaged cellular lipids for healthy ones to ensure the proper structure and function of the cells. We have used oral lipid replacement therapy in many Lyme-MSIDS patients with fatigue and elevated levels of mold, and have found it to be effective.

We can use LRT to support mitochondrial function by using supplements such as NT factors/ATP Fuel (glycosylated phospholipids, such as those from Researched Nutritionals), three tablets two times per day for two months, followed by three per day, which helps repair damaged mitochondrial cell membranes. NT factor is most often prescribed with other supplements that support mitochondrial function, such as acetyl-L-carnitine (which transports fats into the mitochondria), CoQ10, NADH (which is part of the electron transport chain that creates energy), and occasionally, D-ribose (which acts as a fuel for energy production but needs to be limited in patients with metabolic syndrome and diabetes who have elevated levels of glycation). When individuals have elevated levels of mold toxins, we have found that adding 3 grams of phosphatidylcholine with liposomal glutathione, NAC, alpha-lipoic acid, N-butyrate, and toxin binders (cholestyramine, bentonite clay, and/or charcoal, taken several hours away from food and supplements) also has effectively lowered levels of mold. Recent clinical trials have shown that lipid replacement therapy (LRT) plus NADH and CoQ10 can also prevent excess oxidative mitochondrial membrane damage and restore mitochondrial and other cellular membrane functions, which reduce fatigue. It was shown to be safe and effective in treating intractable chronic fatigue, fibromyalgia, and unresolved Lyme disease. If you are actively treated for babesiosis with Mepron or Malarone, do not take CoQ10 with LRT. Atovaquone's action is on the mitochondrial electron transport chain in parasites, and CoQ10 inhibits its action.

DAVID'S MITOCHONDRIAL DYSFUNCTION AFFECTED HIS HEART

David was fifty-eight when he first came to me complaining of severe fatigue, muscle and joint pains, swelling of the legs, significant shortness of breath, and worsening memory and concentration problems. His past medical history was significant for hypertension, hyperlipidemia, atherosclerotic heart disease, and a cardiomyopathy. He had already seen a cardiologist, who sent him for an echocardiogram, which showed that the muscles of his heart were weak and not functioning properly. His ejection fraction (the volume of blood pumped from the heart) was 28 percent on the echocardiogram, which is the equivalent of having severe congestive heart failure. His doctors assumed it was from a combination of heart disease and a probable viral infection, causing a viral myocarditis and cardiomyopathy. They treated him with standard cardiac regimens of Lanoxin, Lasix, Aldactone, ACE inhibitors, and a statin drug, Mevacor, for his elevated cholesterol. His cardiac function did improve a bit with this medication regimen, but he was still complaining of being quite tired with significant shortness of breath.

David remembered being bitten by a tick years earlier. He did not notice an unusual rash but did remember feeling flulike symptoms several days after the bite. Those eventually disappeared, but he never felt the same afterward. Now that his heart issues were mostly under control, he didn't know if his fatigue, intermittent joint and muscle pain, and poor memory were just old age or Lyme disease that had gone untreated.

I had David fill out the HMQ, and we administered a physical exam, which revealed a normal blood pressure and no abnormal heart sounds. I picked up some faint crackling in the lungs (signs of fluid overload) and a slight edema of the lower extremities, again consistent with his history of congestive heart failure. We sent off a Lyme Western blot with a full tick-borne co-infection panel and a fungal and viral panel, and did a CBC, a CMP, vitamin levels with his MTFHR gene status and homocysteine levels, checked his mineral levels, as well as hormone panels for thyroid, adrenal, and sex hormone deficiencies. We also sent off bloods for a HbA1c for metabolic syndrome, did a high-sensitivity CRP, and fibrinogen levels with a full lipid panel; finally, we checked him for food allergies, gluten sensitivity, and heavy metals.

David's Western blot came back strongly positive, confirming past exposure to Lyme disease, with positive tests for ehrlichiosis and Rocky Mountain spotted fever. His heavy metal tests revealed significant exposure to mercury, lead, arsenic, and cadmium, as well as to small amounts of uranium, even though he couldn't recall any type of toxic exposure. His food allergy tests revealed IgG-delayed food hypersensitivity reactions to dairy, wheat, and corn, and his adrenal function as well as his mineral levels were low. He had a normal serum magnesium but a low red blood cell magnesium level (implying total body magnesium deficiency) and a low zinc level. His CRP was high, consistent with inflammation, and his HbA1c was 6.0, confirming that he was prediabetic and suffered from metabolic syndrome. His hyperlipidemia was controlled on his statin drug, as he had an LDL of 72, but now he was diagnosed with elevated blood sugars and inflammation, which were all separate risk factors worsening his underlying cardiovascular disease. He was also found to be MTHFR positive, with an elevated homocysteine level at 16. This is another cardiac risk factor that could have been responsible for the development of his atherosclerotic heart disease.

Based on these test results, there were multiple reasons why he was not feeling energetic, and could also explain why he continued to suffer from muscle and joint pains and memory problems. We started David on Plaquenil and minocycline for his Lyme and co-infections. He was given adrenal support with low-dose Cortef and adrenal supplements. We recommended that he follow a very low-carbohydrate diet, having small frequent meals that would treat his metabolic syndrome, and told him to avoid his allergic foods. He was given a multivitamin with B_6, methyl B_{12}, activated folic acid for his elevated homocysteine level and MTHFR status, and nystatin tablets to control yeast overgrowth.

We also discussed trying mitochondrial support. I suggested using four different types of supplements that together would hopefully improve his energy level and help treat the cardiomyopathy. His high CRP alerted us to chronic inflammation, and since mitochondrial cell membranes have no protection against free radical stress, there was a high likelihood that they had been damaged. The first supplement used was enzyme CoQ10, which is an essential nutrient in the mitochondrial pathway necessary for proper heart muscle function (statin drugs, like the one he was taking, have been shown to deplete CoQ10 from the body). The second supplement was acetyl-L-carnitine, which provides a transport mechanism to get fatty acids into the mitochondria to make ATP. The third was NT factor, which may indirectly help heart function by helping the muscles of the heart operate more efficiently. Finally, he was given adequate amounts of minerals, such as zinc and magnesium, in which he was deficient. The zinc could help decrease his cytokine levels and improve his immunity, and the magnesium would support his heart muscle function.

A month later David reported that his energy level and his joint and muscle pain were better. His stamina had increased, his shortness of breath had decreased, and I suggested that after six months on this regimen, he recheck his echocardiogram to see if his heart muscle function had improved. He agreed, and after six months of rotating through several antibiotic regimens, chelating his heavy metals, taking hormonal support for his adrenals, shoring up his mineral deficiencies, and giving him mitochondrial support, he returned to see us with his new echocardiogram report in hand. His ejection fraction had increased to 42 percent, roughly a 30 percent improvement in cardiac function. He was no longer winded with exertion and wasn't waking up in the middle of the night with shortness of breath. His lungs were clear, and the edema of his lower extremities had improved, all signs that his congestive heart symptoms and cardiomyopathy were resolving. In short, treating David's Lyme disease and multiple abnormalities on the MSIDS map, including mitochondrial dysfunction, improved his energy, cardiac functioning, and overall well-being.

TWELVE

Lyme and Hormones

ormone deficiencies and imbalances are some of the most commonly overlooked causes for the failure of antibiotics in MSIDS, and I often find that by treating them I can restore my patients' health. Sometimes adrenal function is low, and they aren't producing enough of the hormones necessary for an adequate response to stress (i.e., cortisol), contributing to chronic fatigue and resistant symptomatology. Others have abnormal patterns of cortisol secretion, where the cortisol level is high at night, interfering with sleep. They can also have anti-thyroid antibodies, as Lyme frequently causes autoimmune manifestations, with associated clinical hypothyroidism. Or, they may have low levels of sex hormones: I often see young men, even those in their twenties and thirties, whom I diagnose with andropause (low testosterone), or women occasionally present with amenorrhea (lack of menstrual cycles), irregular cycles, or early menopause, who are in their late thirties or early forties. A large percentage of American men and women also have insulin resistance, with hypoglycemia and metabolic syndrome. Often several hormonal abnormalities coexist, which can increase the severity of symptoms and contribute to the underlying disease process.

Most often, patients who have clinical hormone imbalances complain of an increase in fatigue and a lack of stamina. Low adrenal and low thyroid hormones (T3, T4), low growth hormone and sex hormones (testosterone, affecting men and women), and insulin resistance with low blood sugars can all cause fatigue.

Hormonal imbalances also cause problems with maintaining or losing weight. With hypothyroidism (low thyroid function), patients gain weight, and in hyperthyroidism (high thyroid function), they tend to lose weight. Polycystic ovarian syndrome (PCOS) is characterized in women by multiple ovarian cysts; irregular menses; high levels of male hormones, causing acne and/or abnormal hair growth; and is oftentimes associated with high-cholesterol and type 2 diabetes and/or high insulin levels with insulin resistance. These women will gain weight and have great difficulty taking it off. Insulin resistance is a precursor to type 2 diabetes, in which cells do not respond to the normal action of insulin, causing blood sugar levels to rise, and it is a factor in metabolic syndrome. Researchers recently identified a set of somatic symptoms, which are present in the majority of those suffering from Lyme and associated co-infections (i.e., fatigue, joint and back pain, headaches, dizziness, shortness of breath, and insomnia), which are premonitory signs of type 2 diabetes long before clinical recognition. Lyme causes inflammation and can be associated with weight gain and hyperinsulinemia.

Hyperinsulinemia often coexists with insulin resistance and may contribute to many inflammatory conditions, including vascular disease, type 2 diabetes, nonalcoholic fatty liver disease, and obesity, as well as certain cancers and dementias like Alzheimer's. It also affects cytokines and other hormones including leptin, adiponectin, and estrogen. Resistance to leptin (the hormone from fat that regulates appetite and metabolism) can occur simultaneously with high levels of insulin, further increasing the difficulty in losing weight. Women with these conditions usually require a medication such as Glucophage to stop gluconeogenesis—the production of sugar in the liver—and to help with insulin resistance, and/or go on a strict Paleo-type diet with healthy fats, high protein, and very low carbohydrates (below 60 grams/day) to help with weight loss. Cushing's disease (an overactive adrenal gland) and high cortisol secretion will increase weight, whereas low cortisol with adrenal insufficiency (Addison's disease) usually results in a loss of weight. Low testosterone levels can contribute to weight loss through the loss of muscle mass, and it may cause body fat to shift toward the abdominal region, increasing abdominal girth, as it may with insulin resistance. Low testosterone, elevated levels of the hormone prolactin (one with many functions, including milk production), and slightly elevated levels of cortisol can also be seen in weight loss syndromes, such as in AIDS patients, who lose weight rapidly.

Pain and inflammation are also part of the symptom complex of endocrine conditions. Various chronic inflammatory conditions, auto-immune diseases, such as rheumatoid arthritis and lupus, as well as CFS/SEID and fibromyalgia, can all result in immune disorders and neuroendocrine abnormalities. Autoimmune diseases are more common in women than in men, and in the case of rheumatoid arthritis and lupus, estrogen levels can accelerate and androgens, such as DHEA, can inhibit the development of the disease. Hormonal manipulation by lowering prolactin levels in some autoimmune eye diseases like uveitis and iridocyclitis can even lead to the remission of autoimmune symptoms.

Growth hormone and prolactin also play important roles in regulating inflammatory reactions. Scientific studies have shown that they both increase resistance to bacterial infection, and therefore may be important factors in fighting chronic infections. This could explain, in part, the resistant symptoms seen in patients with growth hormone deficiency.

Other hormonal abnormalities that may contribute to autoimmune diseases are caused by defects in the hypothalamic-pituitary-adrenal (HPA) axis. The hypothalamus and the pituitary gland are located in the brain, and the adrenal gland is located right above the kidneys. The HPA axis is the master controller of hormones, via a feedback loop. The hypothalamus monitors the levels of hormones in the blood and then sends out a message to the pituitary gland (via hypothalamic releasing hormones) to increase or decrease its secretion of hormones. The pituitary then secretes "stimulating" hormones, which affect the production of other hormones, such as thyroid hormones (TSH, thyroid stimulating hormone); adrenal hormones (ACTH, adrenocorticotropic hormone); sex hormones (LH, luteinizing hormone, and FSH, follicle-stimulating hormone, which affect testosterone and estrogen levels); growth hormone (GH); hormones associated with autoimmune diseases and pregnancy (prolactin); and influences melanocyte-stimulating hormone (MSH), which affects melanocyte production (darkening of the skin), appetite, and sexual arousal. Inflammation from multiple sources, such as Lyme, associated co-infections, and environmental toxins (like mold), can all affect the hypothalamic-pituitary-adrenal (HPA) axis and potentially lead to hormonal deficiencies.

The hypothalamus has many other roles, including controlling body temperature and sleep, regulating hunger and thirst, as well as having an effect on our immune system. When functioning well, the HPA axis helps suppress excessive cytokine production and inflammation through a feedback loop. However, cytokines themselves can also affect the HPA axis and thereby affect hormone levels, especially the production of stress hormones, such as cortisol. Cortisol is the main brake in the production of inflammatory cytokines. Although cortisol production is enhanced by cytokines, shutting down the production of cytokines will only take place if there is no cortisol resistance, and cortisol resistance can be seen in fibromyalgia and Lyme disease.

Defects in the HPA axis due to trauma, infections, and stress all have been reported in the medical literature in patients with both fibromyalgia syndrome and Lyme disease. Similarly, defects in the functioning of the HPA axis show up in autoimmune diseases such as rheumatoid arthritis, where the immune and inflammatory reactions are supposed to raise the levels of steroids in the blood to control inflammation, but do not, due to inflammatory cytokines causing dysfunction in the secretion and function of hormones from the pituitary gland. These abnormalities lower adrenal, thyroid, and sex hormone production by decreasing the pituitary hormones ACTH, TSH, and HCG. This causes abnormal growth hormone and prolactin secretion, with decreased activity of prolactin, higher basal levels of insulin (which leads to metabolic syndrome), furthering inflammation, with diminished serum levels of endorphins, adversely affecting pain control. The cytokines produced in rheumatoid arthritis are therefore able to lower endorphins and multiple hormones simultaneously through their effect on the HPA axis. The result is an increase in fatigue and joint pain.

The endocrine abnormalities that are seen in CFS/SEID, fibromyalgia, as well as in Lyme disease, are linked to cytokine production affecting the HPA axis. It is not sufficient to just treat the symptoms, treat the infections, or give hormonal therapy alone. The underlying problem with cytokine production must be addressed. Once we have addressed all of the causes of inflammation, we will have a better chance of getting the HPA axis to work correctly, although we will often need to rebalance the hormones through hormonal support.

DO I HAVE ISSUES WITH THYROID HORMONES?

Thyroid problems are commonly found in Lyme patients. Some of these problems are from an overactive or underactive adrenal gland affecting thyroid function (high cortisol for example, interferes with conversion of the thyroid hormone T4 into its active form, T3), but often there is an overlapping autoimmune thyroid problem, such as Hashimoto's thyroiditis. In this disease, the thyroid is attacked by antibodies made by an over-stimulated immune system, causing bouts of hyperthyroidism (elevated thyroid hormones) and/or hypothyroidism (low thyroid hormones). In both Lyme disease and Hashimoto's thyroiditis, antithyroid antibodies are produced, such as antithyroglobulin antibodies (anti-TG ABs) and, less frequently, antithyroid peroxidase antibodies (anti-TPO ABs), which may or may not be associated with clinical hypothyroidism. Although Hashimoto's disease can be genetic in origin, infections like Lyme disease can trigger this autoimmune reaction by the process of molecular mimicry, where the immune system tries to attack the infectious agent but instead attacks your body's own tissues. Some integrative practitioners have also seen a link between Hashimoto's thyroiditis and other infectious agents like herpes viruses (i.e., Epstein-Barr and cytomegalovirus), as well as GI pathogens like *Helicobacter* and *Yersinia enterocolitica*, and they have found that treating these infections in combination with gluten-free/Paleo-style (anti-inflammatory) diets can be helpful.

It is important to test thyroid antibodies and all of the thyroid functions when doing the initial MSIDS workup, as the thyroid regulates our general metabolism and energy levels. The initial screening thyroid panel should include tests for anti-TG and anti-TPO antibodies, T4, T3, free T3, and reverse T3 with thyroid-stimulating hormone (TSH). I also usually include a serum iodine level and occasionally selenium level, since we have found that roughly 25 percent of all of our chronically ill patients are deficient in iodine and other trace minerals. Iodine is necessary in the production of T3 and T4, and selenium is necessary in the deiodinase enzyme that converts T4 to T3, so low iodine and selenium may contribute to low thyroid function. In certain predisposed individuals, iodine deficiency combined with too much fluoride in the diet (fluoride antagonizes the effects of iodine) may also lead to a thyroid dysfunction and goiter. Iodine deficiency is also now considered to be a contributing factor that increases the pain of fibrocystic breast disease.

The classic symptoms of hypothyroidism include fatigue, weight gain, dry skin, dry hair, constipation, cold intolerance, and memory and concentration problems. These symptoms may not improve until the levels of T3 and T4 are in the top third of the reference range, with a TSH below 1. Reference ranges are usually established for healthy populations and may not reflect the needs of chronically ill individuals. Some require a TSH level just above the lower range of normal (reflecting improved thyroid function) before they notice a clinical improvement.

Clues that you may be suffering from a low thyroid, apart from the above clinical symptoms, include loss of the external third of the eyebrows, swelling around the ankles (nonpitting edema of the lower extremities), swelling around the eyes/orbits (periorbital edema), scalloping of the tongue, and a delayed Achilles tendon reflex. Basal body temperatures may also be low upon awakening in the morning (around 96 degrees to 97 degrees Fahrenheit).

Hyperthyroidism that accompanies Lyme-MSIDS is usually due to an acute thyroiditis (inflammation of the thyroid from an infection), Graves's disease (autoimmune hyperthyroidism), or hyperfunctioning thyroid nodule(s) with a multinodular goiter, in which independent nodule(s) on an enlarged thyroid gland over secrete thyroid hormones. It is not as frequently seen as hypothyroidism but should always be considered if you have sweating, anxiety, tremors, palpitations, and diarrhea with weight loss. Some of these same symptoms are seen in Lyme disease with coinfections like babesiosis or brucellosis and should always be considered in the differential diagnosis with other hormonal problems, such as the carcinoid syndrome or a pheochromocytoma. Carcinoid tumors can produce a variety of biologically active messenger molecules, such as prostaglandins, serotonin, and histamine. They commonly produce flushing and diarrhea, which can be confused with hyperthyroidism. A pheochromocytoma is usually a benign tumor of the adrenal gland that can also mimic the symptoms of hyperthyroidism through the production of elevated levels of catecholamine hormones, such as epinephrine and norepinephrine. Testing with a full thyroid panel, checking urinary

Vanillylmandelic acid and metanephrines in the urine to rule out a pheochromocytoma, and assessing urinary 5-HIAA levels to rule out carcinoid syndrome will help to differentiate among these illnesses.

There are new reference ranges for thyroid functions established by the American Association of Clinical Endocrinologists. These ranges are usually not included on the standard laboratory reports sent to most medical offices. The new range for TSH is 0.3 to 3.0, and in some patients, TSH levels need to be on the lower end of the spectrum (i.e., a TSH close to 0.3) to see a significant clinical improvement. TSH and T4 also may not be a reliable predictor of other thyroid hormone levels, since both may be suppressed by cytokines. Monitoring levels of T3, free T3 (active thyroid hormones), and using replacement therapies that include T4 and occasionally adding T3 (i.e., Synthroid or Levothroid with Cytomel or Tirosint) or certain desiccated thyroid extracts (Armour Thyroid, Nature-Throid, Westhroid) from bovine or porcine thyroid glands are the most commonly used therapies. Responses to these therapies differ greatly and must be individualized. Certain medications may interfere with thyroid absorption (like proton pump inhibitors [PPIs], H2 blockers, multivitamins with minerals, cholestyramine, and/or charcoal), as can diet (taking them with a meal, high fiber, espresso, soy products, and/or grapefruit), or drugs that increase clearance (like rifampin), so speak to your healthcare provider about your diet and medications, which play a role in determining the efficacy of replacement therapy.

DO I HAVE ADRENAL DYSFUNCTION OR ADRENAL FATIGUE?

The next most common endocrine abnormality that occurs for MSIDS patients is adrenal dysfunction. At least 40 percent to 50 percent of my patients coming in for an initial consultation have adrenal dysfunction, which explains in part their resistant symptoms.

In medical school I was taught that there were two main forms of adrenal disease: Addison's syndrome, which is adrenal failure, and Cushing's syndrome, which is due to an overactive adrenal gland. One could recognize Addison's disease by its major clinical features of fatigue, weight loss, loss of appetite, gastrointestinal complaints of nausea, vomiting, and occasional diarrhea, with hyperpigmentation, low sodium (hyponatremia), and mildly elevated potassium levels. Cushing's disease, on the other hand, is due to elevated levels of cortisol and is responsible for obesity, hypertension, diabetes, hyperpigmentation (similar to the pigmentation seen in Addison's disease), acne, hirsutism (increased hair growth), memory problems, and decreased resistance to infection. Yet we now know that there is a spectrum of adrenal dysfunction that lies between these two diseases, which is what typically presents in Lyme-MSIDS patients.

During times of extended or extreme stress, the adrenal glands go into a "fight or flight" mode and secrete high levels of hormones, such as DHEA, aldosterone, and cortisol. Cortisol's main functions include a proactive mode, in which it helps coordinate circadian rhythms, such as sleeping and eating, and processes involved in attention, learning, and memory. Yet it also has a reactive mode, which enables us to adapt to and cope with stress. We know that Lyme patients are under huge amounts of stress, both mentally and physically. The stress can be caused by their physical health along with its consequences on their jobs, families, and friends. Our patients often have elevated levels of cortisol, either throughout the day or at night, when they are desperately trying to get to sleep. These interfere with their already disturbed sleep patterns, worsening their insomnia. Taking phosphatidylserine at night (and up to three times per day) with adaptogenic herbs during the day such as rhodiola, ashwagandha, and ginseng, as well as B vitamins, vitamin C, and pantothenic acid, will help lower the stress response and support and rebalance the adrenal glands.

Chronically elevated levels of cortisol eventually may lead to adrenal fatigue and burnout, which is associated with recurrent clinical depression, post-traumatic stress disorder, and mild/moderate cognitive impairment. When cortisol levels are chronically too high or too low, the hippocampus, the center for memory and attention, is affected and may be associated with the breakdown of the blood-brain barrier. People with adrenal fatigue are not only tired, they experience salt cravings, hypoglycemia, low blood pressure with dizziness while standing (postural hypotension, seen with POTS/dysautonomia), low libido, nonregenerative sleep, mood changes, and memory problems, many of the same symptoms commonly seen in those with Lyme-MSIDS. Chronically low cortisol levels also interfere with immune functioning, and the MSIDS patient with low cortisol may have chronic infectious symptoms that are resistant to antibiotics. We often need to give our patients adrenal support and rebalance their adrenal hormones, or their chronic symptoms may persist.

Testing and Treating Adrenal Issues

There are several methods for testing adrenal hormones. Blood tests, such as an 8:00 A.M. fasting cortisol level (checking the adrenal hormones first thing in the morning), may give a rough indication of the patient's adrenal status, but it is only a snapshot of the hormone levels, which change throughout the day. A twenty-four-hour urinary cortisol test would be a better indicator of the total production of cortisol throughout the day, and if the levels are in the bottom third of the "normal" range, we would suspect decreased adrenal functioning.

The most specific method of testing for low adrenal function is to do an ACTH challenge. Adrenocorticotropic hormone (ACTH) is the hormone produced by the pituitary gland that stimulates cortisol secretion (as well as other adrenal hormones, such as aldosterone and DHEA sulfate). We can give a patient ACTH and measure the amount of cortisol that is produced. It is considered to be a positive test for low adrenal function if the cortisol levels are less than two times normal after the patient receives a bolus of ACTH. The easiest, simplest, and most practical method, however, is to perform a DHEA/cortisol salivary test. This procedure has been validated as a reliable marker of cortisol levels, reflective of tissue levels of the hormone in the body. There are many good laboratories performing the tests, including Genova, Labrix, and Diagnostek.

There are three phases of adrenal dysfunction associated with chronic illness. Phase I is where there is an acute "fight or flight" response associated with elevated levels of cortisol and early adrenal fatigue, with an elevated or high-normal cortisol level in the morning. If cortisol levels are elevated at night, when it interferes with sleep, we can use phosphorylated serine mixed with melatonin. Vitamins B_5, B_6, and C are also useful in combination with lifestyle modifications that help reduce stress, such as meditation, yoga, deep breathing, exercise, and a healthy diet. Phase II is where there is evolving adrenal fatigue, with normal or low morning cortisol levels and/or low levels during various times of the day. Phase III is established adrenal fatigue, with significantly low cortisol levels throughout the day. In Phase II adrenal fatigue, we often add adaptogenic herbs to the B and C vitamins, such as rhodiola, ashwagandha, ginseng, and

Cordyceps (a medicinal mushroom), and consider an adrenal glandular supplement while continuing to try and achieve better stress management. In Phase III adrenal fatigue, associated with significantly low cortisol levels and a decreased functioning of the HPA axis (where adrenal glandular supplements are usually insufficient), Cortef needs to be added. Although prednisone is generally contraindicated in those with active Lyme and co-infections like Babesia (due to immunosuppressive effects and potential severe relapses), Cortef is safe and effective and can significantly improve health and overall functioning. The hormone DHEA may also be added at this stage, or at any time when levels are low, as DHEA does not just function as a precursor for testosterone and estrogen but also plays a role in stress management. It is secreted in response to ACTH stimulation, as is cortisol, and has been shown to help with mood stability during stressful events. DHEA elevates mood, calms emotions, increases alertness, and helps improve memory. Pregnenolone, the DHEA precursor helping to make cortisol and sex hormones, is also sometimes necessary for patients with chronic stress, as they have a "pregnenolone steal," using it to make adrenal hormones, instead of sex hormones. Adrenal balancing with pregnenolone, DHEA, and cortisol is a foundation of all endocrine balancing, and is often necessary in the Lyme-MSIDS patient.

LARRY WAS AFFECTED BY LOW ADRENAL HORMONES

Larry was forty-five years old when he first came to my office with a history of Lyme disease. He had been sick for nearly thirteen years and had seen multiple physicians for his illness, which started with grand mal seizures. His initial workup at a major medical center in New York City did not reveal a cause for his seizures. Instead, he was told that they were "idiopathic," meaning no clear cause could be discovered. He was placed on Depakote to control them but would still have occasional breakthrough seizures, despite the medication.

Larry had already been to see a host of specialists to treat his vast array of symptoms: drenching night sweats; teeth-chattering chills; recalcitrant insomnia, with associated restless leg syndrome and nocturia (getting up to urinate at least five times per night); irritable bowel symptoms, with alternating constipation and diarrhea; light and sound sensitivity; fatigue; joint pain and low-back pain, with associated neuropathy; and severe memory and concentration problems, with overwhelming depression. Larry was completely homebound due to his illness, as he was in the bathroom for up to four hours a day trying to relieve his bowels and constantly urinating. He became so forlorn over his resistant symptoms that his depression worsened and led to thoughts of suicide.

Another physician had diagnosed him with Lyme disease based on his history of multiple tick bites, even though his Lyme ELISA was negative and his Western blot was not CDC-positive. The physician initially prescribed high-dose amoxicillin, which only gave him minimal improvement in his physical symptoms. His memory and concentration problems were so severe that he was then prescribed IV Rocephin to get better penetration into the central nervous system, along with Flagyl and Zithromax.

He had a severe Jarisch-Herxheimer reaction two weeks into the IV medication, but then started to feel better. His bowel symptoms improved, as did his memory and concentration. Yet despite these medications, he was still severely affected by his illness. He continued to have drenching sweats; severe fatigue and cognitive problems; severe depression and mood swings, including paranoid episodes and occasional hallucinations; as well as double and blurry vision; facial twitching; almost constant nausea; intractable constipation, and nocturia, which compounded his poor sleep patterns. That's when he decided to get another opinion.

When Larry came to see me we sent off a full range of blood tests, including a CBC, CMP with mineral levels, a prostate-specific antigen (PSA), vitamin levels (B_{12}, folate, methylmalonic acid, and homocysteine), a co-infection panel (testing for *Babesia microti* and *duncani,* and Bartonella, Mycoplasma, chlamydia, Rocky Mountain spotted fever, Q fever, tularemia and Brucella, EBV, CMV, HHV-6, and West Nile). We also tested his immunoglobulin levels and subclasses, complement studies, an antigliadin antibody and TTG with a food-allergy panel (IgE and IgG), an ANA, RF, ESR, cytokine panel and high-sensitivity C-Reactive protein (HS-CRP), and studies to evaluate the thyroid, growth hormone, and sex hormones. He was also sent home with a salivary adrenal test kit to check his adrenal hormones, and a six-hour urine DMSA challenge, to check for heavy metal exposure.

The tests clearly showed that he continued to suffer from multiple tick-borne infections, including Lyme disease, with severe neurological involvement and babesiosis. There was also laboratory evidence of possible brucellosis (which may have been responsible, with Babesia, for the drenching sweats and teeth-chattering chills), possible Bartonella (which might explain his seizures and severe neurological involvement), and evidence of very low white cell counts, which may have contributed to his low immune status. We also suspected autonomic nervous system involvement causing his constant nausea, constipation, and bladder difficulties (implying possible vagal nerve problems), and postural orthostatic tachycardia syndrome (POTS) with low adrenal function based on his symptoms and prior blood tests. At the end of his history and physical, when I reviewed the stacks of records he had brought in from prior physicians, I noticed an adrenal test done years earlier showing a low cortisol level that had never been repeated.

We then designed an initial antibiotic regimen and herbal protocol to help him with his resistant symptoms. A round of oral medications had already failed, as had IV Rocephin, so I asked him if he had ever had Bicillin injections. He said no. I then asked him if he liked pain. He smiled and said no, but he was willing to do whatever it took to get better. Since Bicillin is one of my most effective regimens for persistent Lyme disease symptoms, with twenty-four-hour killing power, we put him on it as my cell-wall drug, and on grapefruit seed extract to address the cystic forms of borrelia. We waited on starting other cystic drugs, such as Plaquenil (until he had an eye exam for his history of blurry vision and double vision), and didn't start Flagyl or Tinidazole right away, as he had a history of GI problems and severe Jarisch-Herxheimer reactions. I gave him minocycline with Zithromax as a double intracellular regimen and added nystatin tablets with meals to keep down yeast in the gastrointestinal tract. This was on top of a sugar-free, yeast-free diet with three different probiotics. He was told to order the herb cryptolepis to treat his babesiosis, and Florinef was prescribed for his POTS, with a high-salt diet, drinking at least two to three liters of fluid per day to help increase his blood pressure. Zofran was prescribed for his nausea, with Lyrica at bedtime to help him sleep, as well as Detrol LA, a drug used for urge incontinence. He was also to add herbs such as valerian root if he still had difficulty falling asleep or frequent awakening.

Finally, we asked him if he had ever had a shot of glutathione. He asked if it was as good as a shot of whiskey. (I saw a glimmer of humor come out after he had been in our office for three hours and we had worn him down.) He read and signed the consent form, and we started him on a glutathione trial.

The next morning Larry called to schedule another shot. He let us know that his response to the glutathione was no less than a miracle. Within several hours of getting home from our medical office, his energy level started to improve, he felt much calmer, and his mind had started to clear up for the first time in years, with greatly improved mental clarity. Prior antibiotic regimens had been ineffective in helping these resistant symptoms. Glutathione had probably helped remove some of the neurotoxins that were responsible for his symptoms, and Larry had hope for the first time in years.

The only positive clinical improvement we saw after the first month was with his drenching night sweats and chills: They were significantly better on the cryptolepis for the Babesia, which was interesting, because he was not yet taking a classical drug regimen for babesiosis. Otherwise Larry was still feeling extremely ill, and very depressed. I decided to add Deplin to his regimen. This is a form of activated folic acid that helps to augment the efficacy of other antidepressants. I also reminded Larry to send off his salivary adrenal test.

I got the DHEA/cortisol salivary test result back two weeks later, and I nearly fell off my chair when I saw the results. Larry had virtually no cortisol production in the morning, and his cortisol graph was essentially flat for the rest of the day. His only minimally normal cortisol level was at night. The normal range for this test is 0.15 to 0.5 ng/ml nanograms per milliliter between 10:00 P.M. and 2:00 A.M., and he was just above the low-normal range in the evening. I'd seen low cortisol levels before, but I had never seen anything like this. Larry was clinically in full-blown adrenal insufficiency, which would explain his resistance to standard treatment regimens.

I hurriedly got on the phone with him and his wife to explain the results and discuss treatment options. My first choice was Cortef. It is the bioidentical equivalent to the cortisol naturally made in the adrenal gland, and it is the standard treatment for adrenal insufficiency. He let me know that he had tried steroids one time but he didn't like them, because they made him confused and agitated. That reaction was so severe that he refused to take a steroid like Cortef ever again. I suggested a natural product called Adrenal Complex instead, which is a glandular adrenal extract from New Zealand I had used in the past with good results. Larry agreed to take the Adrenal Complex at the maximum dosage, and made another appointment to see me two weeks later.

The next time I saw Larry he had a big smile on his face. He looked like a new person. Within one week of starting the adrenal supplements he started feeling so well that he stopped his antibiotics, and he let me know that he had more energy than he had felt since the beginning of his illness thirteen years earlier. If that wasn't enough, his bowel movements were now normal for the first time in years! His bladder symptoms had also improved—80 percent! He no longer was getting up at night, and his sleep was better. His joint pain had completely resolved, as well as his chronic low-back pain, and he no longer had any neuropathic symptoms. His memory and concentration were also much better, and he was happy. This was the same man who had been close to suicide several months before, when he felt he had no hope.

I was close to tears as he described his newly found good health. I have seen patients respond to adrenal support in a positive fashion, but what he told me was certainly one of the most telling stories regarding the importance of the adrenal gland with Lyme-MSIDS. For Larry, his low adrenal function had interfered with his body's response to the antibiotics used to treat the Lyme and co-infections. We see this problem (although usually not in this severity) in at least 40 percent of our patients with Lyme-MSIDS. Without properly addressing the underlying adrenal issues, patients with MSIDS will not fully recover.

HORMONE REPLACEMENT THERAPIES FOR MEN

Treatment resistance can also occur in some patients because of low levels of sex hormones. My view of hormone replacement has changed radically over the years as I have learned more about hormone replacement therapy from colleagues at major medical centers, and as new studies have emerged. For example, we learned in medical school that testosterone can cause prostate cancer, yet a study of one-quarter-million medical records of white men, presented at the annual meeting of the American Urological Association in San Diego, California, May 2016, showed that testosterone therapy does not raise the risk of aggressive prostate cancer, and that it improved sexual functioning and mood. The science is continuously changing, yet there are conflicting results in different groups of men regarding the safety and health benefits of testosterone. At the 2012 Integrative Healthcare Symposium conference in New York City, at which I was a speaker, I learned about the importance of hormone levels for adult health and the cardiovascular benefits of testosterone. In an article published in 2006 in the *Archives of Internal Medicine*, mortality levels were 88 percent higher in men with low testosterone ("low T") compared to men who had normal levels of testosterone. Low testosterone contributes to degenerative diseases of aging that involve chronic inflammation, and testosterone is cardio-protective. Men who receive testosterone replacement therapy have a slower progression from metabolic syndrome to diabetes or cardiovascular disease. This is because testosterone increases insulin sensitivity and helps to regulate blood pressure and lipid levels in the body. Declining levels of testosterone are also linked to rises in markers of inflammation, such as C-reactive protein (CRP). This elevated level of CRP is due to low levels of testosterone that, in conjunction with other stress hormones (epinephrine and cortisol), alter protein synthesis in the liver, increasing the production of inflammatory cytokines. Abdominal obesity, which results from testosterone deficiency, actually pumps out increasing levels of inflammatory cytokines, which is one of the reasons why low testosterone has been shown directly, in multiple scientific studies, to increase the risk for atherosclerosis. Yet in two other recently published studies, men with a history of cardiovascular disease treated with testosterone were significantly more likely to have a heart attack in the first ninety days after starting the medication, and another study found testosterone therapy in older men was linked with an increased risk for death, myocardial infarction, or ischemic stroke. How can we make sense of these seemingly conflicting results?

There are multiple cardiovascular risk factors that can affect overall mortality, which were not controlled for in all studies. For example, when pregnenolone and DHEA sulfate (DHEA-S) levels drop with age, we see an increase in cardiovascular mortality. Pregnenolone is the precursor to DHEA production in the body, which subsequently is converted into androstenedione and then into testosterone. Chronic stress can initiate a "pregnenolone steal," which is when the body begins to make more cortisol from pregnenolone instead of making sex hormones, thereby lowering DHEA and sex hormone levels. A low serum DHEA(-S) level has been shown to be associated with a higher death rate from all causes, including cardiovascular disease and ischemic heart disease. This association remained after adjusting for CRP, circulating estradiol, and testosterone levels. The effects of testosterone therapy also vary among different populations of men depending on their levels of oxidative stress. Research published in the *Journal of Alzheimer's Disease* in 2014 showed that high levels of oxidative stress (as measured by elevated homocysteine levels) determined whether testosterone therapy would increase the risk of dementia, whereas in men with low oxidative stress, testosterone had beneficial effects. The cardiovascular risks and benefits of testosterone replacement in men may therefore vary depending on race, underlying history of cardiovascular disease, levels of pregnenolone and DHEA, and oxidative stress levels. Checking a homocysteine level and oxidative stress markers is important before starting therapy, although we still need large clinical trials to be completed to evaluate the full long-term effects. We certainly see men with unresolved Lyme disease who also have low T feel significantly better with hormone rebalancing.

Testosterone is necessary for energy, mood, libido, sexual function, prostate growth, muscle and bone mass, muscle strength, red blood cell production, proper sleep, and cognitive health. Its deficiency is associated with a decline in energy, low libido, anemia, insomnia, a decreased sense of well-being, low mental energy, difficulties in short-term memory, depression and anxiety, loss of muscle mass, an increase in abdominal fat (increasing the risk of metabolic syndrome), osteoporosis, an increase in prostate size with benign prostatic hyperplasia (BPH), and decreased sperm production.

Testing and Treating Low T

Men experience a decline in hormone production as they age, in a similar fashion to a woman's menopause. This is referred to as andropause, or as I like to call it, "manopause." The symptoms of andropause described above are very similar to those we see in many young men suffering with Lyme disease, co-infections, and MSIDS. Therefore, our physical examination for men in whom we suspect low T focuses on the amount of body hair, muscle mass, breast enlargement or tenderness, and the size and consistency of the testicles, as well as the size of the penis. Preliminary testing includes a luteinizing hormone (LH), total testosterone level, bioavailable and free testosterone level (unbound hormone), estrogen level, sex hormone–binding globulin (SHBG), the carrier protein for testosterone in the blood, and DHEA-sulfate. Although serum total testosterone levels of 300 ng/dl to 1,000 ng/dl are considered normal, these can vary between laboratories. What's more, normal values are based on statistical values of healthy individuals. Many men with symptoms of low T may be in the bottom third of the normal range. Morning measurements around 8:00 A.M. are recommended, when levels are usually the highest, but certain medications, poor nutrition, and illness can temporarily reduce levels.

Laboratory tests showing a total testosterone level of less than 300 ng/dl, bioavailable testosterone of less than 70 ng/dl, and free testosterone of less than 50 pg/ml are considered proof of andropause. Screening tools such as the ADAM questionnaire (Androgen Decline in the Aging Male), the AMS (Aging Male's Symptoms) scale, and the MMAS (Massachusetts Male Aging Study) questionnaire can also be used to assist in evaluating symptoms.

There are four basic medications that can be used to increase testosterone: beta-human chorionic gonadotropin (β-HCG) and Clomid (clomiphene) in the younger male, and testosterone replacement by cream or injection in men over forty, with or without aromatase inhibitors. β-HCG and Clomid will preserve sperm generation, and are therefore preferred for younger men who may wish to have families. Testosterone cream is easy to administer, but absorption through the skin may decrease over time, and injections may yield more consistent blood and tissue levels. Aromatase inhibitors, such as Arimidex, stop the conversion of testosterone to estrogen (and are therefore also used in women with estrogen-receptor-positive breast cancer) and help maintain testosterone levels.

Elevations of estrogen levels are not uncommon while trying to replace testosterone using the above medications, and it also happens in men who are overweight, so following estrogen levels is important when placing men on hormone replacement therapy.

There are also natural ways to increase testosterone. Cardiovascular exercise, as well as strength training, can increase levels of testosterone and free testosterone. It is essential that men exercise regularly, lifting weights or using other forms of strength training to maintain hormone levels. Since some men are also deconditioned (as are the majority of MSIDS sufferers), starting an exercise regimen slowly and gently is fine, gradually increasing the level of difficulty.

Getting proper sleep is also crucial to maintaining proper testosterone levels. Sleep reduction drastically reduces the levels in healthy young men, according to a study published in 2011 in the *Journal of the American Medical Association*. The effects of sleep loss on testosterone became apparent after only one week without adequate sleep. Researchers found that getting only five hours of sleep per night decreased testosterone levels by 10 percent to 15 percent. That is a big drop, and unfortunately, the majority of my Lyme patients do not sleep well. When I'm lecturing, and I tell men that Lyme disease can lead to low T and that they won't be able to make love, that usually is the clincher for them to go and get tested. They also seem to take note when I tell them that certain nutraceuticals, such as Vitamin D, mung bean extract, zinc, high-protein diets, soy, and fish oils will also have a positive effect on increasing testosterone levels.

All hormone therapies need to be carefully monitored, especially for men taking testosterone. Side effects to watch for include:

- Testicular atrophy (due to decreased luteinizing hormone production)
- Benign prostatic hypertrophy with lower urinary tract symptoms
- Gynecomastia (breast enlargement due to increased aromatization to estrogen)
- Increased edema in those with preexisting cardiac, hepatic, or renal disease
- Worsening of sleep apnea
- Polycythemia (an increase in red blood cells)

Follow-up testing should include CBCs, liver functions, PSAs, luteinizing hormone (LH), total and free bioavailable testosterone levels, estradiol levels, sex-hormone-binding globulin (SHBG), dihydrotestosterone, androstenedione, and DHEA-S levels after the first month of treatment. These tests should be repeated every three months afterward for several cycles, until the target goals are reached, or more frequently if any abnormalities are found. Then, testing CBCs, liver functions, and hormone levels every four to six months is usually adequate, while also checking PSAs twice a year, with intermittent prostate exams.

HORMONE REPLACEMENT THERAPIES FOR WOMEN

Women also are affected by a lowering of DHEA, cortisol, and testosterone, but it is, of course, estrogens and progesterone that play the major roles in maintaining a woman's health. It is easier to see the effects of hormones in women, as Lyme symptoms are frequently affected during the fluctuations in estrogen and progesterone that take place during the menstrual cycle. Many women report that right before, during, or after their menses (when estrogen and progesterone levels drop off), their Lyme symptoms flare up and get much worse, and they subsequently improve as they move into the first part of their cycle. In women who are well/asymptomatic most of the month without any Lyme symptoms, but flare up primarily around the menstrual cycle when the bacteria are active, I find pulsing antibiotics (with a cell wall, cystic, intracellular drug, and biofilm busters) to be an effective method to address the bacteria during a cyclical flare and help women to continue to get better. Four pulses, modeled after the work of Kim Lewis (every other day, or Monday/Wednesday/Saturday/Monday) with high-dose probiotics is one way to try and lower down the total load of Lyme bacteria in the body, as we're only treating when they are active. This pulsed regimen also keeps down antibiotic use, with a minimal effect on the microbiome of the gut, although probiotics should be continued post pulse therapy. The efficacy of this approach can be measured by the length and intensity of symptom flares over time, and whether the flares continue to decrease around the menstrual cycle.

There are three major estrogens—E1, E2, and E3—present in women, and the ratios change as they get older. Women who suffer with MSIDS often have an estrogen dominance or estrogen deficiency with or without early menopause. Estrogen dominance refers to an excess of estrogen with insufficient levels of progesterone, causing a poor estrogen/progesterone balance. Signs and symptoms of estrogen dominance include irregular and/or heavy menses, increased ovarian cysts, fibrocystic breasts with breast tenderness, uterine fibroids, weight gain, bloating, irritability, anxiety with mood swings and hypersensitivity. It is also associated with an increased risk of blood clots, gallstones, breast cancer, and metabolic syndrome with high triglycerides. Causes include a poor diet, stress, adrenal fatigue, luteal-phase deficiency with lack of ovulation, erratic cycles, and, in postmenopause, a decline in estrogen production by as much as 60 percent, with levels of progesterone dropping to nearly zero and causing the imbalance of estrogen to progesterone.

Iodine deficiency and xenoestrogens will also contribute to estrogen dominance. Lack of adequate levels of iodine, apart from affecting thyroid function, result in increased estrogen receptor activity in the breast. We have found that replacing iodine, combined with lowering caffeine intake, helps to decrease fibrocystic breast disease in women who are estrogen dominant.

Estrogen dominance is now common in many women because of the load of xenoestrogens that regularly enter the body from industrial pollution, although in women with polycystic ovarian syndrome (PCOS), high levels of bisphenol A (BPA) have been associated with insulin resistance and high testosterone. Chemical xenoestrogens such as PCBs, dioxins, plastics, pesticides, heavy metals, and bisphenol A, due to their chemical structure, may act like estrogen in the human body. They have been associated with various forms of cancer such as breast cancer, ovarian cancer, uterine cancer, prostate cancer, lung cancer, thyroid cancer, and colon cancer. Unless we make a conscious effort to avoid plastics, eat organic foods, and avoid pesticides, we are exposed to a regular diet of environmental endocrine disruptors and estrogen-containing compounds every day. This would explain the significant lowering of men's sperm counts over the last fifty years. Detoxification of xenoestrogens can be accomplished through the regular use of far-infrared saunas (FIR). Eating cruciferous vegetables, such as broccoli, cauliflower, brussel sprouts, kale, and garlic, with the use of broccoli compounds such as DIM and sulforaphane (broccoli sprouts) can also help to transform unhealthy estrogens into healthy estrogens in the body. It can also be beneficial in trying to reduce the risk of breast cancer and prostate cancer. In addition, they support the phase I and phase II detoxification enzymes necessary to remove these foreign-based chemicals, and sulforaphane results in antioxidant response element (ARE) gene activation, which enhances detoxification, decreases inflammation, and inhibits cancer growth. If we want to try and further reduce our risk, we should be avoiding all simple sugars and eating a very low-carbohydrate diet, as cancer researchers in 2016 found that high HbA1c levels within the nondiabetic range have been associated with an increased risk for cancer.

Many women in perimenopause and menopause complain of symptoms of estrogen/progesterone imbalance, such as fatigue, low libido, hot flashes and sweats, memory and concentration problems, and brain fog. These symptoms of hormonal deficiency also overlap those symptoms of Lyme disease with babesiosis, and they should be differentiated with proper blood testing. Apart from tick-borne testing, we will check follicle-stimulating hormone (FSH), luteinizing hormone (LH), estradiol, progesterone, testosterone, free testosterone, pregnenolone, and DHEA levels in women complaining of these symptoms. Elevated levels of DHT should be checked in women complaining of hair loss. It is also advisable to check a CBC, a CMP, salivary hormone levels, serum iodine levels, 25 (OH) Vitamin D levels, thyroid functions, HbA1c, and a lipid panel (cholesterol, triglycerides) with Apo E, HDL sub fractions, Lp(a), fibrinogen, and PLAC testing to evaluate for associated hormonal dysfunction, metabolic syndrome, and increased cardiovascular risk. Since Lyme disease can affect the HPA axis in women just as it does in men, younger women should also be evaluated for hormonal imbalances if presenting with low libido (which may be due to testosterone deficiency), symptoms of estrogen deficiency, such as unusual sweats, fatigue, or brain fog, or symptoms of estrogen dominance.

PMS can also be due to estrogen dominance, and the symptoms of fatigue, headaches, joint pain, depression, and irritability (with bloating and breast tenderness) can overlap with symptoms of unresolved Lyme disease. Again, it is necessary to check a full hormone panel for these women, because of the effects of Lyme disease on the HPA axis, which can cause an imbalance in the sex hormones. Overlapping factors can include adrenal fatigue and mineral deficiencies. Diet and lifestyle changes, with progesterone supplementation, can sometimes help to balance the effects of the excess estrogen in PMS, and occasionally SSRIs like Prozac are necessary to help patients with severe mood disorders and associated depression.

Hormone replacement therapy needs to be considered for some women who suffer from severe symptoms of estrogen deficiency, progesterone deficiency, and/or testosterone deficiency. Women who experience vaginal dryness and atrophy can be treated with estriol cream, an estriol (E3) suppository, or vaginal DHEA. If a woman complains of severe fatigue, unrelenting night and day sweats, worsening brain fog, mood swings, and evidence of osteoporosis, which are symptoms of severe hormone deficiencies, then she should be treated more aggressively. Various treatment options exist, but many integrative practitioners use compounded Biest or transdermal patches, such as Climara or Vivelle-Dot. Oral estradiol is also available but is not used as commonly. Since these treatments have both benefits and risks, they should be discussed with your healthcare practitioner.

Finally, progesterone at bedtime, either in a cream or orally, may help women who have severe insomnia as part of their clinical picture of Lyme-MSIDS. Progesterone stimulates GABA receptors in the brain and helps women sleep.

Replacing DHEA Benefits Men and Women

Supplementation of DHEA can be considered when levels are low. Since approximately 50 percent of DHEA converts into testosterone, this is another way to boost hormone levels. It is important, however, to follow the levels of DHEA, estrogen, and testosterone, since it converts differently in individuals, and this may significantly elevate levels of estrogens in overweight women. Both blood and salivary levels may be used.

Rule 5 of the Action Plan is "Provide Internal Balance." Balancing cytokines and hormones can be an important key to your healing. Endocrine abnormalities, with hormone deficiencies and hormonal imbalances, are some of the most commonly overlooked causes for the failure of antibiotics in MSIDS, and men and women often feel much better when these are properly addressed.

THIRTEEN

Lyme and the Brain

L yme disease frequently affects the central nervous system (CNS), as borrelia travels from the site of the initial infection into the bloodstream, past the blood-brain barrier and into the brain and surrounding tissues. When this happens, we refer to the associated symptoms as neurological Lyme disease.

Neurological symptoms of Lyme disease include memory and concentration problems, difficulties with processing new information, word-finding problems, mood disorders (such as depression), and anxiety, as well as a host of psychiatric manifestations, including the potential for mental health disorders such as obsessive-compulsive disorder (OCD) and even schizophrenia. It can also include neurodegenerative problems, when borrelia affects various nerves in the body. The central nervous system and peripheral nervous systems are preferred sites for borrelia to establish an infection, and Lyme disease can cause both subtle and severe neurological complications. For example, my patient Larry had severe neuropsychiatric symptoms from the Lyme spirochetes that invaded his central nervous system as well as autonomic neuropathy, which caused fatigue, dizziness, constipation, and urinary difficulties.

The list of neurological Lyme symptoms includes:

- Autonomic nervous system disorders (such as palpitations and anxiety)

- Bell's palsy and/or other cranial nerve abnormalities
- Changes in hearing
- Changes in vision
- Dizziness and balance problems
- Headaches and migraines
- Insomnia
- Light and sound sensitivity
- Memory and concentration problems
- Mood disorders
- Movement disorders (such as tics, tremors)
- Neurodegenerative disorders (like Alzheimer's), or motor neuron diseases such as amyotrophic lateral sclerosis (ALS/ Lou Gehrig's disease)
- Pain disorders affecting the face
- Psychiatric disorders
- Seizures

The brain is attached to the body through the spinal cord and floats in a cushion of cerebral spinal fluid encased in the meninges, a sac that encloses the brain and the spinal cord. When the sac surrounding the brain is affected, it causes meningitis-type symptoms, and you may complain of a stiff neck, a headache, and light and sound sensitivity. When borrelia invades the brain tissue, it can cause encephalitis, which manifests as memory and concentration problems with or without dementia, a broad range of psychiatric symptoms, and in rare cases, levels of decreased consciousness. When it affects the cranial nerves it can cause abnormalities in the function of each of these nerves, resulting in optic neuritis (loss of vision) and eye movement disorders, vestibulitis, and hearing loss (due to effects on the eighth cranial nerve, which controls balance and hearing), and Bell's palsy.

The spinal cord connects to the rest of the body through the peripheral nervous system. These nerves begin at the spinal cord and end in your extremities: arms and legs, fingers and toes. Affected peripheral nerves lead to symptoms of a radiculitis (inflammation in the nerve root coming out of the spinal column) and/or peripheral neuropathy, which causes symptoms such as tingling, numbness, burning, stabbing sensations, and hypersensitivity of the skin.

There are four principal patterns of peripheral neuropathy that we see when Lyme disease invades the brain and peripheral nervous system:

- Mononeuropathy: A single nerve is affected.
- Mononeuritis multiplex: Multiple nerves are affected in varied parts of the body, asymmetrically (i.e., left arm and right leg). This leads to a loss of sensory and motor function in the individual nerves.
- Polyneuropathy: Many nerve cells in the body are affected, often in a symmetrical fashion (i.e., both hands and/or feet). It can affect the axons (distal axonopathy), the myelin sheath surrounding the nerves (which help conduct electrical impulses for proper nerve function), or the cell body of the neuron, and therefore the sensory nerves (sensory neuropathy) or motor neurons that control voluntary muscle activities, such as walking, speaking, swallowing, and breathing. In severe cases, this type of neuropathy causes motor neuron diseases such as progressive bulbar palsy, in which you may experience difficulty with speech and swallowing; primary lateral sclerosis, in which only the upper motor neurons are affected, causing balance problems and spasticity; and ALS, which is caused by the degeneration of both the upper and lower motor neurons. ALS is the most severe of the motor neuron diseases and often leads to disability and death. While we can't say that Lyme is the sole cause of these motor neuron diseases, as environmental toxins (such as organophosphate pesticides, PCBs, and brominated flame retardants) have recently been found to be significantly associated with ALS, this severe type of neuropathy is occasionally seen in the Lyme-MSIDS patient.
- Autonomic neuropathy: A form of polyneuropathy that affects the involuntary nerves of the autonomic nervous system. This affects the functioning of internal organs, such as the digestive tract (causing constipation), bladder muscles (causing difficulties with urinating, such as incontinence or urinary retention), and the cardiovascular system (causing problems with blood pressure control and heart rate). One form of autonomic nervous system (ANS) dysfunction is postural orthostatic tachycardia

syndrome (POTS), in which low blood pressure occurs when standing (postural orthostasis) with compensatory high heart rates (tachycardia), often causing resistant fatigue, dizziness, anxiety, and cognitive problems. This will be further discussed in detail in Chapter 15.

NEUROPSYCHIATRIC COMPLAINTS

Apart from physical symptoms, many Lyme disease patients complain of mood disorders, especially severe anxiety, depression, and post-traumatic stress disorder. Typically, their physicians have told them that these feelings and emotions are psychiatric in nature and unrelated to their physical health, since the physicians were unable to find a cause for their illness. This pronouncement is often devastating. Truthfully, I find it to be equally upsetting, because I've found that treating Lyme disease and associated co-infections often improves psychiatric symptoms.

As we've discussed, Lyme disease is a multiple systemic disorder, and can therefore affect any part of the body, including the brain. Lyme disease, with or without co-infections like Bartonella, which can also worsen neurological and neurocognitive dysfunction, can mimic every psychiatric symptom and can cause numerous psychiatric and neurological presentations. In fact, it is often underdiagnosed in the psychiatric community. Lyme disease has been discussed in the psychiatric literature as being "the great imitator" just as it has been in other medical specialties. Psychiatric case reports have linked Lyme disease to paranoia, thought disorders, delusions with psychosis, schizophrenia (with or without visual, auditory, or olfactory hallucinations), depression, panic attacks and anxiety, obsessive-compulsive disorder, anorexia, mood lability with violent outbursts, mania, personality changes, catatonia, and dementia. Other psychiatric disorders in adults due to Lyme disease include atypical bipolar disorder, depersonalization/derealization, conversion disorders, somatization disorders, atypical psychoses, schizoaffective disorder, and intermittent explosive disorders. In children and adolescents, Lyme disease can also mimic specific or pervasive developmental delays, attention-deficit disorder (inattentive subtype), oppositional defiant disorder, mood disorders, obsessive-compulsive disorder (OCD), anorexia, Tourette's syndrome, and pseudo-psychotic disorders.

A 2010 review of the medical literature by Dr. Brian Fallon, published in the journal *Neurobiology of Disease*, suggests that psychiatric problems can be a prominent feature of Lyme borreliosis. In one study, 33 percent of patients with Lyme disease were clinically depressed, and controlled studies show much more depression among patients with late Lyme disease than among normal controls. It is therefore incumbent on mental health professionals to always keep Lyme-MSIDS in the back of their minds, since patients may well have it in the back of theirs.

Some physicians do their best to treat psychiatric manifestations by prescribing a range of psychiatric medications and recommending psychotherapy. However, by treating complaints without finding a common root cause, these physicians have overlooked the fact that psychiatric manifestations are often the result of a physical health problem. Microbes, as well as toxins, free radical stress, immune dysfunction/autoimmune disorders, an improper diet, lack of exercise and sleep, hormonal dysregulation, and imbalances in the microbiome, as well as mitochondrial dysfunction, can all impair mental health.

For example, one young man came to see me with a history of schizophrenia, which started suddenly in his early twenties. We did a broad differential diagnosis using the sixteen-point MSIDS map, and his test came back positive for Lyme disease. Working with his psychiatrist, we were able to improve his psychiatric functioning by eliminating his antipsychotic drug (Risperdal) and replacing it with a tetracycline antibiotic (i.e., doxycycline). When he stopped the antibiotic, his thought disorder and hallucinations returned. I have seen others with schizophrenia with evidence of Lyme and co-infections like babesiosis respond to antiparasitic medications like Coartem or Dapsone, where they started to speak and act normally, having failed many traditional antipsychotic therapies. How can we explain this?

A 2015 study, published in the *American Journal of Psychiatry*, found that immune cells are more active in the brains of people at risk for schizophrenia as well as those already diagnosed with the disease, raising the possibility that infections like Lyme disease, as well as associated co-infections and multiple overlapping factors on the MSIDS map, are increasing inflammatory cytokines in the brain, worsening psychiatric manifestations. This is scientifically plausible, as research on drugs like minocycline have shown that they help symptoms in early-phase schizophrenia, and omega-3 fatty acids, which have an anti-inflammatory effect, have been shown in a randomized, placebo-controlled study of eighty-one teenagers and young adults at high risk for schizophrenia to significantly decrease the risk of conversion to psychosis twelve months later. Inflammation, as we previously discussed, is a common denominator in many chronic illnesses, and it can worsen neuropsychiatric manifestations.

With these severe types of psychiatric symptoms, Lyme disease treatment should be closely monitored and coordinated with a psychiatrist. Without understanding MSIDS and the map of chronic illness, it would be impossible to discover the multiple causes for neuropsychiatric symptoms in a chronically sick individual, as they can occur in the following conditions:

- Autoimmune disorders (such as *Lupus cerebritis*)
- B_{12} and/or folic acid deficiency
- Carcinoma of the brain or pancreas
- Chronic inflammation resulting from infection with *Borrelia burgdorferi* and co-infections such as Mycoplasma and Bartonella
- Defects in mitochondrial function, which can cause disorders of the central nervous system, such as schizophrenia, bipolar disorder, and anxiety
- Endocrine abnormalities, including type 2 diabetes with hyperinsulinemia
- Endogenous toxins, such as quinolinic acid from borrelia
- Environmental toxins, including mercury, lead, aluminum, pesticides, and phthalates (BPA)
- Inadequate detoxification systems, which allow neurotoxins to accumulate in the brain (chloral hydrate, ammonia, quinolinic acid)
- Temporal lobe epilepsy
- Viral encephalopathies
- Wilson's disease with copper overload

If you are experiencing psychiatric disturbances along with the multisystemic signs of Lyme disease, then the odds are that the Lyme disease has or is also affecting your brain. The following features have helped to make or support a diagnosis of Lyme disease:

- Atypical features of a psychiatric disorder (e.g., absence of typical early signs or symptoms, unusually acute onset without new traumas or life challenges, and an uncharacteristic constellation of symptoms)
- Absence of a family history of psychiatric disorders
- Presentation of a psychiatric disorder at an older or younger age than is typical (e.g., autistic behavior at age six, forgetfulness at age thirty-five, first manic episode at age forty-five)
- Lack of expected response to psychotropic medication
- Adverse response to previously well-tolerated psychotropic medication
- Lack of expected correlation of symptoms to psychological triggers (e.g., mood lability without apparent cause)

Signs that a tick-borne infection could be the cause of a psychiatric disorder would include symptoms of meningitis, encephalitis, cranial neuritis, and radiculoneuropathy early in the illness. We also know that *Borrelia burgdorferi* can rapidly disseminate to the central nervous system, and antibiotics given early in the illness are not necessarily curative. The organism may then lie dormant and reemerge months or even years later, producing neuropsychiatric symptoms at any point in the life span, regardless of when the initial tick bite occurred. You may also be exposed to new tick bites, and sudden neurological deterioration or new psychiatric symptoms should be evaluated with repeat tick-borne titers and PCRs with culture if appropriate, given the limitations of the tests.

Cognitive issues can manifest as mild, moderate, or severe memory and concentration problems that can be mistaken for early Alzheimer's disease or other forms of dementia, especially if other illnesses have been ruled out, such as B_{12} deficiency, gluten sensitivity, or hypothyroidism. You might reverse numbers and letters and have word-finding problems, and occasionally be so confused that you get lost driving, unable to remember familiar streets and signs. Researchers published in the *Journal of Alzheimer's Disease* in 2014 that pure Lyme dementia exists, which can be mistaken for Alzheimer's disease (AD), and that it is advisable to do Lyme serology in demented patients (recognizing limitations of the tests), as they had a good outcome with antibiotics. It is also important to remember that patients with early AD can get a tick bite, worsening symptoms, as activated microglia in the brain are seen in both Lyme and Alzheimer's, with inflammatory cytokines contributing to neuropsychiatric manifestations in both diseases. Blockade of microglial proliferation and addressing inflammation from multiple sources (i.e., stress, insomnia, a sedentary lifestyle, a high glycemic diet eating allergic/sensitive foods, leaky gut with imbalances in the microbiome, mineral deficiencies, environmental toxins, borreliosis, and co-infections), while using targeted nutritional therapies (such as omega-3 fatty acids, resveratrol, and broccoli seed extract), exercise, and ketogenic diets to lower inflammation, has been proven in multiple scientific studies to have beneficial effects on neurocognitive function.

It is important to address increased inflammation from multiple sources, since insomnia is a common complaint among Lyme patients, which contributes to inflammation, worsening their already profound fatigue. This may be accompanied by light and sound sensitivity, headaches, with a stiff neck, dizziness, visual difficulties, with blurry vision, and an associated neuropathy or radiculopathy. Women may experience an exacerbation of psychiatric symptoms around their menstrual cycle (when the estrogen and progesterone levels drop, women often experience Jarisch-Herxheimer flares), and mental health symptoms may also be exacerbated while taking antibiotics for another infection (i.e., sinusitis, upper respiratory infection), which then subsequently improves.

We see a similar improvement in psychiatric symptoms in children who have been exposed to group A beta-hemolytic streptococcal infections who develop pediatric autoimmune neuropsychiatric disorders associated with streptococcal infections (PANS/PANDAS). These children develop obsessive-compulsive disorders and/or tic disorders after being exposed to a bacteria (beta hemolytic strep), and these symptoms improve when the streptococcus is treated, but the children often relapse when the antibiotics are stopped. Some of these children (and adults with Lyme/co-infections) also have an autoimmune encephalitis, contributing to ongoing symptoms, identified by markers on a blood test called the Cunningham panel. This measures human serum immunoglobulin G (IgG) levels by an ELISA assay directed against five important receptors in the brain (i.e., dopamine receptors D1 and D2, gangliosides, tubulin, and calcium/calmodulin-dependent protein kinase II) which control mood/motor control. If one or more of these five assay values is elevated, it may indicate a clinically significant autoimmune neurological condition, where auto-antibodies cross-react and are directed against selected neuronal targets in the brain which are involved in neuropsychiatric and/or motor functions. Like Lyme disease, PANDAS and PANS are clinical diagnoses based upon defined clinical characteristics, and results from the Cunningham panel help to diagnose an overlapping autoimmune encephalitis, where IV immunoglobulin therapy (IVIG) may be necessary to improve neurological function. It is clear that antibodies can damage the brain and initiate or aggravate different neurologic conditions, as brain-reactive antibodies have been found to increase symptomatology in both auto-immune and infectious diseases.

We have seen similar autoimmune manifestations after exposure to Lyme and co-infections like Bartonella (i.e., OCD and tics) worsened by exposure to toxins like mold, where antibiotics and detoxification combined with IVIG helped both resistant neuropathy and neuropsychiatric symptoms. Microbes, toxins, detoxification problems, immune dysfunction with autoimmunity, an improper diet, nutritional deficiencies, deconditioning, sleep, and mitochondrial and endocrine disorders are just some of the physical causes of psychiatric symptoms. The enormous stress of being diagnosed with a long-term illness that many in the medical community are still skeptical about may also make you feel anxious or depressed. Yet when we treat all of the underlying physical and emotional causes of the illness, patients often get better.

IDENTIFYING THE MEDICAL CAUSES OF NEUROPSYCHIATRIC ILLNESS

Failure to recognize a medical illness causing psychiatric symptoms is not uncommon in medicine. In one study, nearly 20 percent of psychiatric outpatients had a medical condition causing their symptoms, and these conditions had been missed by the referring physician in approximately one-third of the cases.

There are some scans and other tests that can be performed to help confirm that the brain has been affected. These include functional brain imaging, using MRI studies, single-photon emission computed tomography (SPECT) scans, and positron emission tomography (PET) scans, as well as performing a spinal tap and administering neuropsychiatric testing. Unfortunately, these are not sensitive nor specific enough to confirm a diagnosis of Lyme disease, or that Lyme has caused these problems. For example, MRI scans of the brain can reveal nonspecific white-matter abnormalities that are commonly found in Lyme patients, although it is not specific enough for establishing a diagnosis or causation. Similarly, an abnormal SPECT scan result simply tells us that there are problems with the blood flow to parts of the brain, but these defects can result from a variety of causes, including vascular problems (vasculitis), metabolic problems, and cellular dysfunction due to the indirect effects of cytokines. Tulane researchers in 2015 demonstrated that ongoing cytokine activation in the central nervous system can contribute to persistent symptoms of fatigue, pain, and cognitive dysfunction; but we see an increase in brain cytokines in many inflammatory diseases, such as autoimmune disorders, autism, Alzheimer's, and neurological Lyme disease, so we cannot use the SPECT scan as a stand-alone test to make an accurate diagnosis.

The typical PET scan is more specific, and in the right clinical circumstance it can be more useful, since it reflects changes in the brain's regional metabolism. PET scans are valuable to neuropsychologists as a tool to evaluate the effect of various drugs on cerebral metabolism. Lyme disease is known to cause changes in the brain's metabolic pathways, which can affect memory, concentration, and moods. This was demonstrated in the NIH clinical trial conducted by Dr. Brian Fallon at Columbia University, where Lyme disease patients with chronic encephalopathy were retreated with antibiotics to see if their cognitive problems improved. PET scans did show an increased metabolism in the brain in the group treated with antibiotics, with associated improved physical symptoms of fatigue and pain, and improvements in cognition. Rocephin improved chronic Lyme patients' physical and neuropsychiatric symptoms as compared to their matched controls, and this improvement was verified via PET scan.

In 2012 the FDA approved a new radiopharmaceutical agent to be used during PET scans to assist clinicians in differentiating the cognitive impairments caused by Lyme disease from other diseases, such as Alzheimer's. This drug, Florbetapir F18, is different than the one used in Dr. Fallon's study to evaluate the metabolic changes in the brain with Lyme disease. It binds to amyloid plaques in the brain, a specific finding commonly seen in Alzheimer's, and it helps determine the amount of amyloid present. A negative Florbetapir scan would help rule out AD, and would inform the clinician that he or she should intensify efforts to look for another cause of the cognitive decline. This test should be considered for patients with an undetermined cause for their neurocognitive impairment after an extensive workup has been performed. Researchers are evaluating specific biomarkers in saliva ("salivary metabolomics") to detect Alzheimer's disease, but today, brain MRIs with FDG-PET scans, combined with Tau, p-tau, and Beta amyloid (Aβ42) concentrations in the cerebral spinal fluid (CSF), looking at apoE genotypes, may be helpful in differentiating the two diseases.

Since MRIs, SPECT scans, and PET scans of the brain are not able to definitively determine if a patient has neurological Lyme disease, physicians will occasionally perform a spinal tap and look at markers in the spinal fluid to determine if *Borrelia burgdorferi* has invaded the CNS. Unfortunately, spinal taps also have their limitations. Although increased antibody production in the spinal fluid can be seen in early Lyme disease with a lymphocytic meningitis or encephalitis, late-stage neurological Lyme patients can have normal cerebrospinal fluid (CSF) antibody studies. For example, in a 1990 study of thirty-five patients with the specific Lyme antigen (Osp A) in their cerebrospinal fluid, 43 percent had no evidence of antibodies to Lyme in their CSF testing, and 47 percent had otherwise normal routine CSF analyses. Sixty percent of these patients were also seronegative for Lyme disease when tested with standard blood tests, implying that a patient can have Lyme disease despite a negative blood test and a negative spinal tap. The authors concluded that "neurologic infection by *B. burgdorferi* should not be excluded solely on the basis of normal routine CSF or negative CSF antibody analyses."

If antibody tests in the spinal fluid are so unreliable, what about conducting a PCR study on the spinal fluid to demonstrate the existence of the Lyme disease spirochete by DNA analysis? In children with known Lyme meningitis, Lyme CSF-PCR had a sensitivity of only 5 percent and a specificity of 99 percent. This means that we will only be able to diagnose

Lyme meningitis by PCR in five out of one hundred children who have contracted the disease. A positive test can make the diagnosis, but a negative test result cannot rule it out. However, one test performed on the spinal fluid that may be useful in differentiating patients with neurological posttreatment Lyme disease (nPTLS) from patients with other illnesses, such as chronic fatigue syndrome (CFS), is to look at certain specific proteins in the spinal fluid. A recent study performed by Dr. Steven Schutzer and colleagues used a technique known as proteomics, which examines the entire complement of proteins in the cerebral spinal fluid. They found specific protein profiles in Lyme patients that varied from patients with CFS, supporting the hypothesis that these are two distinct disease processes. In 2015, researchers also found distinct plasma immune signatures in CFS early in the course of the illness. As we have shown, many of the cytokine profiles increasing inflammation in CFS, FM, Alzheimer's, autism spectrum disorder, and Lyme disease are similar, yet there are still distinct differences between these disease processes.

Since laboratory testing for tick-borne disorders is imperfect, and neuroimaging studies are nonspecific, the last commonly used test to help establish the diagnosis of neurological Lyme disease is neuropsychiatric testing. This is usually administered by a psychologist who has been trained in administering a specific battery of tests—including the Minnesota Multiphasic Personality Inventory (MMPI), Patient Health Questionnaire-9 (PHQ-9), Beck Depression Inventory, Mini-Mental State Examination (MMSE), Alzheimer's Disease Assessment Scale–Cognitive Subscale (ADAS–Cog), and Severe Impairment Battery—that determine the severity of mood and cognitive disorders present. Neuropsychiatric testing can help determine the extent of a patient's disability, as well as how much underlying depression and anxiety is interfering with their cognitive processing. Fifty percent to 60 percent of patients with chronic neurological Lyme disease have objective evidence of impairment on neuropsychological tests. A multisystemic illness, high score on the HMQ (with good and bad days, and especially migratory pain), positive tests for Lyme (ELISA, C6 ELISA, borrelia-specific bands on a Western blot, PCR, positive antigen testing [Nanotrap, Lyme Dot Blot], culture, ELISPOT), and/or evidence of tick-borne co-infections with significant abnormalities on neuropsychiatric testing (having ruled out other common causes of neurological disorders), help to confirm the clinical diagnosis.

There are patterns seen in neurocognitive testing that are often found in patients suffering from Lyme disease and co-infections. These include verbal fluency and word-finding problems, memory and concentration problems, dyslexia (number and letter reversals), problems with executive functioning (including an inability to make decisions), and problems with perceptual motor functioning (with spatial disorientation). These objective cognitive deficits can be seen on neuropsychiatric testing, while other studies, such as an MRI of the brain, EEG, or cerebrospinal fluid results are completely normal.

LYME CAN MAKE PSYCHIATRIC PROBLEMS WORSE

Lyme disease can exacerbate underlying psychiatric symptoms, no matter what the cause. The increase in neuropsychiatric symptoms seen with Lyme disease is due in part to lipoproteins on the outer surface of the organism causing ongoing proinflammatory cytokine production. These cytokines contribute to frequent complaints of fatigue, pain, depression, anxiety, and cognitive problems that tend to come and go in severity. Symptoms often remit and then relapse again when the lipoproteins that stimulate cytokine production change over time. Some appear on the surface of the organism (up-regulation) and others disappear from the surface of the organism (down-regulation), depending on environmental conditions, such as the temperature and pH of the host. Certain lipoproteins are also more inflammatory than others, contributing to an increase in the severity of symptoms. For example, the inflammatory reaction seen with *Borrelia burgdorferi* in the United States is stronger than some borrelia species (*B. afzelii* and *B. garinii*) in Europe, where U.S. strains secrete higher levels of cytokines and chemokines. An increase in neuropsychiatric symptoms also takes place when a patient has contracted co-infections, such as babesiosis, which can exacerbate underlying Lyme disease symptoms, including depression.

Other co-infections also can influence psychiatric symptoms. Ehrlichiosis can cause central nervous system symptoms, as can viruses and intracellular infections with Mycoplasma spp. and *Chlamydia pneumonia*, which are frequently found in MSIDS patients. Often the ones with the worst neurological symptoms have Lyme disease, Mycoplasma, and/ or Bartonella simultaneously (three intracellular persister bacteria), with or without other co-infections. This is especially true in patients who present with severe neuropathy and encephalopathy.

Bartonella henselae, the organism that causes cat scratch fever, exacerbates many of the neurological and neuropsychiatric symptoms we see with Lyme disease, and has been linked to anxiety disorders and depression, as well as various central nervous system abnormalities. These include encephalomyelitis (involving inflammation in both the brain and spinal cord, leading to difficulties with cognition and motor function); transverse myelitis (inflammation and demyelination of the spinal cord, leading to difficulty walking); spastic paraparesis (stiffness and spasm in the lower extremities, affecting walking); seizures, with hemiparesis (weakness on one side of the body); cerebellar syndromes (primarily defined by symptoms of dizziness and poor balance); and movement disorders (which can cause a variety of symptoms, including spasms, twitching, and involuntary movements). Like Lyme disease and babesiosis, Bartonella can also be transmitted to a fetus. Therefore, resistant neuropsychiatric symptoms in children might be linked to maternal transmission of various organisms, and it should be suspected if you are living in a Lyme-endemic area, and/or have had exposure to ticks, fleas, lice, and biting flies.

Some patients with Bartonella have other severe neurologic manifestations with ophthalmologic involvement, such as inflammation of the eye manifesting as optic neuritis, episcleritis, conjunctivitis, uveitis, or iritis. Bartonella can also cause an oculoglandular syndrome with preauricular adenopathy and conjunctivitis, neuroretinitis, branch retinal artery occlusion, and vision loss. Bartonella should therefore be considered if you are experiencing particularly severe ophthalmological symptoms.

The profile of cognitive deficits, depression, headaches, ongoing muscle and joint pain, poor sleep, and persistent marked fatigue is also seen in chronic fatigue syndrome (CFS), previously known as myalgic encephalomyelitis, because it was affecting brain function and the musculoskeletal system. Chronic fatigue syndrome has now been redefined as systemic exertional intolerance disease (SEID), and the Institute of Medicine's diagnostic criteria include profound fatigue, of new or definitive onset (not the result of ongoing excessive exertion, and not substantially alleviated by rest), post-exertional malaise, unrefreshing sleep, and either cognitive impairment and/or orthostatic intolerance. Symptoms of light and sound sensitivity, with symptoms of autonomic nervous system (ANS) dysfunction, such as low blood pressure, tachycardia (rapid heart rate), and digestive disturbances also have been reported with CFS.

The symptom complex used to define CFS overlaps those seen in Lyme disease and associated co-infections, like Bartonella. One of the primary ways to differentiate these diseases is that the symptoms of persistent Lyme disease tend to come and go, and the pain migrates, improving or worsening with antibiotics, with positive blood tests. *Erythema migrans* rashes (bullseye or spreading solid red rashes after a tick bite) as well as classical Bartonella rashes ("unexplained stretch marks" that can be perpendicular to skin planes) also help to differentiate CFS/fibromyalgia from Lyme and associated co-infections.

Treating Lyme and Psychiatric Symptoms

The primary modes of treatment for the Lyme patient with neuropsychiatric illness involve a combination of antimicrobial therapies, psychotropic medications, herbal and vitamin therapies, detoxification, and various forms of psychotherapy and stress reduction techniques, including yoga, meditation, and neurofeedback.

Antimicrobial therapies do not differ from what has been previously discussed, but certain guidelines should be observed when there are severe central nervous system (CNS) symptoms. Some of these treatment-resistant patients require several months of IV and oral antibiotics, rotating the regimens to achieve a significant clinical improvement:

- Intravenous Rocephin should be strongly considered in patients with severe neuropsychiatric manifestations from Lyme disease who have failed oral therapy. Although I usually start with dosing five to seven days a week in severe CNS disease, several patients who plateaued have responded to pulsing a cell-wall drug like Rocephin, 2 grams, three days a week (Monday, Wednesday, Saturday), with a cystic drug (i.e., Tindamax) and intracellular medication (Minocin), which all have good central nervous system penetration. I include Actigall to decrease the possibility of gallstone formation/sludge, biofilm busters (Stevia, Serrapeptase, Lauricidin), other cystic drugs (Plaquenil, grapefruit seed extract), and nystatin with a sugar-free, yeast-free diet with high doses of probiotics.

- Intravenous Clindamycin should be considered in patients with severe overlapping babesiosis who have failed oral Babesia regimens, as well as Dapsone (which can be used in combination with Clindamycin, macrolides, and Mepron or Malarone with antimalarial herbs, like Artemisia or cryptolepis). Oftentimes the full dose of Dapsone is necessary with Malarone and/or other meds/herbs in patients with ongoing sweats, chills, flushing, air hunger, and a cough who have failed multiple antiparasitic protocols.
- Intravenous vancomycin is surprisingly effective in a small group of patients who have failed other treatment regimens. IV Daptomycin, discussed in recent studies from Johns Hopkins as a persister drug for Lyme (which is normally used in vancomycin resistant infections), caused significant Herxheimer reactions in the few patients who could afford to use it, and did not appear to be "curative" after one month of therapy in combination with cephalosporins and tetracyclines. Treatment-resistant patients usually require several months of IV and oral antibiotics, rotating the regimens to achieve a significant clinical improvement, while addressing overlapping abnormalities on the MSIDS map.
- Macrolides such as azithromycin or clarithromycin may be used alone or in combination with these drugs, but caution must be exercised in patients being treated with certain psychiatric medications, such as carbamazepine (Tegretol) or SSRIs, such as Celexa, Prozac, and Paxil. In the case of SSRIs, macrolides may increase the levels of the psychiatric drugs and subsequently increase the risk of mania, delirium, and serotonin syndrome (a potentially life-threatening drug reaction affecting the autonomic nervous system). SSRIs like Zoloft, which have the least effect on the cytochrome P450 3a/4 enzymes, are therefore safer choices. Proton pump inhibitors (PPIs) like omeprazole also interact with macrolides like Biaxin, increasing levels with potential QT interactions on the electrocardiogram. Caution is therefore advised. Recent scientific studies have shown that there may be an association of PPIs with the risk of dementia, and certain statins (pravastatin, not atorvastatin) have also been associated with memory impairment, so the risk/benefit of using these drugs should be discussed with your healthcare provider.

- Rifampin, a useful drug for intracellular infections such as Lyme and Bartonella, which also has an effect on biofilms, can change the drug metabolism in the body of many medications, so caution needs to be taken with its use.
- Quinolones (Cipro, Levaquin, Avelox, and Factive) can also be very helpful in cases of resistant neurological Lyme disease with associated bartonellosis, but attention needs to be paid to possible drug interactions and side effects (including tendon problems with fluoroquinolone toxicity). Patients with encephalopathy, neuropathy, and severe musculoskeletal pain who have failed other regimens may respond to a quinolone, and the higher the generation, usually the better the clinical effect. Now that we have had good initial success in resistant patients with the Horowitz Dapsone protocol, we don't use quinolones as much as in years past.

Treating Mood Disorders with Medication

Psychotropic medications may be needed if a mood disorder does not improve on antibiotics or professional therapy. Treatments that are commonly found to be of benefit in our practice include SSRIs such as Lexapro, Celexa, Paxil, Prozac, and Zoloft. Paxil is particularly useful in treating severe anxiety disorders. Cymbalta may be a better choice if there is a weight problem with low libido associated with depression, since those are more common side effects of the other class of SSRIs. Cymbalta also has effects on associated fibromyalgia symptoms and neuropathy, which makes it a very useful drug in the MSIDS patient who suffers simultaneously from those two symptoms.

Augmentation therapy with Wellbutrin, which stimulates dopamine receptors, may be useful in patients not adequately responding to an SSRI. It is also weight neutral, and can be helpful as an activating agent in the morning for those with significant fatigue and ADHD. Pharmacogenetic testing (individual genetic analysis to identify which treatments have the greatest likelihood of success) through a laboratory like Genomind (www.genomind.com) can be helpful if the above approaches are inadequate.

Helpful Nutritional Support:

Treatments that are commonly found to be of benefit in our practice include herbs such as St. John's wort, and 5-hydroxytryptophan (5-HTP helps make serotonin). Some resistant patients will also respond to the following nutritional approaches:

- Activated folic acid with a medication such as Deplin can help to augment the mood effects of other antidepressants. Deplin is essential for detoxification of certain hormones and heavy metals as well as for improving neuronal cell health and regeneration. It is also helpful as extra folate support in those on Dapsone if there are no methylation defects causing overmethylation (i.e., too much methylation with resulting irritability/anxiety).
- S-adenosinemethionine (SAMe) is useful as a nutritional supplement, because it both decreases joint pain and improves mood, while supporting methylation.
- Other treatments to be considered for severe and resistant neuropsychiatric symptoms include the use of oral liposomal and IV glutathione, which assists detoxification; low-dose naltrexone (LDN) and other pharmaceuticals and nutraceuticals that decrease the production of cytokines (i.e., curcurmin, green tea extract, resveratrol, sulforaphane, and alpha-lipoic acid); or help eliminate neurotoxins from the body (bile acid sequestrants such as Questran or WelChol, supplements such as Chlorella, clay/charcoal compounds, Pekana drainage remedies, lymphatic drainage). We occasionally see miraculous results using these treatments, especially when we use glutathione, which may remove some toxins that affect mood and brain function, although this line of thinking has not been researched directly. However, we do know that while borrelia increases inflammation in the brain, microglial cells (immune cells of the central nervous system) are activated by free radicals and proinflammatory cytokines. These in turn release more proinflammatory cytokines, which leads to increasing fatigue and reduced physical activity, muscle pains (myalgias), joint pain (arthralgias), enhanced perception of pain, impaired learning, and depression. This inflammation, created by oxidative stress, damages our cell membranes, mitochondria, and nerve cells. It is therefore crucial that we have an adequate antioxidant reserve to protect the brain and nerves from this free radical stress (using

supplements such as alpha-lipoic acid, which is water soluble and fat soluble and penetrates the brain well), while shutting down the production of these inflammatory cytokines, and opening up the detoxification pathways to remove toxins that may cause neuropsychiatric symptoms such as depression.

WHY AM I SO ANXIOUS?

The vast majority of my patients have acute and chronic anxiety. Some handle it better than others, but I have seen many cases where anxiety levels are as high as those experiencing post-traumatic stress disorder (PTSD). Some of it is due to simply dealing with their physical symptoms. Other times I notice that they are anxious to get better and are continually worrying about their health status, which in turn makes them more anxious, and Lyme and co-infections exacerbate underlying anxiety issues. Jarisch-Herxheimer reactions are also known to cause anxiety as well as lack of sleep, which can increase anxiety. Whatever the cause, my patients often benefit from learning how to relax, and I typically prescribe stress reduction techniques such as a mindfulness-based meditation, Shamatha (calm-abiding meditation), deep-breathing techniques, Tai Chi, yoga, home biofeedback monitors (HeartMath.com) as well as neurofeedback training.

Drugs such as the benzodiazepines (Valium, Ativan, and Xanax), BuSpar, SSRIs such as Paxil, and trazodone at bedtime can be helpful when relaxation techniques are insufficient, but benzodiazepines can be addictive and their effects tend to wear off over time. If the anxiety symptoms are mild, drugs may not be necessary, and appropriate herbs can be used instead, or in combination with pharmaceuticals. For example, valerian root is helpful for anxiety during the day, with associated insomnia at night. GABA (gamma-Aminobutyric acid, an inhibitory neurotransmitter) and L-theanine, a green tea extract, can also be useful for anxiety and assisting with sleep. Inositol helps with obsessive-compulsive disorder symptoms in adults and children. Some patients will also respond to Bach flower remedies such as Rescue Remedy, or an individualized homeopathic remedy, such as Kali Phos 6 X, or Psystabil, which is a combination of different homeopathic remedies in varying dilutions.

You may need to see a therapist to help with significant depression, anxiety, trauma, and PTSD. I have found that my patients with a history of trauma and abuse will have an exceedingly difficult time healing from Lyme disease without professional mental health services. The mind and body do not function separately, and when there has been trauma or abuse, or if you have suffered a loss, the unresolved conflict usually has a deleterious effect on your immune system. Some people (often on an unconscious level) feel that they are somehow responsible for the event and have often lost the will to be well, believing that they need to suffer. It is as if the guilt, shame, and grief that are experienced from their emotional trauma acts as a signal to the immune system to fail.

Skilled psychotherapy and techniques of restructuring memories and painful emotional experiences through cognitive behavioral therapy (CBT), EMDR, the Journey technique (Brandon Bays), the emotional freedom technique (EFT; www.tapping.com), and body-centered therapies (i.e., Rosen Method Bodywork) can be helpful in shifting frozen emotional memories that are stuck in the body, affecting our mood and immunity. Family systems therapy and couples work may also be necessary, as the stresses of chronic illness can take a toll on relationships.

NEURODEGENERATIVE DISORDERS: ALS, ALZHEIMER'S DISEASE, AND LYME

Amyotrophic lateral sclerosis, or ALS, is a disease of the nerve cells in the brain and spinal cord that control voluntary muscle movement. It is also known as Lou Gehrig's disease, and it is the most common motor neuron disease. This is one of the most devastating illnesses, as it leads to progressive weakness and atrophy of the muscles of the extremities, leading to difficulty walking, speaking, swallowing (associated bulbar palsy) and, ultimately, death. As the illness progresses and the respiratory muscles are affected, there are also problems with breathing. Early physical examinations often reveal fasciculations (twitching) of the muscles of the extremities and tongue, with slurring of speech and difficulty walking and grasping objects: a common early sign is the loss of muscles in the thenar eminence, at the base of the thumb.

Approximately 2 percent of ALS cases are linked to genetic factors. A mutation in the superoxide dismutase enzyme (SOD 1) that helps control oxidative stress has been identified as one possible cause of familial ALS. Other factors may include systemic mycoplasmal infections and higher than normal levels of glutamate in the blood and spinal fluid, which might play a role in motor neuron degeneration. However, none of these factors has been shown to adequately explain the cause of the disease or its progression. A recent article published online in *JAMA Neurology* in 2016 found persistent environmental pollutants to be associated with ALS (which increases oxidative stress) and we know that Lyme disease can mimic ALS, where a small number of cases in our practice respond to antibiotics, detoxification, and mitochondrial regeneration with improvement in neurological functioning. Infections and toxins drive inflammation, and we must not only shut off the multiple sources of inflammation but also heal the damage that has taken place. Stem cell therapies may represent the new frontier in healing.

Of the twelve-thousand-plus patients I have treated in the last twenty-nine years, I have seen approximately fifty to sixty ALS patients. A combination of genetics, chronic infections, environmental toxins, inadequate detoxification pathways, and oxidative stress with free radical damage may all be implicated. Many of my ALS patients have told me of significant environmental exposures, especially to pesticides and volatile organic solvents. Perhaps ALS patients are more sensitive to these environmental chemicals.

Lyme and associated co-infections also seem to be associated with neurodegenerative symptoms. *Mycoplasma fermentans*, the organism associated with Gulf War syndrome and found in ticks carrying Lyme disease, has also been implicated with several neurological diseases, such as MS and ALS. Ticks have recently been found to contain filarial organisms, and Dr. Alan MacDonald reported in a 2016 abstract that he found larval nematode filarial worms in the cerebrospinal fluid of an MS patient at autopsy. Helminthic infestation of the brain, spinal cord, and, eye have been described in the literature, and may contribute to demyelination.

One of my colleagues, Dr. David Martz, was diagnosed with ALS and then discovered he had Lyme disease. He is still alive more than fourteen years after the diagnosis, having treated himself for Lyme disease with long-term IV antibiotics, even though he still has neurological symptoms, with some weakness of the lower extremities and balance problems. However, these symptoms have not progressed, and he is still able to function after being diagnosed years ago with what should have been a life-threatening illness. I am treating another physician with the same diagnosis and presentation who continues to show slow clinical improvement year after year. Yet, if Lyme disease, co-infections, and environmental toxins were the sole cause of ALS, I would expect to see even more of these patients coming in with the disease.

It is possible that people with a genetic predisposition to ALS are exposed to the same wide array of environmental toxins affecting all of us, and that they also contract Lyme disease and associated co-infections, which then exacerbate their original neuronal insults? Perhaps they also have nutritional deficiencies, sleep disorders, leaky gut with food allergies, and/or imbalances in their microbiome, increasing inflammation and worsening mitochondrial and neurological function. As we know, Lyme disease and co-infections cause inflammation and free radical stress in the central nervous system, which certainly may exacerbate and quicken the neuronal cell death seen in ALS and other neurodegenerative diseases. A small percentage of ALS patients respond positively to antimicrobial therapies combined with antioxidants, while lowering overlapping sources of inflammation, and increasing detoxification and mitochondrial support, lending an endorsement to the theory that there may be a multiplicity of factors at work underlying the pathology of this and other neurodegenerative disorders, like Alzheimer's disease.

In the last three years there have been nine factors on the Horowitz Sixteen-Point MSIDS Map, all of them published in the scientific literature, that have been proven to be associated with Alzheimer's disease, apart from genetic influences. These factors are affecting the neurocognitive functioning of large numbers of the general population.

1. Infections: bacteria: *Borrelia burgdorferi*, other spirochetes (*B. miyamotoi*, denticola spirochetes in the mouth); similar spiral-shaped organisms (*Helicobacter pylori*); *Chlamydia pneumonia*; *Porphyromonas gingivalis*; viruses (HSV-1, cytomegalovirus); and possibly fungal infections. The higher the load of infections (i.e., infectious burden, or IB), the greater the risk. Infections

like borrelia have also been found within biofilms in the brains of AD patients, which co-localize with β amyloid, activating Toll-like receptor 2 in the same areas. The subsequent inflammatory reaction contributes to neuronal death.

2. Immune Dysfunction/Autoimmunity: Brain-reactive autoantibodies are nearly ubiquitous in human sera and may be linked to pathology in the context of the blood-brain barrier (BBB) breakdown. The BBB breakdown is a common finding in AD brains, and Alzheimer's patients were found to have brain-reactive ABs in their brains, which can damage brain tissue and initiate or aggravate multiple neurologic conditions. Lyme increases autoimmune phenomena, as do multiple environmental toxins.

3. Inflammation: The Framingham Study found inflammation and an increase in inflammatory cytokines to increase the risk of Alzheimer's disease. Lowering inflammatory cytokines like TNF-alpha (a pro-inflammatory cytokine) has been shown to not only improve cognition in AD but also to reduce amyloid plaques and tau phosphorylation, hallmarks of the disease.

4. Environmental Toxins and Neuroimmunotoxicology: In 2014, *JAMA Neurology* reported that levels of the pesticide DDE were 3.8-fold higher in those with AD. When we expose human neuroblastoma cells to DDT or DDE, we get increased levels of amyloid precursor protein. Other environmental toxins like ozone and small-particulate matter have also been linked to Alzheimer's dementia. Most people are exposed to multiple toxins and pesticides, which use up glutathione, leading to a potential shortage and inability to detoxify other chemicals. This further leads to increased toxicity and oxidative stress, damaging DNA, and disabling DNA repair and expression enzymes in the periphery and the brain.

5. Diet: Lipid-based diets effectively combat Alzheimer's disease in the mouse model, and increases in dietary intake of either flavonoids (blueberries) or the omega-3 FA (DHA) in fish enhances neurogenesis and memory.

6. Sleep disorders: Lack of sleep contributes to elevations in inflammatory cytokines like IL-6, microinfarcts in the brain, metabolic

syndrome, and diabetes, with neurocognitive deficits. Midlife type II diabetes has been linked to cognitive decline with aging.

7. Hormonal Dysregulation: Numerous studies have documented a strong association between diabetes and Alzheimer's disease (AD), and suggest that avoiding excess insulin and supporting insulin-degrading enzyme (IDE levels) may help prevent and lessen the impact of the disease.

8. Rest and Restore: Meditation may reduce hippocampal-volume atrophy in mild cognitive impairment (MCI), while having a positive impact on brain regions most related to dementia.

9. Exercise: increases the size of the hippocampus and improves memory while attenuating age-related biomarker alterations in preclinical Alzheimer's disease.

So how do we ensure that we are maintaining a healthy brain? Based on all of the scientific research that shows multiple overlapping factors on the MSIDS map can impact cognitive function and neurological disease, we need to effectively treat Lyme disease and persister co-infections, immune dysfunction and autoimmunity, and all overlapping causes of inflammation; detoxify environmental toxins and upregulate glutathione; keep a healthy diet and normal weight (especially by eating healthy fats and avoiding simple carbohydrates); get eight hours of sleep; exercise regularly; and engage in some form of stress reduction like meditation. In short, follow my Action Plan. If we do all these things, we will be supporting and optimizing our neurological function for long-term health.

FOURTEEN

Lyme and Sleep Disorders

People who suffer from Lyme-MSIDS do not sleep well. My patients either have problems falling asleep or complain of frequent awakenings during the night. They also complain of *hypersomnolence*: sleeping for twelve to fourteen hours. Yet, despite sleeping for long periods of time, they often report that they are still extremely fatigued. Worst of all, they often experience these problems despite more and more adults using classical sleep remedies like over-the-counter Benadryl, prescription Ambien, or Lunesta. These sleep aids just don't work for many of my patients; the medication doesn't put them to sleep as it is supposed to, and/or it can take several hours to work, or they aren't able to stay asleep.

Chronic sleep disorders are a major source of morbidity and mortality in the United States. I was a speaker at the 2016 Institute for Functional Medicine conference, which focused on sleep, exercise, rest, and regeneration, and the conference highlighted the scope of the problem and health consequences of inadequate sleep. Dr. Mark Hyman and Dr. Phyllis Zee pointed out that more than a third of adults do not get at least seven hours of sleep per night, and between 50 and 70 million Americans have chronic sleep and wakefulness disorders, which are significantly associated with a broad range of chronic diseases. These include an increase in autoimmune disorders, metabolic syndrome and type 2 diabetes, mental disorders (like depression and anxiety), accidents, cognitive dysfunction with or without Alzheimer's disease and dementia, as well as increased mortality from heart attacks, strokes, obesity, and cancer.

Sleep deprivation is one of the primary reasons that you may remain chronically ill, because impaired sleep directly correlates with impaired immune function and, subsequently, inflammation. Sleep loss increases inflammatory markers like C-reactive protein (CRP) and interleukin-6 (IL-6), leading to increased fatigue, pain, and mood and cognitive difficulties, whether related to Lyme or other chronic diseases. Lack of sleep can also increase blood pressure, activate the sympathetic nervous system, and increase cortisol levels, prothrombotic factors (PAI-1) increasing risks of strokes, while lowering testosterone and leptin levels. We even need proper sleep to clear toxins from the brain, so getting to the source of a sleep disorder is crucial, whether it is a direct effect of *Borrelia burgdorferi* and co-infections and/or due to overlapping medical problems, such as associated sleep apnea (affecting 22 million Americans), restless leg syndrome (RLS), mood disorders, medications, diet, nocturia (getting up to urinate), or hormonal dysregulation.

Insomnia can cause fatigue, daytime sleepiness, and increased pain perception as well as irritability, mood disorders, and memory and concentration problems. These same symptoms occur both for those sleep-deprived "normal" healthy individuals and for those with unresolved Lyme disease. What's more, these symptoms mimic the disease states of fibromyalgia and CFS, making it exceedingly difficult to differentiate which symptoms are due to one particular disease and which are caused by the resulting sleep deprivation, especially since the blood tests for Lyme disease are unreliable. This may be one of the reasons why so many Lyme sufferers are misdiagnosed with CFS/SEID and fibromyalgia. Luckily, once you are able to sleep, your symptoms will often lessen: One study of rheumatoid arthritis sufferers who used sleep medication reported less joint pain, even though their illness was still active.

Aside from inflammation and immune disorders, there are many medical conditions associated with significant insomnia. These include:

- Acute viral illnesses and HIV
- Adrenal hormone imbalance, in which cortisol is high at night
- Caffeine: too much caffeine can delay sleep onset, reduce total

sleep time, and alter stages of sleep (decreased slow-wave sleep and REM sleep)
- Cancer: different types cause sleep problems
- Chronic bacterial infections
- Chronic fatigue syndrome/SEID: inflammatory mediators interfere with sleep
- Chronic pain conditions: pain and/or medication used (narcotics) can affect REM sleep
- Circadian rhythm disorders: these can be transient disorders (i.e., jet lag, or a change in work schedule); a chronic disorder such as advanced sleep phase syndrome (ASPS), seen in the elderly/depressed, with an early sleep onset (6:00 to 9:00 P.M.) and early wakeup; or delayed sleep-phase syndrome (DSPS), frequently seen in Lyme disease, where it can take hours to fall asleep and awaken at socially accepted times, and peak alertness is in the late evening and night
- Depression and anxiety
- Electromagnetic field (EMF) exposure: EMFs have been reported to cause widespread neuropsychiatric effects including depression and insomnia
- Environmental factors/toxins: e.g., an increase in ambient noise as well as mercury
- Endocrine disorders, such as hypo/hyperthyroidism, low sex hormones, high insulin secretion with hypoglycemia, hypercortisolism, and elevated growth hormone (acromegaly)
- Fibromyalgia
- GI reflux (may cause coughing, choking, or asthmatic symptoms in the middle of the night)
- Lyme-MSIDS: borrelia and multiple co-infections affect sleep
- Medication: various medications can interfere with sleep (e.g., stimulants with a long half-life)
- Menopause (secondary to hormonal changes): decreases in estradiol, progesterone, and testosterone, with increases in follicular stimulating hormone (FSH) have been correlated with sleep difficulties
- Narcolepsy with excessive daytime sleepiness and/or cataplexy

- Nocturia (having to get up several times per night to urinate): multiple causes are possible, including low hormones (ADH), elevated blood sugars (diabetes), fluid overload (congestive heart failure, cirrhosis, nephrotic syndrome), benign prostatic hypertrophy (BPH, which can be worsened with antihistamines), and drinking too much fluids after the evening meal or taking diuretics too close to bedtime
- Non-Lyme-MSIDS: co-infections and multiple factors on the MSIDS map can increase inflammation and interfere with sleep
- Obstructive and restrictive lung diseases: any lung disease decreasing oxygen saturation and impairing breathing can adversely affect sleep patterns (i.e., Emphysema/COPD, asthma, pulmonary fibrosis)
- Renal disease: advanced stages of renal disease from multiple causes (i.e., polycystic kidney disease, autoimmune disease, diabetic/IgA nephropathy, stones, contrast agents)
- Restless leg syndrome: an irresistible urge to move the extremities (not just the legs), increased with relaxation, varying with clear circadian rhythms. May be associated with low iron/dopamine in the central nervous system as well as hypoglycemia, antidepressants (tricyclics, SSRIs), antihistamines, medication withdrawal (benzodiazepines, narcotics)
- Shift worker syndrome (SWS): those who work atypical hours (i.e., 4:00 P.M. to midnight, or midnight to morning shifts) have an increased risk of cardiovascular disease, diabetes, obesity, depression, accidents, and cancer
- Sleep apnea: approximately 6 percent of the U.S. population suffers from sleep apnea

COMMON MEDICATIONS THAT INTERFERE WITH SLEEP

Many over-the-counter stimulants such as Sudafed can affect sleep, especially if they are taken as a twenty-four-hour, slow-release preparation (the same is true for Claritin D 24 hr, Allegra D 24 hr, Zyrtec D 24 hr). If you have to take Sudafed for sinus congestion, I recommend the short-acting form (30 mg) taken up until 5:00 P.M., at a maximum dose of 120 mg per day, or a maximum of one twelve-hour, slow-release formulation per day (120 mg total of Sudafed, as in Claritin D-12 hour, Allegra D-12 hour), taken early in the morning. This way the effect of the drug wears off before bedtime.

Individuals with ADD/ADHD may also be taking stimulants to help them concentrate, which may interfere with sleep. These include Vyvanse, Ritalin, and Adderall XR. Vyvanse is particularly problematic for individuals with sleep disorders, due to its long half-life. I suggest changing to shorter acting medication when possible.

Other stimulants that may interfere with sleep are Provigil and Nuvigil, which are medications taken in the morning to help with resistant fatigue from sleep apnea, or from shift worker syndrome, in which sleep cycles are affected by getting to bed late every night. Although helpful to stay awake, it is best to choose the minimum effective dose.

Certain foods can also have a stimulant effect. For example, some people cannot tolerate caffeine, or even chocolate, especially in the afternoon, since the stimulant effect may keep them up at night. We want to address all the potential overlapping etiologies responsible for sleep deprivation, including the common causes of nocturia we regularly see in our practice, since it can lead to increased fatigue, daytime sleepiness, mood changes, impaired work productivity, cognitive dysfunction, and an increased risk of accidents. Older individuals often fall (occasionally breaking their hips), and 25 percent of these falls occur while waking up to void.

DO I NEED A SLEEP STUDY?

If it is unclear which factors may be responsible for causing insomnia, a sleep study can be useful. Sleep studies (also known as polysomnography) are performed overnight, during which your sleep patterns are monitored, evaluating brain wave patterns (EEG), eye movement patterns (EOG), changes in heart rhythm (EKG), as well as the quality and duration of sleep. Important measurements include the number of apneic and hypopneic events (when people stop or have decreased breathing during sleep), decreases in oxygen saturation, and evaluating for restless legs. Some companies offer sleep studies that can be done at home (Accusom), offering a more natural environment to evaluate sleep patterns.

Sleep studies are particularly useful for determining a condition known as sleep apnea, which typically affects overweight individuals, but it can also affect young, thin women who deny snoring. It can contribute to the daytime fatigue and headaches that we often see in the MSIDS patient. Patients with severe sleep apnea may have many episodes during the night where they stop breathing for several seconds at a time, while simultaneously the oxygen saturation in their blood drops. This is particularly important to diagnose, because low oxygen levels in the blood during sleep apnea can adversely affect the heart, leading to heart attacks and arrhythmias in those with underlying heart disease.

Some MSIDS patients also suffer from narcolepsy, falling asleep suddenly in the middle of the day, having excessive daytime sleepiness and/or cataplexy, where there is a sudden loss of voluntary muscle control. In cataplexy the signs can be obvious (dropping objects, dropping to the knees, or falling down with sudden strong emotions, such as laughter, anger, fear, or orgasm), or there can be subtler manifestations, such as a slackening of the facial muscles and a dropping of the head or jaw. These different conditions are best evaluated with a different type of sleep study, known as an MSLT (multiple sleep latency test). Although cataplexy is rare, it happens in about 70 percent of people with narcolepsy, and can also be present as a side effect of the discontinuation of an SSRI like Prozac.

One of my favorite patients is a pastor who has a very challenging congregation (he is certain they all have Lyme disease), and whenever he gets angry with them, he falls to his knees. Everyone thought he was praying to the Lord for help (which may have been true), but we discovered with an MSLT that he had cataplexy.

Sleep Medications That Work for MSIDS

Controlling and balancing inflammatory cytokine levels are essential if we are to feel energetic and get a good night's sleep. An analogy that I often use with my patients to explain this process is that of a faucet and a sink. If we have a running faucet (the ongoing production of cytokines) as well as a clogged drain (poor detoxification pathways), we are going to accumulate abnormal levels of these inflammatory molecules. We therefore need to control cytokine production by "shutting down the faucet" (i.e., decreasing their overproduction) and "opening up the drain" (eliminating them from the body), as well as eliminating associated toxins, if we are to feel well.

Many sleep medications share the same liver detoxification pathways, so it is important to check for drug interactions, as they may have additive effects and cause excessive daytime drowsiness if one drug interferes with the excretion of another from the body. Since we often use combination therapy to treat resistant insomnia, I find it essential to use the trusty *Physicians' Desk Reference* (known as "the PDR") to check for drug interactions when combining medications.

General treatment guidelines to deal with resistant insomnia and fatigue, after doing a full differential diagnostic evaluation, include using activating agents, which are drugs with a stimulating effect in the morning and sleep-promoting agents in the evening. Activating agents include medications such as Provigil and Nuvigil; stimulants like Ritalin, Vyvanse, and Adderall; and Wellbutrin, noradrenergic agents, and the SSRIs.

Provigil can be effective for those who are unable to stay awake during the day, and for whom classical therapies for insomnia have failed. It must be used with caution if there is an associated anxiety disorder and/or heart palpitations, since it can increase these symptoms and also interfere with sleep if taken late in the day or in too high a dose.

Wellbutrin is a much easier drug to use. It augments the efficacy of other antidepressants, such as SSRIs, improving patients' moods, and inhibits the neuronal uptake of the excitatory brain chemicals dopamine and norepinephrine. This helps patients be more alert in the morning. I have generally found Wellbutrin to be a very well-tolerated medication with fewer drug interactions than many of the commonly used antidepressants on the market. Other options include balancing neurotransmitter levels (i.e., low serotonin) with 5-HTP.

Sleep agents that promote deep, slow-wave sleep include Lyrica, trazodone, Gabitril, Seroquel, and Xyrem. These drugs are typically used for other conditions (except Xyrem) but have been proven very effective for getting people to sleep. However, a typical internist would not normally consider them, since we are primarily taught in medical school to use sleep drugs such as Ambien, Lunesta, and benzodiazepine derivatives (Valium, Restoril). Yet these other drugs have certain distinct clinical advantages. For example, Lyrica is commonly used for neuropathic pain in both diabetics and postherpetic neuralgia (pain experienced after getting shingles). Up to 70 percent of persistent Lyme disease patients have peripheral neuropathy. Similarly, Lyrica is approved for use in fibromyalgia. I have therefore found that my patients suffering from insomnia, neuropathy, and FM may benefit from the use of this drug if standard sleep medications have failed. Since the drug can cause drowsiness, dizziness, visual changes, and confusion, we generally need to keep the doses of this medication on the lower side during the day, since the side effects mimic the same symptoms seen in our MSIDS patients. Many of our patients are also on antidepressants, and the combination of Lyrica and antidepressants may increase the risk of central nervous system depression, leading to a decreased level of consciousness, so this also needs to be kept in mind.

Gabitril, like Lyrica, is an antiseizure medication. It stimulates the brain's GABA receptors, which help induce sleep. Like Lyrica, it can cause central nervous system depression as well as other possible side effects, including fatigue, dizziness, and impaired concentration. It can be used alone or in combination with other drugs that hit GABA receptor sites in the brain that help induce sleep, such as benzodiazepines like Valium. Some patients who have failed trials of standard sleep medications, such as Ambien (which also interacts with GABA-benzodiazepine receptors), find that they finally fall asleep taking Gabitril, even at low doses with or without benzodiazepines. Since benzodiazepines are addictive, their use should be limited if possible, as their effect will wear off over time and require higher and higher doses to be effective. I usually will combine natural products with GABA (GABA pills, creams) with Gabitril or Lyrica instead of benzodiapines, and find it to be effective. Progesterone at bedtime also hits GABA receptors, and can be used in women going through menopause to help get them to sleep, versus using SSRIs like Paxil or Lexapro, which may help decrease hot flashes and insomnia while helping associated mood disorders.

Trazodone is helpful if there is significant overlapping depression and anxiety. I find it to be a useful addition to standard sleep medications or when used alone. It may cause drowsiness, fatigue, headaches, and dizziness, and possibly serotonin syndrome or neuroleptic malignant syndrome. Serotonin syndrome is a potentially life-threatening drug reaction, affecting the autonomic nervous system and leading to high temperatures (hyperthermia), sweating, nausea, diarrhea, elevated heart rates (tachycardia) with elevations in blood pressure (hypertension), tremors, and muscle twitching (myoclonus). It can also affect cognition, causing agitation and confusion, and can even lead to a coma. Careful attention, therefore, needs to be paid to using drugs that affect serotonin pathways simultaneously. I have never seen a case of serotonin syndrome in all of my years of practice, but it should always be kept in mind, as MSIDS patients also often suffer from autonomic nervous system dysfunction.

Remeron is an antidepressant that I did not frequently prescribe prior to treating patients with Lyme disease. Although its exact mechanism of action is unknown, it seems to increase the efficacy of serotonin receptors and block the excitatory neurotransmitters like norepinephrine and epinephrine, therefore allowing the brain to quiet down and induce sleep. At its lowest dose, it has the greatest effect on putting one to sleep. Although the PDR lists a whole range of possible side effects for Remeron, we generally have found the drug to be well tolerated with minimal side effects.

Seroquel is used by many Lyme-literate psychiatrists as an adjunct for sleep, especially for those with overlapping psychiatric problems such as schizophrenia or bipolar disorder. I generally avoid it because of my concern that it may cause extrapyramidal symptoms (movement disorders) and affect the endocrine functioning of the thyroid (hypothyroidism) and pancreas (increased risk of diabetes).

Xyrem should be considered when most other drug and herbal regimens have failed. It is indicated for excessive daytime sleepiness, cataplexy, narcolepsy, or shift-work sleep disorders (SWS). One of the advantages of Xyrem is that it is metabolized in the liver but primarily excreted through the lungs as carbon dioxide, with a very short half-life of thirty to sixty minutes. The short half-life is why the drug needs to be given twice a night, right before bedtime and then four hours later. An abnormal sleep study indicating narcolepsy and/or cataplexy, and a history of excessive daytime sleepiness or SWS, is usually necessary to get insurance approval. Potential adverse effects include somnolence, confusion, and attention disturbances the next day, as well as sleep walking and sleep paralysis, so watching carefully for side effects is important.

Newer sleep medications that have been released in the past few years include melatonin receptor agonists (e.g., tasimelteon [Heltioz], which is only for a circadian rhythm disorder known as non-24 sleep disorder in blind patients), and orexin receptor antagonists (e.g., suvorexant, Belsomra) in those with insomnia characterized by difficulties with sleep onset and/or sleep maintenance, who have failed traditional therapies. Belsomra is contraindicated in those with narcolepsy, and it can impair daytime wakefulness with a CNS depressant effect that can last for up to several days after discontinuation. It therefore has to be used very carefully, especially if mixed with other medications that are central nervous system depressants. It is a controlled substance usually only prescribed by sleep specialists. Belsomra was given to one of my patients in the Southwest who had a circadian rhythm disorder with delayed sleep phase syndrome (DSPS) who couldn't fall asleep until 5:00 or 6:00 A.M. every morning for years, and it was the only drug that helped get her to sleep. Due to severe side effects, however, the treatment for DSPS is usually trying chronotherapy first, for instance, moving bedtime and rising later and later each day until the circadian rhythm is back within the normal range. For those with ASPS (i.e., elderly patients, who may be depressed), chronotherapy or behavior modification can be helpful, but bright light therapy, especially for those with SAD (seasonal affective disorder) is suggested as the primary therapy.

Other medications for sleep that we have found to be useful include some of the older tricyclic antidepressant drugs, such as Elavil, and muscle relaxers such as Flexeril. Elavil has similar indications as Lyrica: It is a neuroleptic drug that can be used for neuropathic pain, postherpetic neuralgia, as well as migraine prophylaxis. Therefore, it can be useful for those with Lyme disease and Bartonella who suffer from an associated neuropathy, with or without a history of frequent migraines. I usually find low doses (10–20 mg) are effective at night, but all of these drugs must be used with caution in the elderly who may be sensitive to their CNS depressant effect. Elavil was a commonly used drug for depression until SSRIs emerged. It can cause QT interval changes on the electrocardiogram, and the PDR drug interaction checker should be used when combining medications.

Many people who suffer from Lyme-MSIDS with associated insomnia also experience muscle pain and spasm that in turn may further interfere with sleep. A magnesium supplement at bedtime may be helpful. I tend to use magnesium malate and glycinate, but magnesium L-threonate (200 mg PO HS) is a newer form that has been shown to have good CNS penetration. Flexeril is the drug that is classically used for muscle spasm. I have generally avoided its use during the daytime because of its significant side effect of drowsiness, but if it is used as a nighttime aid for sleep, it may be effective, even in low doses (5 mg PO HS).

Frequently prescribed sleep drugs such as Ambien were created and approved for the short-term treatment of insomnia; however, some need it for longer periods of time if no other medications have been effective. One of the serious side effects of Ambien is that it can cause complex sleep-related behavior, such as sleepwalking. There are stories in the medical literature of people eating or even driving their car and not remembering their actions the next morning. Similarly, it can cause memory loss, not a desired side effect in the Lyme patient who may already suffer from severe neurocognitive deficits, and a recent study indicated other potential serious side effects with long-term use (every night for years). Taking a drug-free holiday may be important when it is difficult to determine whether certain symptoms are due to the disease or to the drug that you are taking. I no longer prescribe Ambien and encourage my patients to find other solutions if they need a long-term sleep aid.

Lunesta is a sleep medication that has been approved for longer-term use. We have generally not seen significant side effects in our patients who use Lunesta. However, as with Ambien, side effects of drowsiness, hallucinations, and confusion have been reported. Once again, it is important to be sure that you are not experiencing a drug side effect that resembles the symptoms of disease.

Herbal Remedies Worth Trying

I find certain herbs and nutraceuticals to be useful for treating insomnia, and many have been validated scientifically. If one regimen is ineffective, these herbs and nutraceuticals can be combined, helping to increase their efficacy. What's more, combining herbs and medications means that less prescription medication can be used, with generally less drug interactions and side effects.

Valerian root has been extensively reviewed by the German Commission E, a governing body in Germany that created a therapeutic guide for licensed medical professionals prescribing herbal medicine. It has been shown to have a relaxing effect and can be used for the treatment of anxiety and stress-related disorders during the day, and at night to help you get to sleep and stay asleep. It comes in drops (Amantilla, NutraMedix) and capsules. I generally prefer the drops, as the dosage can be adjusted much more easily and because (according to my patients) the capsules smell like old socks.

GABA-L theanine comes in creams, powders (Xymogen), and capsules. L-theanine is a derivative of green tea, which has a relaxing effect on the body, and also affects glutamate reuptake in the brain. The GABA-L theanine cream can be applied to the temples and on the back of the neck before bedtime, and when combined with inositol, can be helpful in treating obsessive-compulsive disorder, or for individuals who can't shut off their thinking at night. I have used this combination in both adults and children, and it has definitely been effective without the associated side effects of more traditional OCD drugs, such as Anafranil.

Melatonin is commonly used for sleep disorders, especially DSPS. It is an essential hormone produced by the pineal gland that helps regulate circadian rhythms to elicit sleep, and whose production tends to decrease as we age. There are controlled-release, long-acting formulations that may also help decrease frequent awakening in the middle of the night. The dosage needs to be properly adjusted, however, because too much melatonin can cause a hangover effect in the morning. One of the advantages of melatonin is that it functions as a powerful antioxidant, decreasing oxidative stress and protecting the CNS as well as mitochondrial and nuclear DNA. It also decreases production of TH17, a pro-inflammatory cytokine. Melatonin can be mixed with other supplements or medications to improve efficacy.

Phosphatidylserine (PS) affects dysregulated adrenal hormone production. An overstimulated adrenal gland produces excess cortisol, which can contribute to sleep problems. PS helps to decrease the overproduction of hormones from the pituitary gland, which subsequently leads to lower levels of cortisol, helping to regulate the stress response and relax the body. It is insufficient as a stand-alone supplement to regulate sleep, but it can be helpful when excess production of cortisol is identified as one of the causes of insomnia. Magnesium at night may also be helpful, especially in those with restless leg syndrome.

Some of the Bach Flower remedies, such as Rescue Remedy, and homeopathic remedies like Kali phos have been prescribed as sleep aids by naturopathic doctors, and they can help when you wake up in the middle of the night and can't fall back asleep.

Chinese doctors who treat Lyme disease with traditional Chinese herbs also have formulas that include herbs such as *Ziziphus jujuba*, *Schisandra Chinensis*, *Paeonia lactiflora*, and *Rehmannia glutinosa*.

Finally, for those who get inadequate results from classical sleep medications and herbal therapies, and are very sensitive to ambient noise, snoring spouses, and/or noisy neighbors, we find sound soothers, noise cancelling devices, and earplugs may be helpful.

MICHELLE COULDN'T SLEEP

Teenagers are some of the best sleepers, yet my patient, Michelle from Vermont, couldn't get to sleep. At just eighteen years old she complained of severe fatigue, migraines with light and sound sensitivity, dizziness, joint pain that would migrate around her body, GI problems, vaginal itching and discharge, day sweats, chills, flushing, lack of a regular period for years, anxiety and palpitations, moderate to severe memory and concentration problems, and severe insomnia: She had difficulty falling asleep and also was complaining of frequent awakening. She was diagnosed with Lyme disease a year before she came to see me, after suffering with these symptoms for years, and was referred to a Lyme-literate doctor for treatment. She underwent one year of antibiotics before coming in, but she was still only functioning at about 30 percent of normal. A gynecologist placed her on birth control pills, as her estrogen and progesterone levels were all found to be in the very low range, yet she still was not having regular periods. She had also been seen by a cardiologist and an endocrinologist because of her palpitations. She had a negative workup, including a negative echocardiogram and Holter monitor, with normal norepinephrine and VMA levels in her urine.

We sent off a CBC, a comprehensive metabolic profile; B_{12}, folate, methylmalonic acid, and homocysteine levels with a methylenetrahydrofolate reductase (MTHFR) test; as well as a comprehensive co-infection panel, which included a Babesia FISH test, Bartonella titer and PCR, Mycoplasma titer and PCR, rickettsial panel for Rocky Mountain spotted fever, typhus, and Q fever; and tularemia and Brucella titers for her chronic fatigue, sweats, joint pain, and severe memory problems. We also performed hormonal studies and checked Vitamin D levels, sex hormone levels, thyroid functions (T3, free T3, T4, TSH with antithyroid antibodies), adrenal function (DHEA/cortisol levels by saliva), and an IgF-1 level to rule out growth hormone deficiency. We also tested for mineral deficiencies (magnesium, iodine, and zinc), checked autoimmune markers, and expanded her GI workup by sending off an *H. pylori* test, an antigliadin antibody and TTG with an IgE and IgG food allergy panel (for her chronic digestive complaints), with a Genova Diagnostics GI Effects panel with a Comprehensive Digestive Stool Analysis (CDSA).

After drawing blood, we gave her an injection of 2 gm of IV glutathione, since it has been effective in so many patients with fatigue, muscle and joint pain, and cognitive problems. Michelle felt better within fifteen minutes of the injection, with a significant decrease in her fatigue, headache, and cognitive problems.

One month later Michelle came back for her test results. She was positive for babesiosis, Bartonella, very low adrenal function, with cortisol levels below range in the morning but high at night (which may have interfered with her sleep), a low free T3, other thyroid functions within range, low sex hormone levels (low estradiol and progesterone levels), a positive antigliadin and negative TTG, positive food allergies by both IgE (shrimp, hazelnuts) and IgG (milk, wheat, beef, and eggs being the highest) with a low Vitamin D_3 and a slightly low B_{12} level. Her CDSA showed infections with two parasites. In other words, not only did Michelle suffer from Lyme disease, she had MSIDS. The overlapping factors that were contributing to her illness included Babesia and Bartonella, intestinal parasites, various hormonal abnormalities including adrenal dysfunction, gluten sensitivity with food allergies, vitamin deficiencies, and detoxification problems. No wonder Michelle was so tired all the time!

Due to the yeast and the severity of her GI symptoms, Michelle did not want to try antibiotics or antiparasitic drugs right away. We started her on supplementation to treat her adrenal fatigue. Phosphatidylserine was prescribed to be taken at night for her elevated cortisol and her difficulties with sleep, with pregnenolone in the morning to give her further hormonal support for low adrenals and sex hormones. She was told to liberalize the salt and fluids in her diet and also take licorice, which supports adrenal function and helps raise blood pressure.

She was placed on a strict hypoglycemic diet because many of her symptoms were worse after eating carbohydrates, especially the wheat products we now knew she was allergic to. I also recommended a yeast-free diet that might help her mitigate her GI symptoms of gas and bloating, vaginal itching, and discharge. It was important that she follow a strict yeast-free diet, since Candida symptoms can mimic Lyme symptoms (except the pain usually doesn't migrate).

We started her on an herbal protocol for Lyme disease with Samento and Cumunda instead of antibiotics, which would have exacerbated her Candida problem, and gave her Malarone with Artemisia for the babesiosis. She was also given NAC, alpha-lipoic acid, and glycine to support her own glutathione production after we saw how effective the IV glutathione was in relieving her headache and brain fog. Finally, she was given Amantilla (valerian root in liquid form) for her anxiety, palpitations, and difficulty sleeping.

At her next visit Michelle reported that her energy swings were more stable when she followed a hypoglycemic/yeast-free diet, and her migraines and GI symptoms had improved. Her joint pain initially flared from the herbs that she was taking to treat the Lyme disease, but it eventually improved; the sweats and chills decreased with the antimalarial therapy for Babesia. However, she still complained of resistant fatigue, brain fog, and insomnia. We reviewed the sleep medications she had tried that had failed before coming to see me. Standard sleep medication such as Lunesta and Ambien had failed, as well as benzodiazepines such as Valium, Xanax, and Restoril. She had also tried Lyrica, trazodone, Gabitril, Elavil, Flexeril, and Remeron, and multiple natural products, including melatonin, and now she was on valerian root and phosphatidylserine, but nothing made her sleep. Michelle was barely sleeping four hours per night and couldn't go to school, as she was exhausted most of the time.

The next logical choice for Michelle was Xyrem. I gave her a DVD that instructed her on how to take it. She would have to be in bed when she took the initial dose, then wake up four hours later to take the next dose. I told her to call if she had any side effects. We started with 3 gm (6 ml) twice a night, as I had found that the lower doses can cause confusion and disorientation. If 3 gm didn't work after a week, and she tolerated it without side effects, she was instructed to try increasing the dose to 4 gm (8 ml) twice per night, four hours apart.

Michelle returned a month later. She was sleeping soundly for the first time in years! Xyrem was the answer. She had no side effects from the drug and felt a sense of wellness that she had not experienced in a long time.

She was now sleeping eight hours per night and was able to go back to school. Michelle told me that without getting her to sleep none of the other interventions would have made a significant difference. Even though balancing hormones, bringing up her blood pressure, stabilizing her gut, and treating the infections were all beneficial, she only turned the corner once she finally got some sleep.

FIFTEEN

Lyme and Autonomic Nervous System Dysfunction/POTS

One disease process that is often missed in MSIDS, which can mimic some of the most frequently reported Lyme symptoms and explain a poor response to traditional therapies, is Postural Orthostatic Tachycardia Syndrome (POTS), a form of autonomic nervous system (ANS) dysfunction. If you suffer from unexplained fatigue, dizziness, brain fog, anxiety, and/or palpitations, then you may have POTS/dysautonomia.

An ANS dysfunction (also known as autonomic dysfunction, or dysautonomia) describes any disease or malfunction of the nerves that control blood pressure, heart rate, sweat glands, bladder, and bowel function. An ANS dysfunction can develop as a symptom of Lyme disease, but it may also occur with other diseases that affect the nervous system, such as diabetes or Shy-Drager syndrome (the degeneration of nerve cells in the brain). In Chapter 13 we learned that there were four types of neuropathy that can affect the nervous system in patients with Lyme disease. One of them is autonomic neuropathy, a form that affects the involuntary nerves of the autonomic nervous system. The ANS involves elements of the central nervous system (brain/hypothalamus and spinal cord), the peripheral nervous system, with its sensory motor branches, and the enteric nervous system, made up of nerve fibers that go to the bladder and gastrointestinal tract (including the pancreas and the gallbladder). The ANS performs its duties by acting through two main branches: the orthosympathetic (OS) and parasympathetic (PS) nervous systems.

The particular ANS symptoms seen in Lyme-MSIDS patients will depend on which part or parts of the system have been affected: If it's the brain/hypothalamus you may experience temperature dysregulation; if it's the peripheral sensory nerves you may feel burning, tingling, numbness, stabbing, or crawling sensations (one or several of these symptoms that usually comes and goes with Lyme disease) as well as problems with sweating. If either the parasympathetic or orthosympathetic system has been affected, you may have symptoms affecting your heart rate and blood pressure, as well as bladder and bowel function.

Postural orthostatic tachycardia syndrome (POTS) refers to symptoms resulting from the impaired functioning of the autonomic nervous system, when we are unable to maintain our vascular tone. The OS nervous system regulates the contraction and expansion of blood vessels. Proper regulation of vascular tone is crucial, for we need to be able to remain in an upright position and maintain a normal blood pressure in order to accomplish many of our daily activities. When the ANS fails to function properly, whether through failure of other organ systems (congestive heart failure or either renal or hepatic disease), systemic illness (strokes), endocrine abnormalities (hypothyroidism, or a pheochromocytoma, an adrenal tumor that secretes excessive catecholamines), or other causes of autonomic neuropathy, then blood pressure and cerebral blood flow will be compromised and POTS can result.

This syndrome leads to low blood pressure when standing and/or changing position (postural orthostasis). The heart tries to compensate for the low blood pressure by beating faster, thereby causing palpitations. This acute lowering of the blood pressure causes dizziness, fatigue, exercise intolerance, and difficulty concentrating due to poor cerebral blood flow. These findings were seen in a 2007 Mayo Clinic study, one of the largest clinical studies on this syndrome to date. This study was of particular interest, because many of the participants also had symptoms we commonly see with Lyme disease.

Patients with POTS may also suffer from an autonomic neuropathy. This can affect several different nerves in the body, causing a wide variety of symptoms.

- The autonomic small nerve fibers of the skin impact our sensation of temperature as well as the functioning of the sweat glands. Patients with POTS therefore may not sweat (anhidrosis) or sweat too much (hyperhidrosis), depending on how these nerve fibers are affected. Small-fiber neuropathy would explain the abnormalities seen on sweat testing in patients with ANS dysfunction (the quantitative sudomotor axon reflex test and thermoregulatory sweat testing), in which certain patients with POTS have regional, global, or mixed patterns of sweat loss or hyperhidrosis.
- The peripheral nerves are also affected. This can cause symptoms of burning, tingling, numbness, stabbing, or crawling sensations of the skin (small-fiber neuropathy), as well as contributing to the pooling of fluids in the lower extremities, lowering blood pressure.
- The vagus nerve can be affected, and thereby our heart rate. A normal pulse rate is 72 beats per minute, although there are variabilities depending on how physically fit we are, and we see a loss of heart rate variability in those with signs of vagal nerve involvement. This also explains the varied gastrointestinal and urinary complaints in POTS, as the vagus nerve activates and controls the gastrointestinal (GI) and genitourinary (GU) systems. This can interfere with our ability to properly move our bowels and bladder.
- Baroreceptor reflexes can be affected. These are specialized nerve cells in arteries (the carotid sinuses and aortic arch) that monitor our blood pressure and send the information to the brain (brain stem) and autonomic nervous system. They also help us maintain a stable blood pressure. For example, if the blood pressure starts to decrease too much, it would cause the heart rate to increase, raising the blood pressure. This homeostatic feedback loop does not work well in those with POTS. The result is blood pressure swings without a compensatory increase in heart rate necessary for maintaining blood pressure.
- Nerve fibers of the internal organs can be affected by autonomic neuropathy, further affecting hormonal systems that regulate blood pressure. One of the functions of the kidneys, apart from filtering toxic waste, is the production of hormones such as erythropoietin, which stimulates red blood cell production,

increasing the intravascular volume and raising blood pressure. The kidneys also produce the hormone renin, which raises blood pressure through a hormonal feedback loop known as the renin-angiotensin-aldosterone system. If the kidneys are affected by ANS dysfunction, less renin is produced and blood pressure is lowered. Lower renin levels decrease aldosterone, leading to less effective salt retention, which then decreases the production of angiotensin II, another hormone that increases blood pressure through the constriction of blood vessels. Low plasma renin levels are seen with those who have POTS, whereas normally we would expect a high renin level for those with low blood volume (hypovolemia).

- Autoimmune autonomic neuropathy is another mechanism that is occasionally seen with POTS. Autonomic ganglia contain the cell bodies of the autonomic nerves that connect neurological structures such as the peripheral and central nervous systems. In the same study done at the Mayo Clinic, specific autoimmune markers, antiganglioside antibodies, were seen in 10 percent of the 152 patients studied who had POTS. Other studies have similarly described autoantibodies against ganglia in autoimmune neuropathies. We find the same autoimmune markers in many of our Lyme patients who have ANS dysfunction and POTS, especially if they also have associated peripheral neuropathy.

DO I HAVE POTS AND LYME?

If you are experiencing symptoms of low blood pressure and lightheadedness, with weakness/dizziness upon standing or changing position, and have generalized profound resistant fatigue and/or episodes of nearly passing out (pre-syncope) or passing out (syncope), you may have POTS. If your history suggests autonomic hyperactivity, such as unexplained anxiety and palpitations, and have experienced hyperhidrosis (too much sweating) or loss of sweating in parts of the body (anhidrosis), then POTS is a likely diagnosis. Similarly, people with resistant gastrointestinal symptoms of nausea, vomiting and/or chronic constipation, and/or urinary difficulties with voiding, may have vagal nerve dysfunction from an autonomic neuropathy. Gastroparesis is one particularly rare and severe manifestation of POTS/dysautonomia, causing delayed emptying of the stomach with associated abdominal pain with nausea, vomiting, and an inability to eat.

According to a 2008 study published in *Current Rheumatology Reports*, POTS has been associated with chronic fatigue syndrome and fibromyalgia, but it has not been linked with Lyme disease in the medical literature. Yet I believe, as others do, that POTS may be one of the reasons individuals with Lyme disease continue to experience chronic symptoms. I see many patients with confirmed POTS and Lyme who have positive tilt-table tests and positive tests for ANS dysfunction by a board-certified neurologist. I have also seen patients come in with early signs of POTS, including high resting-heart rates, before they experience any significant drops in blood pressure. Other doctors may mistake this sign for an anxiety or panic disorder if the full clinical picture is not recognized, or think that their patients are excited to see them (mine are, or at least that's what they tell me when I ask).

On physical examination, patients with POTS often have elevated resting heart rates in the high 80s, 90s, and occasionally over 100 beats per minute. This is consistent with the hyperadrenergic state seen in autonomic nervous system dysfunction. Their resting blood pressure, on the other hand, tends to be in the low normal range (i.e., 90–100/60), and will usually drop (mildly, or significantly) when they stand up for several minutes. Checking resting and standing pulse and blood pressure is an easy test for dysautonomia, and it can be performed in a physician's office. We do blood pressure and pulse readings at time zero (sitting for several minutes), and then at 3, 6, and 9 minutes standing. An increase in heart rate of more than 30 beats per minute (BPM), or a total heart rate greater than 120 beats per minute, is more typically seen on a head-up tilt-table testing (HUT) done in the hospital, but we do see those types of elevations occasionally in our office. Mild-to-moderate POTS may cause a slight decrease in blood pressure standing, and heart rate elevations in the 15–25 BPM range. A simple screening blood pressure and pulse check with changing position can help lead the medical detective to the right diagnosis.

In order to diagnose POTS definitively, an individual would be sent to the hospital to have a head-up tilt-table test. This is administered by lying flat on a special table while the heart rate is monitored (by EKG), and blood pressure is checked. The table then is placed in an upright position, usually at 60 or 80 degrees. If there is orthostatic intolerance (a significant drop in blood pressure, with dizziness and/or fainting) and an increase in heart rate (an increase of more than 30 beats per minute, or a heart rate greater than 120 beats per minute within 10 minutes of the test) while going from the sitting to standing position, that is considered to be a positive head-up tilt-table test.

Apart from the tilt-table, other tests used to evaluate POTS/dysautonomia include monitoring the heart rate response to deep breathing and Valsalva maneuvers (pushing on the carotid arteries or increasing intraabdominal pressure by moving the bowels). A second test, quantitative sudomotor axon reflex testing (QSART), which detects abnormal sweating, can also be performed to further evaluate the functioning of the autonomic nervous system.

Neurologists such as Dr. David Younger at NYU and Dr. Amri Katz from Yale have seen many patients with POTS who also suffer with neurological Lyme disease. These patients may present with the classical symptoms of polyradiculoneuritis (inflammation in different nerves coming out of the spine), distal polyneuropathy (neuropathy in the distal nerves), dysautonomia (autonomic nervous system dysfunction), and small-fiber sensory neuropathy. Their complete neurological workup often includes an MRI of the brain, SPECT scans for hypoperfusion, tilt-table testing, quantitative sensory testing (QST) for heat pain perception thresholds, EMGs with nerve conduction studies, and epidermal nerve fiber studies of the thigh and calf to screen for small-fiber sensory nerve dysfunction. They are also sent for neuropsychological studies, which can show significant deficits in memory and concentration, a slowing of processing speed, and problems with executive functioning.

Along with these tests, I also recommend testing for autoantibodies against nerves (antiganglioside antibodies, i.e., IgM and IgG anti-GM1, Mag, and ASI), one of the manifestations of ANS dysfunction, as well as looking into other causes of neuropathy. This would include ruling out common causes such as diabetes, hypothyroidism, pregnancy, carpal tunnel syndrome, and vitamin deficiencies (B_{12}, folate); performing antimyelin antibodies (seen in Lyme and autoimmune disorders); evaluating immunoglobulin levels (IgA, IgM, and IgG levels with subclasses), as some patients suffer from Lyme with overlapping Chronic Variable Immune

Deficiency (CVID) contributing to their neuropathy and resistant symptoms; and also check for heavy metal burdens (mercury, lead, and/or arsenic), and co-infections like Bartonella, *Borrelia miyamotoi*, and Q fever (*Coxiella burnetii*), which can all cause and simultaneously increase neuropathy. Using the MSIDS model, I often find multiple overlapping etiologies driving symptoms.

Lyme disease patients occasionally test positive for antibodies against peripheral nerves, due to a process called molecular mimicry. This is where an immune reaction against the flagellar proteins of borrelia cross-reacts with the myelin sheath surrounding the nerves, leading to neuropathy and the formation of anti-myelin antibodies. We also find antiganglioside antibodies in patients with persistent neurological Lyme disease and associated co-infections, which can be a surrogate marker for autonomic nervous system dysfunction and POTS.

Treatment Options for ANS and POTS

When my patients with chronic neurological Lyme disease complain of tingling, numbness, and burning or stabbing sensations of the extremities (symptoms of peripheral neuropathy), a small percentage will test positive for antiganglioside antibodies, confirming an autoimmune process is overlapping their bacterial, viral, and parasitic infections. Associated environmental pollutants such as elevated heavy metal burdens may also play a role in this process, as mercury is known to act as a hapten on the outside of cells, increasing autoimmune reactions. Similarly, small-particle pollution has recently been found to increase autoimmunity.

Once you are exposed to infections like Lyme disease, and have antiganglioside antibodies with or without CVID, you may require IV immunoglobulin therapy (IVIG) to help with your acquired autoimmune peripheral and autonomic neuropathy. Dr. Younger has found sustained subjective and objective neurological improvement in his patients following this treatment. Gamunex-C and Gammagard are some of the most well tolerated forms of IVIG in my patient population.

I have seen similar improvements in ANS dysfunction in some Lyme-MSIDS patients following this protocol, and some with severe Herxheimer reactions with relapsing infections can greatly benefit from IVIG, but my patients usually require other medical interventions. Those with Lyme and POTS, along with associated severe neuropathy, often require antibiotic therapy for Lyme disease and co-infections such as Bartonella until the neuropathy is better. The Dapsone pilot study that we published in the peer-reviewed scientific literature, which used triple intracellular medications (tetracyclines with either rifampin and/or macrolides with Dapsone, combined with biofilm busters, cyst busters, and cell-wall drugs), helped some with resistant neuropathy who had failed other protocols. Oftentimes, we will follow antibiotics with herbal therapies to maintain progress, with nutritional support (i.e., curcumin, resveratrol, green tea extract, broccoli seed extracts, omega-3 FAs, NAC, alpha-lipoic acid, and glutathione) as well as low-dose naltrexone (LDN) to manage the inflammatory cytokines increasing pain. Shutting down the faucet of the overproduction of cytokines and opening up the drain to remove toxins (using drainage remedies, glutathione, and/or charcoal/clay compounds) is particularly helpful for some with POTS and ongoing inflammation with resistant neuropathy.

Increasing salt and fluids to help expand the intravascular volume and bring up the blood pressure is the first therapy most commonly tried by healthcare providers to treat POTS. You can increase the amount of salt you cook with, or take salt tablets with meals. This is not suggested for those who suffer from high blood pressure and certain medical disorders with fluid overload, such as congestive heart failure and cirrhosis of the liver. Even when it is indicated, this protocol does not always work: One study examined thirty-five adolescent patients with POTS who had chronic fatigue and cognitive impairment and found that volume expansion was only effective in relieving symptoms in two of them. We often use licorice extract (which increases blood pressure) with salt and fluids to improve efficacy.

Drugs such as Florinef, which directly help to raise the blood pressure, are most commonly used as the next line of therapy, with or without associated beta-blockers to control palpitations. Toprol XL is my preferred beta-blocker, because it has a twenty-four-hour delivery system that prevents breakthroughs. Tenormin, another beta-blocker, can be a reasonable substitute, but it may need to be taken several times a day. Florinef with beta-blockers are a mainstay of treatment in patients who do not respond to more conservative measures of aggressive salt and fluid replacement. ProAmatine (midodrine) is another drug that can help raise blood pressure with POTS, and we use this when Florinef fails a patient or when they cannot tolerate it. Supine elevations in blood pressure have been reported with midodrine, but we have generally not seen it, especially when it is mixed with beta-blockers. Like Florinef, midodrine can occasionally cause nausea, and rarely cause a rash, but oftentimes it is well tolerated. For those who have failed Florinef or midodrine, and/or had intolerable side effects (which are rare), a new drug has come on the market in the past few years that can be helpful, called Northera (droxidopa). It is indicated for neurogenic orthostatic hypotension, and works by raising norepinephrine levels. Like midodrine, it has a short half-life and can cause nausea, headaches, and supine hypertension (monitoring supine BP is advisable) by inducing peripheral arterial and venous vasoconstriction.

Other therapies that have been shown to be beneficial in POTS are selective serotonin reuptake inhibitors (SSRIs), which are particularly helpful to MSIDS patients, since many also suffer from overlapping anxiety and depression. This classification of drugs, which has been used in clinical trials for POTS, includes Prozac, Zoloft, and Paxil. They are generally useful in combination with other approaches, such as Florinef, ProAmatine, and beta-blockers, with salt and fluid repletion. Dual reuptake selective serotonin inhibitors such as Cymbalta also have beneficial effects, including decreasing pain with associated fibromyalgia symptoms and neuropathy. While Cymbalta is primarily used for diabetic neuropathy, we have found it to be useful for those patients with neuropathy associated with POTS and MSIDS. It is also more weight neutral than the other SSRIs and has less sexual side effects. The drug should be avoided in patients with significant palpitations and anxiety as well as those with hyperadrenergic POTS, since Cymbalta can increase levels of both serotonin and norepinephrine, which can produce the same symptoms.

I also occasionally treat POTS with Catapres, a centrally acting blood pressure drug that acts on alpha receptors in the brain (brain stem), which results in decreased levels of norepinephrine and epinephrine, which is helpful in those suffering with hyperadrenergic POTS. Since many patients with POTS have high levels of norepinephrine, decreasing this hormone helps to balance out their autonomic nervous system dysfunction.

Other drugs that are occasionally used in the medical literature to treat POTS are Diamox, Mestinon, and IV Procrit therapy. Mestinon is best known for its use in *myasthenia gravis*, an autoimmune disease that causes fluctuating periods of muscle weakness. Muscles contract when the neurotransmitter acetylcholine binds to receptors on the muscles, but in myasthenia there are anticholinesterase antibodies that block the acetylcholine receptors, preventing the muscles from working properly. Mestinon is an inhibitor of the enzyme that breaks down acetylcholine, raising its concentration at the receptor sites. It can overcome a block-ade of acetylcholine by increasing the concentration locally. If patients with Lyme-MSIDS test positively for ganglionic acetylcholine receptor antibodies, they may particularly benefit from Mestinon, especially if they have failed to get adequate results with other treatments. IV Procrit works on a different mechanism to help increase the blood pressure in POTS.

Some patients have low intravascular fluid volume (hypovolemia) due to leakage of fluid from the blood vessels, or from pooling of the blood outside the vascular space. Erythropoietin increases the intravascular vol-ume by working as a hormone at the level of the kidney to produce more red blood cells. This increases the volume circulating in the blood, and erythropoietin also has the ability to constrict blood vessels, thereby rais-ing blood pressure. This is not a commonly used medication in POTS, however, and would only be used as a last resort if the patient has failed all other treatment regimens, since side effects of Procrit include increased risk of a heart attack (myocardial infarction), stroke, phlebitis (venous thromboembolism), and death.

There are also several natural methods that can help with autonomic nervous system dysfunction, including resistance training (to help with poor muscle tone), which can be done at specialized cardiac rehabilitation facilities for those who are severely deconditioned and impaired, as well as using compression stockings to help prevent blood pooling in the lower extremities. Both of these methods may be used in combination with some of the drug regimens discussed. Biofeedback training with medita-tion, to help retrain the autonomic nervous system, has also been helpful in a select group of my patients with POTS. This is especially useful for those with high levels of circulating catecholamines, such as epinephrine and norepinephrine, which can increase palpitations and cause severe anxiety reactions.

Combining natural therapies with medications provides a more com-prehensive approach to help the resistant MSIDS patient with POTS get better. Oftentimes, when the underlying infections in MSIDS are adequately treated, these symptoms and those associated with POTS also improve.

NANCY HAD POTS AND LYME

Nancy was forty-nine years old with a past medical history significant for an elevated level of mercury in the blood, allergic rhinitis, irritable bowel syndrome, and Lyme disease. She was first diagnosed with Lyme back in 1998. Other co-infection testing was negative except for prior *Mycoplasma pneumonia* exposure and a history of viral infections, including EBV, parvovirus, and HHV-6. Although she felt somewhat better after an initial course of doxycycline, she noticed that her health had taken a precipitous decline several years later after having two children in 2000 and 2003.

When I met Nancy she told me that after each of her children were born, she had severe postpartum depression and anxiety with resistant insomnia. Then, in 2007, she developed increased joint pain in the hips, shoulders, knees, and toes (which migrated), with debilitating fatigue and dizziness. She went back to her primary care physician, who did another Lyme test that returned positive, and he placed her back on doxycycline, which was continued for several months, since she also suffered from acne. She felt better physically after the course of the antibiotics but still had some resistant fatigue, and the antibiotics did not help the neuropsychiatric symptoms that had developed. She was still depressed despite going for counseling and taking Prozac, and had developed significant headaches, memory and concentration problems, "vicious" insomnia that no medication helped, and unexplained "tremors" in her brain. She saw another Lyme-literate doctor in 2009, who felt that her symptoms were consistent with active Lyme disease, and tried her on different medication regimens. Unfortunately, when the dose of the doxycycline was increased to get better central nervous system penetration, her stomach couldn't handle the medication. She tried minocycline, but had a severe Jarisch-Herxheimer reaction. By this time, she felt that she could not tolerate any further antibiotics, and went the integrative/complementary route. She clinically improved on Dr. Zhang's protocol of herbs, as 80 percent of her joint pain and palpitations were better, but she still had resistant fatigue, insomnia, and "brain tremors" as some of her worst symptoms.

We sent out a CBC, comprehensive metabolic profile, HbA1c, and vitamin levels for her neuropathy, fatigue, and cognitive issues; co-infection panels to check for associated infections (especially Babesia and Bartonella to determine the cause of her severe neurological problems); an autoimmune panel, immunoglobulin levels with subclasses, hormone levels (thyroid, growth hormone, adrenal function, and sex hormones); as well as mineral levels, food allergy testing, and a parasite panel. She came back positive for certain autoimmune markers. Although her ANA, rheumatoid factor, sedimentation rate, and CRP were normal, she was HLA DR4 positive and had a positive antiganglioside antibody, which I've seen in autoimmune peripheral neuropathy with Lyme and POTS. She also had elevated liver functions with no associated alcohol use, and no clear toxic exposure to explain the abnormality. Her hormone studies came back positive for a low IgF-1, consistent with possible growth hormone deficiency, and significantly elevated levels of cortisol in the morning and at night. The upper limit of cortisol at 10:00 P.M. is normally 0.5. She was 8.54, more than sixteen times above the normal range. This could have accounted for her resistant insomnia.

Her medical work-up for the elevated liver functions was negative. Nancy was placed on nutritional supplements to support the liver detox pathways (NAC, alpha-lipoic acid, magnesium, and milk thistle) and was tried on the herbs Samento and Banderol for her Lyme disease, since she was wary of taking antibiotics. We placed her on Vitamin B_6, methyl B_{12}, and activated folic acid for her positive MTHFR gene status with an elevated homocysteine, as well as trazodone for sleep with L-theanine and phosphatidylserine to decrease the elevated cortisol levels at night.

Nancy returned one month later. Her liver functions remained elevated, although slightly decreased from her initial visit. Her sleep was better with the trazodone, as she went from sleeping two hours to five to six hours a night, but she still did not feel refreshed in the morning and complained of frequent awakening, fatigue, dizziness, agitation, anxiety, depression, and resistant "brain tremors" that would bother her day and night. She was tried on Sonata for the frequent awakening, with Lunesta at bedtime for sleep, and we discussed a stricter sugar-free diet to prevent hypoglycemic swings, which could contribute to her fatigue and insomnia. She was also given oral liposomal glutathione for detoxification, since she had resistant neurological symptoms, and her elevated liver functions could represent problems with detoxing chemicals from the environment.

On her next office visit I noticed something strange. Her blood pressure had always been in the normal range (110/72), but this time it was 98/68 sitting, with a resting pulse rate of 68, and her standing blood pressure dropped to 84/62, with a pulse rate in the low 80s. She also felt slightly dizzy upon standing. This was not a severe reaction by any means, but it did make me question whether Nancy was suffering from a mild case of POTS and autonomic nervous system dysfunction, which would account for some of her resistant symptoms. We discussed going for a head-up tilt-table test at a university center to confirm the diagnosis of POTS, but she was not emotionally ready to subject herself to more tests. We therefore tried adjusting her medication instead. We first discussed changing her trazodone to Lyrica at bedtime to try and help with the sleep. Next, I wanted her to try the herb cryptolepis for her resistant sweats. Her Babesia testing was negative, but she had normal sex hormone levels, and there was no way to easily explain her resistant sweating. Either she had an infection with Babesia (or other piroplasm), which was increasing all of her symptoms, such as the resistant fatigue, sweats, joint pain, memory and concentration problems, and sleep disorder, and/or she suffered from autonomic nervous system dysfunction. This could also account for the resistant fatigue, dizziness, palpitations, anxiety, insomnia, sweats, and cognitive problems. We therefore suggested a trial of licorice and Florinef while increasing her salt and fluid intake (to a minimum of two to three liters per day) and recommended an endocrine consultation to evaluate the low IgF-1 to determine if a growth hormone deficiency was an overlapping factor contributing to her chronic fatigue.

Nancy returned several months later after following this last protocol. She was elated to report that for the first time in years she was feeling great. Almost all of her symptoms were finally gone, and within one week of starting the Florinef, she started to feel better. Her sleep, fatigue, and dizziness improved, and the resistant "brain tremors" that she complained about for years were gone. She also found that two other suggestions made a big difference. The hypoglycemic diet stabilized her energy and improved her concentration, and her sweats were gone after taking the cryptolepis.

Nancy's autonomic nervous system dysfunction was impacting all of her resistant Lyme-MSIDS symptoms. Until she increased the salt and fluids in her diet and took the licorice and Florinef, we were not seeing the clinical improvements that we were hoping for. If you are experiencing ongoing fatigue, dizziness, palpitations, anxiety, and/or cognitive difficulties despite classical treatments, POTS/dysautonomia may be contributing to why you are not getting better.

SIXTEEN

Lyme and Allergies

You may have noticed that many of the patients discussed in the book have been diagnosed with allergic reactions to foods, where these reactions were a contributing factor in their underlying symptomatology. That is because food and food-chemical sensitivities can trigger pro-inflammatory cytokine production, increasing symptoms such as fatigue, joint and muscle pain, headaches, nausea, stomach pain, cognitive problems, and mood disorders. These symptoms overlap many other disease processes, including autoimmune diseases, CFS/SEID, fibromyalgia, environmental illness (EI), and Lyme disease, and they are a common reason why medical treatments are not fully effective. Regular intake of sensitive/allergic foods increases inflammation, and they may be making you sick and hidden from view because symptoms can arise hours to days later, making it difficult to see a cause and effect.

There are five main types of antibodies in our bodies that help protect us from foreign invaders. Allergies may present as two different types of hypersensitivity reactions, known as immediate hypersensitivity reactions (caused by IgE antibodies), or delayed hypersensitivity reactions (caused by IgG antibodies). Food allergies mediated by IgE antibodies play a role in acute, severe reactions to foods. These are called type I allergic reactions and they cause a range of symptoms, from mild to severe life-threatening anaphylactic reactions, including swelling of the tongue and throat, urticaria/hives, and severe asthmatic reactions with airway closure. Some IgE-related food allergies can be life-threatening and affect approximately 1.4 percent of the total population, the most common allergen being peanuts. Unfortunately, IgE testing does not identify all patients with peanut allergies, and there are reports in the scientific literature that some patients can develop adult onset allergies, even if they never suffered from this problem in childhood. Adults with a known history of life-threatening allergies are careful to avoid the offending foods, but sometimes peanuts can show up in spices like ground cumin or cumin powder, contributing to sudden anaphylactic reactions. This happened in 2015 when the FDA forced a voluntary recall of ground cumin and seasoning blends. Food allergies are responsible for up to half of food-related deaths in this country.

An allergic reaction takes place because of the interaction between the allergens, IgE antibodies, and mast cells, which are part of our immune system. These IgE antibodies are found on mast cells, and mast cells remain inactive until an allergen binds to the IgE receptor sites. An allergic reaction is triggered when an allergen binds to IgE antibodies. When this happens, it causes the release of histamines and cytokines from mast cells, causing a dilation of small blood vessels and increasing their permeability, which together causes pain, itching, swelling (edema), redness, and warmth, and attracts other inflammatory cells to the site of release. Some of my patients suffer from Lyme disease and mastocytosis (an increased number of mast cells), or mast cell activation disorder (MCAD), where they have a normal number of mast cells that are hyper responsive, leading to sudden episodes of abdominal pain, diarrhea, nasal congestion, itching, flushing, wheezing, low blood pressure, and dizziness. These patients are severely ill and oftentimes have associated POTS/dysautonomia, common variable immune deficiency (CVID), and/or Ehler Danlos syndrome (EDS). They also have evidence of increased mast cell mediators (N-methyl histamine, tryptase, inflammatory prostaglandins [D2, F2 alpha] and leukotrienes) and require strict avoidance of histamine-releasing foods, mast cell stabilizers (Gastrocrom), H1 and H2 antihistamines (Zyrtec and Zantac), and leukotriene inhibitors (Singulair).

Inside the gastrointestinal tract, an allergic food can come into contact with IgE on the surface of a mast cell and cause an inflammatory reaction that releases histamines as well as inflammatory cytokines. These chemicals can increase intestinal permeability and allow allergens to move into the bloodstream and throughout the body, causing widespread inflammation that leads to anaphylaxis and shock. This entire process can take place within a few minutes of ingesting the offending food, although occasionally it can take several hours for a severe reaction to take place. An example of a delayed anaphylactic reaction several hours after eating an allergic food is seen in those who have a lone star tick bite and subsequently develop an allergy to red meat, known as an alpha-gal allergy. Alpha-gal sugar is found in beef, pork, lamb, venison, goat, and bison, and sensitive individuals can get an anaphylactic reaction four to six hours after eating the offending food, with hives and swelling, shortness of breath, low blood pressure (hypotension), vomiting, and diarrhea. Dr. Robert Valet at Vanderbilt University's Asthma, Sinus and Allergy Program is seeing new cases each week where patients are allergic to the alpha-gal sugar present in red meat. It is believed that the tick has the alpha-gal sugar in its gut and introduces it into the skin with a bite, where the antibody then cross-reacts to the meat, causing the allergic reaction.

A second type of food or chemically related reaction is much more common. This is a delayed hypersensitivity reaction (IgG). It is estimated that 80 percent to 85 percent of food allergy/sensitivity reactions are due to IgG antibodies. These cause a delayed reaction, which occurs between twenty-four and forty-eight hours after ingestion of the offending agent, and therefore may not be recognized as a cause of the symptoms. Most individuals would not suspect that their resistant symptoms can be due to food allergies, which is why it is so important to be tested if you have any of the medical problems discussed below.

Scientific studies have shown that symptoms may include:

- Arthritis
- Bed-wetting associated with childhood hyperactivity
- Bladder pain
- Constipation and/or diarrhea
- Eczema and urticaria (hives)
- Fatigue
- Headaches, as well as migraines
- Indigestion and reflux
- Low blood pressure

- Mood swings, with either anxiety and depression
- Respiratory symptoms, with allergic rhinitis and an increase in bronchospasm and asthma
- Stomach upset with abdominal pain

Food and food-chemical sensitivities mediated by IgG are complex immune-mediated reactions that cause a cellular activation of other cells of the immune system called "basophils." Basophils are a type of white blood cell that also contains granules, like the mast cells. When basophils are in contact with an allergen, they similarly release histamine and other inflammatory chemical mediators, such as leukotrienes and prostaglandins, but part of their cellular reaction also includes the release of inflammatory cytokines. These molecules are released as part of an immune response that causes smooth-muscle contraction and swelling, and increases inflammation and pain. This can further exacerbate symptoms for those with Lyme-MSIDS, who already have ongoing inflammatory responses caused by these same cytokines. That is why we place our patients on an anti-inflammatory diet, test them for possible food allergies, and counsel them to avoid these foods so that they can properly heal.

A good starting point for an anti-inflammatory diet is to avoid sugar and the most common food allergens: wheat, eggs, and dairy, and some patients are also sensitive to corn, soy, (certain) nuts, and shellfish. I have found that just by avoiding these allergic foods, many of my patients feel better. Some notice that their fatigue, headaches, joint pain, and symptoms of allergic rhinitis, eczema, and asthma improve after eliminating their allergic foods (especially wheat, dairy, and sugar).

Avoiding these foods may not only make you feel better, it also may be lifesaving. A 2014 study in *JAMA* showed that patients who consumed 10.0 percent to 24.9 percent of their calories from added sugars have a 30 percent increased risk of mortality from coronary vascular disease, and those who consume 25 percent or more calories from added sugars have an almost threefold increased risk. Sugar consumption has also been linked to increased risks of cancer. Carrying excess pounds around the waist (visceral fat) significantly increases insulin resistance and inflammation. If we then add sugar, trans fats, and fried and processed foods to the mix, these foods are high in advanced glycation end products (glycotoxins), which further increase oxidative stress and inflammation. One study done by researchers at the Mount Sinai School of Medicine showed that patients who were asked to steam, stew, or poach their meals, which produces less glycotoxins than grilling or frying foods, had significantly fewer inflammatory markers and improved cardiovascular and metabolic health.

Some patients have signs and symptoms of significant inflammation, with hot, swollen joints and elevated inflammatory markers in the blood. They also have high levels of inflammatory cytokines as well as elevated levels of other inflammatory mediators, such as arachidonic acid, and they need to be stricter with their diets. Arachidonic acid is produced from consuming foods that are high in omega-6 fatty acids (like red meat), and it is a building block for other molecules that cause further inflammation in the body. These patients need to follow a strict anti-inflammatory diet, decreasing red meats and dairy products while increasing sources of anti-inflammatory omega-3 fatty acids (especially fatty fish, such as sardines and salmon, which have high levels of DHA). Consumption of fish high in omega-3 FAs has been shown to also improve brain function and structure in older adults and decrease the risk of Alzheimer's disease, and was proven in a 2016 study published in the *Journal of Clinical Nutrition* to decrease all-cause mortality. If you have to eat red meat and dairy, choose organic; these choices were shown to have higher levels of omega-3 fatty acids than their non-organic counterparts. Organic soy has been shown to contain higher levels of healthy nutrients and significantly less pesticide residues than conventionally farmed varieties.

Some of my patients also need to avoid the nightshade family of vegetables (potatoes, tomatoes, eggplants, and peppers) because these foods can trigger arthritis symptoms. And for others, although they do not have true celiac disease, we have found that they are gluten sensitive and feel better avoiding grains in their diet, such as wheat, kamut, spelt, barley, rye, malts, and triticale. Gluten is also used as a food additive and thickening agent, and can be found in ingredient labels as "dextrin." Many of my patients with gluten sensitivity do not have positive tests for the specific markers for celiac disease (antigliadin antibodies and TTG), while some are antigliadin positive (low, medium, or high levels of antibodies) and are TTG negative (a specific marker for celiac disease). Anyone who has resistant arthritic symptoms and bowel issues should try a diet free of the most common allergens, including nightshades and gluten, for at least four weeks to see if symptoms improve.

Some people with gluten sensitivities can also be deficient in secretory IgA (sIgA). This antibody is the first line of defense against gastrointestinal pathogens and forms immune complexes with food allergens to prevent them from being absorbed into the body. If you have low levels of secretory IgA (fecal sIgA can be tested, as can salivary levels of it), the GI mucosal barrier may be compromised, where tight junctions between cells are damaged, which allows allergic foods to enter the body more easily. Celiac disease also involves IgA pathology, due to the presence of antibodies against this particular immunoglobulin, further increasing allergic reactions to foods. This will be discussed in detail in Chapter 17.

Foods that contain artificial food dyes, flavorings, and preservatives can also cause food intolerances. Some integrative doctors specializing in pediatrics believe that eliminating artificial food dyes, flavors, and preservatives that are petroleum-based (BHA, DHT, TBHQ) from the diet can be helpful in sensitive children with enuresis (bed-wetting), frequent earaches, sleep disorders, asthma, and neurological symptoms, including ADHD. This elimination diet is referred to as the Feingold Diet. Children are usually the most sensitive to food additives, since food dyes can cross the blood-brain barrier more easily in the younger population. This phenomenon has, however, recently been observed in adults with autoimmune disorders. A study published in *Autoimmunity Reviews* showed that food additives can have an effect on intestinal permeability, resulting in increased tight junction leakage and local and systemic immune stimulation, inducing autoimmune disease.

Some people are sensitive to salicylates (the primary ingredient in aspirin), which can cause all of the above symptoms as well as nasal polyp formation and increased asthmatic symptoms. This occurs in up to 10 percent of the population. These people may need to eliminate (at least initially) salicylate-containing foods. This is difficult, as salicylates are found in most plants, as well as in many preservatives and medications.

A diet free of common allergens is more commonly prescribed, and has been used to treat attention deficit disorder, migraines, and arthritis effectively in adults. Once you remove these foods from the diet, you may find that inflammation significantly decreases, leading to improvement in common chronic health conditions. Many patients in my practice with chronic resistant symptoms of fatigue, headaches, muscle and joint pain, and allergy symptoms, who have failed to find a cause for their symptoms and have failed pharmaceutical drugs, have definitely improved with this approach. In those who also suffer from chemical sensitivity and environmental illness, eliminating chemicals and preservatives from their diet and periodically detoxifying from other chemicals also helps reverse certain resistant musculoskeletal and neurological symptoms.

DO I HAVE FOOD ALLERGIES?

Some allergists will do conventional skin testing with RAST tests to measure IgE-mediated reactions. Although this can be helpful, it cannot identify the delayed, non-IgE-mediated reactions, such as those we see with IgG antibodies. Ordering both an IgE and IgG food allergy panel to test for immediate and delayed hypersensitivity reactions is helpful, as you may have an immediate (IgE) reaction to a food but not have an IgG reaction, or vice versa. Checking for itchy red welts that appear after scratching the skin (dermatographism) and evaluating histamine levels in blood and urine (i.e., N-methyl histamine) with tryptase levels can also be helpful to determine the level of hyper reactivity of mast cells in the skin, and the need for further treatment with a histamine-free diet.

Other tests to consider include a Comprehensive Digestive Stool Analysis (CDSA) to look at the digestion and absorption of foods while also looking at the levels of beneficial or harmful bacteria, yeast, and parasites present in the GI tract. This test can be done through functional medicine laboratories such as Genova Diagnostics and Doctor's Data. An intestinal permeability test can also be used as a means to help diagnose food allergies by doing a simple breath test from approved functional medicine laboratories, along with a salivary or fecal secretory IgA (sIgA) level. Anyone who suffers from inflammation in the GI tract (from Candida, for example) may develop leaky gut (intestinal permeability), where macromolecules of food in the GI tract are directly absorbed into the body, stimulating allergic reactions and increasing sensitivities to foods. We discussed earlier how secretory IgA is necessary to help form immune complexes with food allergens to prevent them from being absorbed into the body. If testing shows both low sIgA levels and high intestinal permeability, then the likelihood of having leaky gut and multiple food sensitivities is much higher. There is also a molecule in the blood called zonulin that can be measured, and which will indicate current damage to the bowel wall and point to leaky gut. Zonulin acts as "glue" between the cells of the lining of the intestine, and its presence can precede the development of food allergies by nearly three years. Eating certain foods like gluten, which contains gliadin (the glycoprotein present in wheat), activates zonulin, leading to increased intestinal permeability, and has been found in those suffering not only from celiac disease, but also gluten sensitivity and irritable bowel syndrome (IBS). Some people with IBS and functional gastrointestinal disorders (FGID) are also sensitive to certain short-chain carbohydrates in the diet, including fructose, lactose, and sorbitol, causing increased gas and bloating, and they need to avoid these sugars in a specialized diet plan (i.e., a FODMAP diet) to relieve their symptoms.

Treating Allergies and Sensitivities

The only effective treatment for food allergies and sensitivities is avoidance. The offending allergens must be removed from the diet for at least three months before they can be added back in, via a rotation diet.

My goal is to correct any imbalances in the microbial flora, heal a damaged intestinal mucosa, and reestablish proper digestion. To maintain bowel health, we usually give high-dose probiotics with Lactobacillus and Bifidobacterium to replace the beneficial bacteria in the gut, as well as using *Saccharomyces boulardii* to help prevent antibiotic-associated diarrhea. We find high-dose probiotics and occasionally the use of prebiotics with fructooligosaccharides (FOS) to be extremely beneficial in maintaining bowel health when patients are on long-term antibiotics for Lyme-MSIDS. I rarely see antibiotic-associated diarrhea if patients are compliant with this regimen.

I also recommend GI nutritional products that support bowel health. These often contain:

- combinations of amino acids (glutamine, glycine)
- vitamins and minerals
- anti-inflammatory herbs, such as turmeric and quercetin
- NAC and sodium sulfate, for detox support

- inulin (from chicory)
- arabinogalactans, to help with the production of short-chain fatty acids, which helps decrease intestinal inflammation
- DGL (D-glycerinated licorice) with aloe vera and glutamine to help heal the stomach and intestines, especially for those with associated leaky gut syndrome. DGL helps to form a mucus barrier in the stomach, aloe vera soothes the stomach, and glutamine helps prevent intestinal mucosal damage and stimulates the repair of the damaged intestinal wall.

I also prescribe enzyme therapies when there is a clear deficiency. Pancreatic enzymes and/or oral betaine hydrochloride will occasionally be needed by those who have associated stomach acid issues, causing poor digestion. A Heidelberg gastric analysis test may be considered if achlorhydria (lack of stomach acid) or hypochlorhydria (decreased stomach acid) is suspected, and a CDSA test may also pick up evidence of pancreatic insufficiency.

After three months of avoiding the allergic foods and allowing the gut to heal, a rotation diet reintroduces foods in a methodical manner. This is done by introducing one previously offending food every three days, keeping a food diary, and recording your health status, so that any adverse reactions can be adequately monitored. Rotation diets can help identify each of the sources of ongoing inflammation that are causing cytokine release and sickness syndrome. You may need to do a trial off common allergens (wheat, dairy, sugar, eggs, corn, soy, certain nuts, especially peanuts, and shellfish), with a Candida-free diet as well as a histamine-free diet to feel well. The Candida diet eliminates malt, vinegar, simple sugars, and carbohydrates (including fruits early on in the treatment), as well as all yeast-containing foods (most breads, cheeses, and mushrooms), and fermented foods (e.g., soy sauce, tempeh, and alcohol). A histamine-free diet also requires avoiding some of these foods, especially aged cheeses, alcohol, citrus, chocolate, and fermented/smoked foods, which cause histamine release. If you have unexplained fatigue, low blood pressure, arrhythmias, anxiety, nasal congestion, headaches, dermatographism with itching and/or hives, wheezing, and/or resistant GI symptoms, you may have histamine intolerance. Many books are available on the subject and Dr. Amy Myers, author of *The Autoimmune Solution*, has compiled a list of foods that release histamine, which are listed on MindBodyGreen.com, which is a good source of natural health recipes.

Once we have initially identified and removed all of the allergens from the diet, the next step is to find a healthy nutritional program that can be followed for life. I recommend an anti-inflammatory Mediterranean diet, rich in fresh fruits and vegetables, with smaller portions of red meat, eggs, and dairy (decreased omega-6 fatty acids); healthy fats (increased amounts of omega-3 fatty acids in fish, and increased amounts of omega-9 fatty acids in olive oil); and low in simple carbohydrates. Increasing the amounts of omega-3 fatty acids in the diet and decreasing the amounts of omega-6 fatty acids is beneficial, since omega-6 fatty acids increase the production of arachidonic acid, increasing inflammation. Lowering the carbohydrate content of meals with a Mediterranean diet or Paleo diet also helps, because sugar in carbohydrates drives insulin production and causes metabolic syndrome, whereby elevated blood sugars and associated insulin resistance increase the inflammatory response. Although there has been debate in the medical community over which diet is best, both the Paleo diet and the Mediterranean diet have been proven to lower inflammation. In a 2016 study published in the *Journal of Nutrition*, circulating concentrations of two related biomarkers, high-sensitivity C-reactive protein (hsCRP), an acute inflammatory protein, and F2-isoprostane, a reliable marker of in vivo lipid peroxidation, were both shown to be lowered with these diets, proving lower levels of systemic inflammation and oxidative stress. Adherence to the Mediterranean diet was also associated with longer telomeres (important for health as telomere length, the nucleotides at the end of our chromosomes, is directly correlated with longevity) and a lower risk of invasive breast cancer. The Mediterranean diet is characterized by an abundance of plant foods, fish, and the consumption of extra virgin olive oil, and in a Spanish multicenter randomized single blind controlled trial published in *JAMA* in 2015, invasive breast cancer was reduced by 68 percent in those who were on a Mediterranean diet supplemented with olive oil.

For those who have been diagnosed with hypoglycemia, metabolic syndrome, and/or type 2 diabetes, I recommend a very low-carbohydrate diet, featuring smaller, more frequent meals. Each meal or snack should aim to have a balance of protein (40 percent), complex carbohydrates (25 percent), and healthy fats (35 percent) to avoid swings of blood sugar with high insulin secretion. Reactive hypoglycemia is extremely common in my medical practice and is frequently a manifestation of metabolic syndrome. Those who suffer from resistant fatigue, headaches, dizziness, palpitations, mood swings, and insomnia often benefit the most. We find that at least half of our patients suffer from reactive hypoglycemia, and its symptoms overlap those of multiple food allergies, as well as those of non-Lyme-MSIDS (especially Candida, with adrenal dysfunction) and Lyme-MSIDS. Lyme disease symptoms are also exacerbated during blood sugar swings. A five-hour glucose tolerance test may be necessary to diagnose reactive hypoglycemia for those with resistant symptoms.

A strict hypoglycemic diet may have other benefits. Keeping the total carbohydrate load below 60 grams/day and doing a ketogenic diet will help to lose weight; improve blood sugar control in type 2 diabetes; assist mitochondrial regeneration (which is important for not only increasing energy production, but also helpful in a broad range of neurological conditions); induce favorable epigenetic changes (how your genes express themselves); and lower inflammation. We have found that many individuals report feeling much better after getting off of simple carbohydrates and grains, as well as allergic foods. Speak to your healthcare provider to see if this is appropriate for you.

Others may need to follow a stricter Candida diet, especially if their CDSA test shows elevated levels of yeast in the colon. Candida can cause inflammation in the colon and lead to a leaky gut and subsequent food allergies. A course of Diflucan, followed by nystatin and high-dose probiotics, and/or using natural supplements like monolaurin (Lauricidin), berberine, oregano oil, and Pau D'Arco may be necessary. Remember that "you are what you eat," and Rule #6, mastering food, is essential if you are to heal and reduce hidden sources of inflammation.

SEVENTEEN

Lyme and Gastrointestinal Health

Gastrointestinal disorders are a frequent health complaint, whether or not they are related to Lyme and associated tick-borne diseases. Digestive disorders have been cited as the second leading cause of absenteeism from the workplace. In the United States, sixty million to seventy million people have diagnosable digestive disorders, and there are over one hundred million outpatient visits every year to gastroenterologists. The most common GI condition is irritable bowel syndrome (IBS), followed by gastroesophageal reflux disease (GERD), gastric and peptic ulcer disease, inflammatory bowel disease (IBD, including Crohn's and ulcerative colitis), and celiac disease (sensitivity to gluten). Yet despite modern advances in medicine—antispasmodics (drugs that decrease spasms in the intestines) for IBS, anti-inflammatory medicines with biological modifiers for IBD (such as Crohn's disease), proton pump inhibitors such as Prilosec (which decrease acid secretion) for GERD, and antibiotic treatment of *H. pylori* for ulcer disease (an infection in the stomach)—many people do not find complete relief with these treatments. What's worse, not only are they not getting to the source of the disorder, some of these treatments, like proton pump inhibitors, have recently been linked to a two-fold increase in cardiovascular mortality and possibly dementia. We have already shown how Alzheimer's disease and dementia have been linked to multiple factors on the sixteen-point MSIDS map, including infections, inflammation, environmental toxins, autoimmunity, hormonal dysregulation, sleep disorders, and lack of a proper diet and exercise. We don't need any further increase in risk factors, especially since scientific researchers reported in *JAMA* in 2016 that the pathogenesis of reflux esophagitis may be cytokine-mediated rather than the result of just chemical injury. Lyme disease, associated co-infections, and several abnormalities on the MSIDS map (including food allergies) can all cause inflammation with cytokine release leading to a wide range of treatable GI complaints.

Patients with Lyme-MSIDS often present with gastrointestinal problems, including intermittent abdominal pain, nausea, gas, bloating, constipation, diarrhea, or reflux disease, with occasional vomiting. Although these symptoms may be linked to the common GI problems mentioned above or due to other causes, such as food intolerances or gynecological issues (i.e., painful ovarian cysts or endometriosis), these symptoms can also overlap with some of the symptoms of Lyme disease and tick-borne disorders. For example, a review of gastrointestinal and liver problems associated with tick-borne diseases found that in 5 percent to 23 percent of those with early Lyme borreliosis, patients presented with varied gastrointestinal symptoms, such as nausea, vomiting, abdominal pain, anorexia with loss of appetite, and hepatitis, and some even had symptoms of an enlarged liver and spleen. Diarrhea was rare, accounting for only 2 percent of cases.

Just as Lyme disease can be the great imitator, we see that other tick-borne co-infections can also present with varied gastrointestinal manifestations:

- *Borrelia hermsii* can cause nausea, vomiting, abdominal pain, hepatitis, jaundice, and an enlarged spleen. Diarrhea occurred in 19 percent of these infections, and vomiting of blood (hematemesis) or bloody diarrhea rarely occurred.
- Ehrlichiosis occasionally presents with gastrointestinal symptoms of nausea, vomiting, abdominal pain, and jaundice, especially in the early stages of the disease. Diarrhea occurs in up to 10 percent of patients with ehrlichiosis, and can even be one of the primary manifestations.
- Rickettsial diseases (Rocky Mountain spotted fever and Q fever) can cause gastrointestinal symptoms early in the course of the

illness, including abdominal pain and tenderness, with vomiting, which when associated with elevations in liver enzymes can be mistaken for other inflammatory diseases of the GI tract such as hepatitis, appendicitis, peritonitis (inflammation in the abdominal cavity), and cholangitis (inflammation in the gallbladder). Often the classical rash on the hands and soles of the feet with RMSF may follow the abdominal complaints, mistaking these symptoms for gastroenteritis. Gastrointestinal hemorrhage has also been reported for RMSF, due to inflammation in the blood vessels.

- Tularemia can present in several common forms: an ulceroglandular form (ulcers on the skin with enlarged lymph nodes), an oculoglandular form (eye symptoms, such as conjunctivitis, with enlarged lymph nodes), a respiratory form, and the typhoidal form. The latter may cause nausea, vomiting, abdominal pain, and diarrhea, which can be severe in up to 40 percent of cases.

THE COMPLEX GI SYSTEM

One of the most important functions of the gut is to help with digestion of foods into essential amino acids, fatty acids, and carbohydrates. The gut also plays an important role in immunity. It is the largest organ of immune function in the body. The GI tract houses 80 percent of our immune system and 70 percent of our lymphocytes, making it the first line of defense against infections. The GI tract also functions as a neuroendocrine organ. Every neurotransmitter from the central nervous system is found in the GI tract. Most of the body's serotonin, which is essential for healthy moods, as well as half of the body's norepinephrine, which is essential for proper functioning of the orthosympathetic nervous system (OS), is found in the gut. At the same time, the gut can hold as many as 100 trillion microbes, referred to as the microbiome. There are ten times more microbial cells than mammalian cells in the body, which means, from a cellular perspective, our bodies are only 10 percent human—and 90 percent microbial! These different bacteria in the microbiome play an important role in many different biological functions. They help to supply essential vitamins; fight dangerous pathogens; keep the immune system in balance and modulate autoimmune disease (like MS and rheumatoid arthritis); modulate hormones, appetite, weight, glucose metabolism, and diabetes; modulate cardiovascular risk, neurological and psychiatric diseases (like Parkinson's and schizophrenia); affect epigenetics; modulate cancer risk and affect inflammatory reactions in the body, including allergies, asthma, Crohn's disease, and colitis. A healthy microbiome appears to hold the key for many of our chronic diseases, so we have to care for it properly.

Doctors engage in warfare against bacteria via antibiotics for common infections—urinary tract, sinus, and upper respiratory—without ever giving a thought to replacing the beneficial bacteria that are also destroyed. Even one dose of an antibiotic can damage the fragile microbiome. This indiscriminate killing leads to common problems such as yeast infections, and it may lead to antibiotic-associated diarrhea, including that of *Clostridium difficile*, which is particularly dangerous for immunocompromised individuals. Worse, once *Clostridium difficile* is established, it precludes broad-spectrum antibiotics for other infections, such as Lyme disease. This is because treating a bacterial infection with certain antibiotics will potentially worsen the gastrointestinal imbalance with an overgrowth of yeast and the clostridial species responsible for the diarrhea. Yet it is not common practice to instruct patients to take high-dose probiotics and beneficial yeast, such *as Saccharomyces boulardii*, during and after antibiotic therapy, even though *Clostridium difficile* can be effectively prevented with just such an approach.

As we discussed earlier, bacteria have been linked to GI cancers, inflammatory bowel disease, and irritable bowel syndrome. Dysbiosis, which is an imbalance of healthy bacteria, yeast, and parasites in the gut, is not a new concept in medicine, but its relationship to many disease processes is now beginning to be understood in new ways. We've known for almost a century that GI flora and increased intestinal permeability were responsible for dermatologic and psychiatric disorders. Then, in the 1980s, it was shown that the GI flora may play a role in the development of arthritis and inflammatory bowel disease. In the late 1990s, a new concept was developed, called "small intestinal bacterial overgrowth" (SIBO), which was found to be one of the causes of irritable bowel syndrome. SIBO was later found to be associated with CFS and fibromyalgia, which, as we have seen, are overlapping syndromes that share similar biochemical and pathological processes to Lyme-MSIDS. Here may be one of the missing links showing how dysbiosis and GI bacteria play an important role in contributing to these seemingly different disease processes that have similar clinical manifestations.

The signs and symptoms of SIBO and dysbiosis include:

- Bloating and flatulence after meals
- Constipation
- Diarrhea
- Fatigue
- Indigestion
- Iron deficiency, with weak or cracked fingernails (poor absorption of minerals)
- Nausea
- Rectal itching
- Systemic reactions after eating with food intolerances
- Undigested food in the stool or greasy stools (suggestive of pancreatic enzyme deficiency)

The clinical workup for SIBO includes a CBC, a CMP, and hormone testing; checking for food allergies (IgG and IgE) and antigliadin antibodies; checking pancreatic enzyme levels (amylase and lipase); antibody testing against common parasites (blood and stool); a stool CDSA (Comprehensive Digestive Stool Analysis); *H. pylori* antibody; and specialized SIBO breath tests. An upper endoscopy and colonoscopy should be considered for patients with chronic resistant symptoms when no clear cause is found. However, overlapping causes for bloating and indigestion with SIBO could also include lactose intolerance, fructose intolerance, or Candida overgrowth.

Many patients with MSIDS and SIBO have positive tests for food allergies and sensitivities that are related to an imbalance in gut microflora. These multiple food allergies may be responsible for increased cytokine production and imply a leaky gut. As we discussed in the prior chapter on food allergies, leaky gut is a term used to describe a loss of the integrity of the GI lining of the gut, where macromolecules of food pass through the intestinal barrier and antibodies against them are formed, as they are seen to be foreign invaders. This loss of integrity of the tight junction system in the gut can also take place when patients have cancer and are exposed to radiation or chemotherapy; have chronic bacterial and/or parasitic infections or significant yeast overgrowth; have taken antibiotics long term, leading to an overgrowth of Candida and other fungi; have certain autoimmune diseases; or have been exposed to a high body burden of mercury, which can adversely affect the tight junctions in between intestinal epithelial cells.

Those who suffer from both food allergies and SIBO can be treated with Betaine hydrochloric acid before meals to increase gastric acidity (and avoid proton pump inhibitors, i.e., PPIs, associated with SIBO), digestive enzymes with meals, and fiber (soluble and nonsoluble, including ground flaxseeds), as well as L-glutamine before, during, and after meals. These patients also need to decrease their intake of carbohydrates and sugars, doing a trial of a FODMAPs elimination diet. Fermentable oligo-, di-, monosaccharides, and polyols (FODMAPs) are short-chain carbohydrates that are poorly absorbed in the small intestine, and some individuals with irritable bowel syndrome (and inflammatory bowel disease like Crohn's) improve off fructose, lactose, and sugar alcohols that are artificial sweeteners (like sorbitol, mannitol, xylitol, and maltitol), although the long-term effects on the microbiome and nutrient absorption have not been adequately studied with this approach. Those with SIBO should also avoid hydrogenated oils, alcohol, nicotine, caffeine, allergic foods, and, when possible, stop antibiotics that can contribute to a Candida overgrowth. Dietary interventions to increase healthy prebiotics include increasing intake of fermented foods, such as sauerkraut, kimchee, pickles, pickled ginger, olives, and kefir (as long as you are not diagnosed with systemic candidiasis or histamine intolerance). Healthy probiotic supplementation should include a minimum of at least 10 billion organisms with a good quality probiotic daily, but higher doses of probiotics are preferable for those with severe dysbiosis, as seen on a CDSA test. We typically use a combination of multiple high-potency probiotics when patients are on antibiotics, and/or suffer from SIBO/IBS/IBD, to achieve an intake of over 200–300 billion beneficial bacteria per day, and find it to be effective.

Phase I of treatment for SIBO and IBS uses the antibiotic Xifaxan, followed by a breath test to confirm if there has been eradication of the small intestinal bacterial overgrowth. Occasionally, phase II treatment for SIBO will be needed, and it will require a low-dose antibiotic, such as erythromycin, to continue to eradicate the bacterial overgrowth if Xifaxan has been unsuccessful, although a recent scientific study published in the *NEJM* showed that Xifaxan works in first-time and relapsed diarrhea-predominant irritable bowel syndrome, and can be used repeatedly with success.

THE CYTOKINE CONNECTION

Gut flora directly impacts the production of inflammatory cytokines, and are therefore silent contributors to Lyme-MSIDS symptoms. The Human Microbiome Project, the most ambitious survey of the human microbiome yet performed, has shown that the microbiomes of bacteria, viruses, and fungi are constantly interacting with our body, affecting our health.

Bacteria in our gut are now thought to be associated with Crohn's disease, ulcerative colitis, and asthma, as certain bacteria have been found to stimulate chronic low-grade inflammation, an integral part of these diseases. Exciting new research has shown that gut microbes may also shape metabolic and immune network activity, and ultimately influence the development of obesity, diabetes, and cancer, as well as autoimmune, cardiovascular, and neuropsychiatric diseases. This may in part be due to bacterial influences on nutrient absorption: They prolong the time food moves through the intestines, and they increase the cellular uptake of triglycerides and their subsequent storage into fat (a primary component of obesity and metabolic syndrome, precursors for diabetes) with altered tissue composition of fats in our body. The microbiome has also been shown to affect methylation patterns, affecting our epigenetics and how genes express themselves, influencing heart disease. Researchers looked at the role of GI bacteria (Bacteroides, Firmicutes, and Proteobacteria) and methylation. Methylation helps to "silence" genes, and the group in which Firmicutes was dominant was linked to an increased risk of cardiovascular disease (as the bacteria affected lipid metabolism, obesity, and the inflammatory response). Other studies are showing that bacteria such as Prevotella and Clostridium species in the GI tract may increase the incidence of rheumatoid arthritis and MS, whereas bacteria like *B. Fragilis* may decrease the incidence of autoimmune disease.

Scientists are now beginning to look at practical applications of this research, and have begun to study the effects of specific probiotic supplementation on different diseases. For example, they found that *Lactobacillus rhamnosus* HN001 increased the cytotoxicity of NK cells and phagocytosis of bacteria, decreasing gut and respiratory tract illness, *Bifidobacterium infantis* was able to decrease depression (*Biological Psychiatry,* November 2013), and other bacteria may help mitigate food allergies and gluten sensitivity. Prescript-Assist, which is a prebiotic-probiotic complex with soil-based organisms, was shown to reduce symptoms of IBS. These bacteria are affecting inflammatory processes and cytokine production, providing novel avenues for treatment.

The roles of bacteria in the gut, and their subsequent effects on cytokine production, even play a role in sleep. At midnight, when cortisol production should be low, bacterial peptides from GI flora stimulate the immune cells of our gastrointestinal tract to increase cytokine production. These cytokines stimulate non-REM sleep (early deep sleep), and later during the night, as IL-1 beta decreases, this helps to initiate the transformation from non-REM sleep to REM sleep. Some severely ill Lyme patients, who have high cortisol levels at night and can't fall asleep, will not produce the right types and levels of cytokines necessary for the induction of deep sleep, or produce too many cytokines, making them drowsy during the day.

The intestinal macrophages and T cells in the gut, and the types of bacteria present in the GI tract, also have an effect on which types of cytokines are produced, affecting sleep and inflammation. Although there are hundreds of different species of bacteria in our GI tracts, there are two major types of intestinal bacteria that are particularly important in cytokine production: Lactobacilli and bifidobacteria. Most strains of Lactobacilli are robust producers of these cytokines, but most strains of bifidobacteria are weak cytokine producers. Bifidobacteria are able to decrease the production of cytokines from Lactobacilli, changing their immunological effects. It is therefore possible that by manipulating the types of intestinal bacteria, we can affect cytokine production, and decrease underlying inflammation.

Diarrhea is known to be caused by several different cytokines: TNF-α and IL-6 directly correlate with both fever and the number of diarrheal episodes, and cytokines in general are directly involved in intestinal injury and the severity of the diarrhea. TNF-α is a central mediator of intestinal inflammation, and it is elevated in inflammatory bowel disease (IBD) as well as in Lyme.

Since inflammatory cytokines have been associated with GI diseases, do Lyme flares worsen the bowel inflammation in IBD by further increasing systemic levels of cytokines? Does IBD with elevated cytokine production conversely worsen the symptomatology of Lyme disease? Down-regulation of cytokines is one of the primary treatments used in the management of Crohn's disease, and LDN (low-dose naltrexone) has now been recognized in the medical literature as being effective in helping to control the intestinal inflammation in Crohn's disease. We also find that LDN is extremely beneficial in controlling the symptoms of fibromyalgia in Lyme-MSIDS patients. It can be dangerous to try and decrease inflammation by giving a TNF-α blocker like Enbrel to a Crohn's disease patient with active Lyme disease, as these drugs may significantly worsen Lyme disease symptoms. However, LDN can help balance the immune response, as can the right types of probiotics, and these have the potential to decrease inflammation in those who suffer simultaneously from both diseases.

GASTROINTESTINAL BACTERIA AND NEUROTOXINS

Gut bacteria can also secrete neurotoxins, like ammonia, which is often found in elevated levels with cirrhosis. These patients require a low-protein diet, since the enzyme urease induced in colonic bacteria, such as Klebsiella, Proteus, and Bacteroides, break down urea to form ammonia, which is increased with a high-protein diet. The ammonia also raises stool pH, which has been associated with a higher risk for colon cancer. We occasionally see elevated levels of ammonia in Lyme-MSIDS patients, even without evidence of cirrhosis.

Other neurotoxins found in gut bacteria include D-lactic acid and octopamine, chemicals that are generated by the action of colonic bacteria on undigested protein. In patients with cirrhosis of the liver, these compounds enter the blood and contribute to the confusion and encephalopathy seen in liver failure. Some people with MSIDS also suffer from detoxification problems, and these chemicals may play a role in increasing cognitive difficulties in those with Lyme disease. Other biotoxins may include chemicals produced by living organisms (such as staph, strep, certain blue-green algae, and mold), those from food (preservatives), and xenobiotics (chemicals such as dioxins and PCBs).

Patients with MSIDS also occasionally suffer from systemic candidiasis, and have been found to have elevated levels of alcohol in their blood even when they did not consume any. The sugar and yeast fermentation in the gut produced acetaldehyde, which was then converted into ethanol, causing them to feel constantly drunk. This was first discovered in Japan and labeled "drunk disease." One of my patients with candidiasis recently reported that she needed to avoid all sugars and eat small frequent meals to avoid that type of a drunk sensation arising from her diet. We need to include the gastrointestinal tract as a possible source of neurotoxins potentially affecting the cognitive symptoms in MSIDS.

Maintaining Normal Gut Microflora

We can increase the healthy bacteria in our gut by not only taking probiotics but also by taking prebiotics with FOS (fructooligosaccharides) and eating fermented vegetables. This can be beneficial for those who are suffering from inflammatory bowel disease with colitis or in patients who do not manage to maintain adequate levels of beneficial bacteria in the gut with the use of antibiotics and probiotics.

For treatment of leaky gut, we suggest glutamine; OptiCleanse GHI (Xymogen), and phosphatidylcholine, to help heal the gut lining; high-dose probiotics; digestive enzymes; gamma-linoleic acid (such as borage seed oil); and avoidance of allergic foods (including histamine-releasing foods in those who are sensitive); followed by a rotation diet. Some patients with Candida and/or mercury affecting leaky gut also need to address these problems to decrease the inflammation in the GI tract. Lauricidin (monolaurin) and Biocidin (Bio Botanical Research) combined with other herbal treatments against Candida (oregano oil, garlic, berberine, Pau D'Arco) can be effective with or without antifungal medication (like Diflucan) with a strict sugar-free, yeast-free diet.

When you are taking antibiotics for Lyme disease, we also recommend taking probiotics with acidophilus (over 200 billion colony-forming units/CFUs) and *Saccharomyces boulardii*, the beneficial yeast that has been proven to decrease the incidence of *Clostridium difficile* diarrhea. According to a meta-analysis that appeared in a 2011 article in the *Journal of Clinical Gastroenterology*, three types of probiotics (*Lactobacillus rhamnosus* GG, probiotic mixtures, and *Saccharomyces boulardii*) have all been shown to significantly decrease the incidence of antibiotic-associated diarrhea, but only *S. boulardii* is effective for the prevention of *Clostridium difficile* diarrhea. Some patients will develop *C. difficile diarrhea*, however, despite taking probiotics, and will need to be treated with a course of antibiotics, such as Flagyl, oral Vancocin, or Dificid. In resistant cases, fecal transplantation may be used to restore a diverse, healthy microbiome in the intestine. As an alternative to fecal transplantation, in order to restore a healthy microbiome, we have tried probiotic enemas using over 500 billion beneficial bacteria, including strains of Bifidobacterium (found in Tru-Bifido, Master Supplements), known to colonize the lower intestine and enhance immunity, decrease inflammation (increasing production of the anti-inflammatory cytokine IL-10), and help with functional bowel disorders (i.e., strains HN-019, BI-04, and Bi-07). A small group of patients reported beneficial effects. A placebo-controlled, randomized study needs to be performed to evaluate the efficacy of this approach.

Probiotics have multiple mechanisms of action that allow them to be especially beneficial for health, as they balance intestinal microflora. They help reduce gut permeability, preventing leaky gut and multiple food allergies. They also have an effect on our immunity; they decrease inflammatory cytokine production and assist the immune system found in the GI tract. This is especially important when we consider the causes of infectious diarrhea. Bacterial and viral infections and certain parasites can cause inflammation and disrupt microflora. Common parasitic infections include giardiasis, amebiasis, cryptosporidium, hookworm, pinworm, roundworm (including filariasis), and strongyloides. We have found that certain patients with resistant symptoms of MSIDS improved once intestinal parasites were discovered and treated. These infections are treated differently and, unfortunately, testing may be unreliable, as is the case with Lyme disease and associated co-infections. It is therefore important that we understand the limitations of standard GI testing and examine other methods for determining the parameters of gastrointestinal health.

Evaluating GI Health Using the Comprehensive Digestive Stool Analysis (CDSA)

There are several methods for evaluating your gastrointestinal health. The most common tests are the Comprehensive Digestive Stool Analysis (CDSA), which evaluates your gut microbiome and markers of intestinal health (available through functional medicine laboratories such as Genova Diagnostics, Doctor's Data, or Diagnos-Techs), and companies like μBiome and American Gut. Unfortunately, perfecting commercial testing of the microbiome, looking at Firmicutes/Bacteroides ratios, is still in its early phases, as different labs use different testing protocols, leading to a lack of reproducibility between studies. Therefore, the gastrointestinal function profile from Genova is the one that we most often employ. It evaluates many of the markers of intestinal health, and although the CDSA is generally not taught to physicians in medical school, I have found it to be invaluable in expanding the GI workup for patients with gastrointestinal disorders that could not be explained by routine testing. It includes testing for:

- Bacteria: The CDSA 2.0 identifies the predominant bacteria in the gut. The test also evaluates for the presence of pathogenic bacteria such as *H. pylori*, Shigella, *E. coli*, Campylobacter spp., and *Clostridium difficile,* which can affect your digestion, absorption of nutrients, pH, and immune status.
- Yeast: An abnormally high overgrowth of yeast on the CDSA can point to possible candidiasis, requiring treatment with antifungal agents.
- Parasites: Parasites can increase the symptoms of Lyme-MSIDS. The majority of our patients are co-infected with Babesia, which can suppress the immune system, allowing other parasitic infections to emerge. Parasites can also cause GI symptoms similar to yeast overgrowth, such as gas and bloating, confusing the clinical picture. They can be difficult to pick up on standard parasite testing, and we have found the presence of hidden parasites on CDSA testing from specialized laboratories when local laboratory evaluations were negative.
- Inflammation: The CDSA looks for signs of inflammation in the colon, checking levels of specialized proteins, including Eosinophil Protein X, lactoferrin, and Calprotectin, an FDA approved biomarker that is found in elevated levels in inflammation and/or infection. It is released in inflammatory bowel disorders such as Crohn's disease and ulcerative colitis, but not in irritable bowel syndrome (helping to differentiate the two).
- Beta-glucuronidase: normal levels are associated with balanced microbial activity. Elevated levels indicate drugs, toxins, and

hormones that are circulating between the intestines and liver, which can increase our risk of breast, prostate, and colorectal cancers.

- Lithocholic: Deoxycholic Acid Ratio (LCA: DCA): abnormal levels indicate the possibility of SIBO, gallstones, and inhibition of an important liver enzyme, glutathione-S-transferase, which, again, increases our risk of breast and colorectal cancer.
- Intestinal pH: The CDSA evaluates the intestinal pH related to pH-lowering organic acids and pH-raising ammonia levels from certain bacteria.
- Essential markers of digestion and absorption: The CDSA evaluates pancreatic enzyme secretion, which, if low, can be a sign of malabsorption. It also evaluates levels of short-chain fatty acids (SCFAs) and long-chain fatty acids (LCFAs). Short-chain fatty acids are produced by the fermentation of foods in our diet (dietary polysaccharides and fiber), and one of their products, N-butyrate, has been shown to lower the risk of colitis and colorectal cancer. Antibiotics can lower N-butyrate levels, as can insufficient fiber and a slow transit time. Low levels of N-butyrate indicate a need to increase fiber, prebiotics, and probiotics in order to reestablish a healthy balance in the colon.

Since the microbiome has been shown to play an important role in digestion, weight control, glucose metabolism, heart disease, neurological disorders, inflammation, immunity, and autoimmune processes, while simultaneously affecting the epigenetics of the body, we must take care of it if we are to maintain proper health.

Many patients with resistant symptoms of Lyme-MSIDS who have not adequately responded to standard antibiotic protocols do, in fact, test positive for multiple abnormalities on the CDSA. Using that information and treating associated yeast overgrowth, dysbiosis, enzyme deficiencies, and/or parasitic infections, while evaluating their levels of inflammation and detoxification, can be a turning point in getting to the next level of wellness.

EIGHTEEN

Lyme and Liver Dysfunction

nother gastrointestinal issue that frequently arises in MSIDS patients is elevated liver functions. This term refers to abnormalities that appear in specific blood chemistry tests that measure inflammation in the liver (tests for aspartate aminotransferase [AST], alanine aminotransferase [ALT], gamma-glutamyl transpeptidase [GGT], or obstruction/congestion in the liver [tests for alkaline phosphatase +/− bilirubin]). Unfortunately, these liver chemistry abnormalities are not always accompanied by symptoms, at least not early in the course of the illness, and are only diagnosed by going to your doctor and getting these blood tests. For example, some liver diseases, such as hepatitis, can be present without symptoms for years, all the while leading to significant damage.

Some diseases can cause inflammation in the liver, while others cause a blockage both in and leading from the liver to the pancreas or the gallbladder. A third issue occurs when there is congestion in the liver, as in the case of congestive heart failure. For example, hepatitis is an inflammation of the liver that occurs without significant congestion. It can cause elevations in AST, ALT, and GGT as well as nonspecific symptoms, including fatigue, poor appetite, weight loss, nausea, and muscle and joint pain. Other diseases, such as cirrhosis of the liver, have a significant congestive/obstructive component. The obstruction causes jaundice and fluid accumulation in the abdomen (ascites), an enlarged spleen, and enlarged blood vessels in the esophagus. Diseases such as pancreatic cancer can cause a bile duct obstruction with minimal inflammation (primarily raising levels of alkaline phosphatase and total bilirubin). Symptoms of pancreatic cancer can include painless jaundice, pale colored stools, itching, poor appetite, weight loss, and upper abdominal pain. It is therefore vital to identify which liver functions are elevated so we can create a proper differential diagnosis and order appropriate follow-up testing. It is also important to differentiate whether these elevated liver functions are directly due to tick-borne diseases, are medication side effects, or are due to other diseases that are not only affecting the liver but also mimicking the symptoms of Lyme-MSIDS.

Some of the diseases that cause elevated liver functions can be fatal, and there may be no clinical signs of illness until the abnormalities become severe. When symptoms do occur, they can include:

- Breast development (gynecomastia) in men
- Confusion or difficulty thinking (encephalopathy)
- Fatigue
- Impotence
- Joint pain
- Loss of appetite
- Nausea and vomiting (with occasional vomiting of blood)
- Nosebleeds, bleeding gums, gastrointestinal bleeding (secondary to esophageal varices, i.e., dilated veins which often bleed in cirrhosis, and coagulation defects)
- Pale or clay-colored stools
- Redness of the palms of the hands (palmar erythema)
- Small, red spiderlike blood vessels on the skin (spider angiomas)
- Swelling or fluid buildup in the legs (edema) and in the abdomen (ascites)
- Weight loss
- Yellow color in the skin, mucus membranes, or eyes (jaundice)

LIVER DISEASE AND LYME

Elevated liver functions are frequently seen in patients with Lyme disease. Patients who present with localized EM rashes have been found to have elevated liver function assays 37 percent of the time. In patients who have disseminated Lyme disease, in which the disease has spread throughout the body, the incidence is even higher. In one study, published in the journal *Hepatology*, 115 patients with EM rashes were evaluated; other causes for abnormal liver functions were excluded (they were not yet on antibiotics), and they found that 66 percent of the patients had elevated liver functions in disseminated Lyme disease. These improved or resolved three weeks after the onset of antibiotic therapy. Cytokines causing inflammation or direct borrelia invasion of the liver were thought to be responsible for the elevation in liver functions.

We see the same elevated liver functions accompanying other tick-borne diseases:

- *Borrelia hermsii* and other relapsing fever borrelia can cause nausea, vomiting, abdominal pain, hepatitis with jaundice, and an enlarged spleen. A *Borrelia miyamotoi* infection can also look like Ehrlichia/Anaplasma (low white cell and platelet counts) with elevated liver functions.
- Ehrlichiosis occasionally presents with jaundice, especially in the early stages. Blood testing on those with confirmed ehrlichiosis or anaplasmosis will often reveal elevated liver functions (with associated low white blood cell counts and/or low platelet counts). These will generally promptly resolve with treatment with tetracyclines. (Although rarely, antibiotics may temporarily raise liver functions, and changing the medication or lowering the dose resolves the problem.)
- The Heartland virus and Bourbon virus (tick-borne viral infections) can both raise liver function tests (LFTs). These viruses have laboratory values that look like ehrlichiosis (leukopenia, thrombocytopenia, transaminitis), but are unresponsive to doxycycline.
- Babesiosis can cause mild elevations of AST, serum bilirubin and/or alkaline phosphatase.

- Rickettsial diseases: Rocky Mountain spotted fever (RMSF) and Q fever are also associated with elevations in liver functions. Q fever may lead to chronic symptoms such as Q fever endocarditis, an enlarged liver, hepatitis with liver enzyme elevations, and rare cases of jaundice.

Other Causes of Liver Injury

Often we pick up elevated liver functions on routine blood testing, or the liver problem may develop and/or appear during treatment, as in the case of a toxic chemical exposure, viral infection, or new medication. There are also many systemic diseases that can affect liver functions:

- **Alpha-1-Antitrypsin Deficiency:** This is a genetic disorder responsible for decreased production of the enzyme alpha-1-antitrypsin. It can cause both liver disease and emphysema.
- **Autoimmune Hepatitis (AIH)**
- **Cancer:** Patients with chronic hepatitis B and C are at risk for developing cirrhosis of the liver, as well as primary liver cancers, i.e., hepatomas.
- **Chemical Exposures:** Certain toxic chemicals like carbon tetrachloride have been implicated in cases of acute liver failure.
- **Connective Tissue Diseases:** Lupus (SLE), juvenile idiopathic arthritis, rheumatoid arthritis, Sjögren's syndrome, scleroderma, and polymyalgia rheumatica (PMR) may all present with liver abnormalities. Patients with SLE and autoimmune hepatitis (AIH) require steroids to prevent disease progression, but a patient with active Lyme disease and co-infections like babesiosis will rapidly relapse on high-dose steroids due to suppression of their immune system, so performing a proper differential diagnosis is essential.
- **Drug-Induced Liver Injury:** The most common over-the-counter drug to cause liver injury is acetaminophen (Tylenol). People who take 3,000–4,000 mg per day on a regular basis may experience a rise in LFT's with hepatotoxicity. Any elevation of liver functions while on Tylenol requires stopping the medication and giving high doses of cysteine (orally or IV in severe cases), which helps detoxify the Tylenol through the glutathione pathway,

preventing liver failure. We suggest keeping the total daily dose of acetaminophen to a maximum of 2000 mg a day (especially in the elderly, or those with liver disease), and using a minimum of 600 mg twice a day of NAC (N-Acetylcysteine) in patients who require acetaminophen for pain.

- **Endocrine Diseases:** Hyperthyroidism, hypothyroidism, hyper-cortisolism (Cushing's syndrome), hypocortisolism (Addison's disease), as well as diabetes may cause elevations in liver chemistries.

- **Fatty liver with/without alcoholism** (NASH, nonalcoholic steatohepatitis): Liver disease can occur without an alcoholic component, as in the case of nonalcoholic fatty liver disease (NASH), which causes elevated LFTs. It can be seen in overweight individuals, and is an unrecognized public health threat. The current theory is that excess deposits of fat in the liver cause inflammation and damage liver cells, which can in some cases trigger liver failure. If no apparent cause of elevated liver functions is found in an individual with obesity, an ultrasound of the liver and gallbladder can be performed to check for fatty infiltration. A liver biopsy is needed to confirm the diagnosis. Approximately 25 million obese adults in the United States suffer from some form of NASH, and they are unaware they have it, making it more prevalent than diabetes. It is expected to eclipse hepatitis C as the primary cause for liver transplants in the next decade.

- **Gallstones:** Gallstones are produced in the gallbladder. They may be asymptomatic or symptomatic depending on their size and quantity and whether they pass into other parts of the biliary tree, causing inflammation and obstruction. Mild gallbladder dysfunction may cause nausea, bloating, and abdominal pain after eating a fat-laden meal, but if they obstruct the bile ducts, symptoms may include severe abdominal pain (in the right upper quadrant) with nausea, vomiting, fever, and jaundice.

- **Hematological Diseases:** Sickle-cell anemia, thalassemia, Hodgkin's disease, non-Hodgkin's lymphoma, different types of leukemia, multiple myeloma, and myelodysplasias may all cause elevated liver functions either through infiltration of malignant cells or through iron overload in the liver.

- **Hemochromatosis:** caused by iron overload in the liver, which can lead to cirrhosis, darkening of the skin with diabetes (brown diabetes), testicular failure, arthritis, and congestive heart failure (cardiomyopathy). Eight percent to 13 percent of the population may be carrying the genes for this disease, and it is one of the most common genetic disorders seen in a medical office.
- **Infectious Diseases:** Viral illnesses such as chronic hepatitis B and C (including all forms of hepatitis: A-E), and other infectious diseases such as GI infections (salmonella, Clostridium, and Campylobacter), fungal infections, mycobacteria (tuberculosis), syphilis, HIV, parasitic infections (amoeba, liver fluke), and fungal infections can all cause abnormalities in liver functions.
- **Inflammatory Bowel Disease:** Ulcerative colitis and Crohn's disease often have abnormal liver functions, especially if the disease is severe enough to require surgery.
- **Pulmonary Diseases:** including pneumonia (acute disease) and cystic fibrosis (chronic disease).
- **Right-Sided Heart Failure:** is manifested by an enlarged liver on physical examination (hepatomegaly), an enlarged spleen (splenomegaly), ascites (fluid in the abdominal cavity) with peripheral edema and fluid in the cavity surrounding the lungs (pleural effusions), as well as occasionally jaundice.
- **Wilson's Disease:** This is a rare disease caused by a defect in the excretion of copper, affecting the liver and brain, causing tremors, problems with speech, and personality changes with severe mood swings. It also causes liver disease with associated hepatitis and cirrhosis, with occasional esophageal bleeding.

TESTING FOR ELEVATED LIVER FUNCTIONS

Since many liver diseases can be silent with long-term health consequences, it is important to have your liver functions checked once a year, and to understand the strengths and weaknesses of the currently available testing. Many of these tests are not specific for the liver yet give us clues that there may be disease processes at work.

- **Aspartate transaminase, AST (GOT):** This is a liver enzyme that measures inflammation in the liver. Normal values are usually less than 35 U/L but will depend on the individual laboratory's reference range. In diseases such as chronic hepatitis, values of AST can be greater than twice the normal range, and in some cases are more than ten times the upper limit of normal, which may reflect severe liver and/or biliary disease. This enzyme may be slightly elevated due to certain drug reactions (such as antibiotics), moderately elevated in those who drink too much alcohol (alcoholic hepatitis, with enzymes in the 200 IU to 300 UL range), and very elevated, as in the case of acute viral hepatitis (above 1,000 UL). AST levels can be elevated during a heart attack and in diseases causing inflammation of the skeletal muscle (myositis), even when there is no liver damage.

- **Alanine transaminase, ALT (GPT):** This is a more specific enzyme test for liver disease with associated bile duct and gallbladder dysfunction (hepatobiliary dysfunction) and will generally not be affected by other inflammatory disease processes, which is why it is considered to be a better marker. Normal values are usually less than 40 U/L.

- **Alkaline phosphatase:** This test identifies an enzyme that is associated with congestion and obstruction in the liver. Normal values are between 33 U/L and 115 U/L (Quest Diagnostics). Elevated levels of alkaline phosphatase may be seen with gallstones; if pancreatic cancer is obstructing the bile duct; with bile duct strictures; with congestive heart failure; with cirrhosis of the liver; and with liver cancer. The highest levels of alkaline phosphatase are usually seen in severe liver disease, with bile duct obstruction that is usually associated with elevated levels of bilirubin. Bilirubin is formed when old or damaged red blood cells are broken down in the spleen, forming the compound unconjugated bilirubin, which is then shuttled to the liver via transporter proteins (albumin). An elevated alkaline phosphatase level together with an elevated total bilirubin level is indicative of liver congestion and obstruction, and can cause jaundice (yellowing of the skin, mucous membranes, and the eyes).

As with AST, isolated alkaline phosphatase levels are not specific for the liver. These enzymes are also present in the bone, intestine, placenta, and white blood cells. An elevated alkaline phosphatase level might therefore suggest a bone disease (such as Paget's), or breast cancer with metastases to the bone. Elevations in alkaline phosphatase levels can also occur during pregnancy and in children during a growth spurt (without an increase in bilirubin).

- **Total bilirubin:** This test can help determine if there is an obstruction in the liver, especially with an associated elevation of alkaline phosphatase. However, isolated levels of total bilirubin without an elevation of alkaline phosphatase are not necessarily indicative of an obstruction. This is usually due to Gilbert's syndrome, a hereditary disorder in which there is impaired bilirubin uptake and storage, due to a decrease in the enzyme that conjugates bilirubin. Although this can produce jaundice, it is completely benign. It affects roughly 7 percent of the total population, and we see Gilbert's syndrome frequently. Dapsone can also cause isolated (and reversible) elevations in bilirubin, which is increased with Gilbert's syndrome. Normal values of total bilirubin range between 0.2 mg/dL and 1.2 mg/dL (Quest Diagnostics).

- **Gamma-glutamyl transpeptidase** (GGT): This is a very sensitive marker for inflammation, but it is not specific for any one disease process. An elevated GGT, with an associated increase in the size of the red blood cells (macrocytosis), may be useful in helping to determine if your alcohol consumption is affecting your liver: Abnormal levels are greater than 30 U/L.

- **Supplemental tests to evaluate liver function—albumin levels, prothrombin time, alpha-fetoprotein levels:** I use these tests if the blood work listed above shows that there are abnormalities in liver functions, or when a patient tells me that they are taking anticoagulants such as Coumadin, or that they have a history of (or are at risk for) liver cancer. Low albumin levels can be seen with chronic disease states and liver damage. Elevated prothrombin times are not specific for liver disease, and they can also be seen in cases of vitamin K deficiency, malabsorption, and use of an anticoagulant medication (Coumadin). Alpha-fetoprotein is a serum protein like albumin that can be elevated in pregnancy and indicate developmental disorders in the fetus; it can also be elevated in people with germ cell tumors, a primary cancer of the liver (hepatoma), and metastatic disease to the liver. Alpha-fetoprotein levels can be monitored in these circumstances to evaluate treatment and tumor progression, as well as in those with chronic hepatitis B or C, to evaluate early development of a hepatoma.

Screening for Specific Liver Diseases

Apart from testing for tick-borne disorders, which is a common cause of abnormal liver functions, I also perform the following blood tests to rule out other causes of liver disease. I recommend that everyone be tested for hepatitis B and C at some point in their adult life, and be screened for hemochromatosis. When cross-referenced with symptoms and a complete patient history and physical, these tests will usually help to differentiate the cause for any liver abnormalities:

- **Antinuclear antibody** (ANA): Elevated levels are seen in auto-immune diseases of the liver, such as lupus.
- **Anti–smooth muscle antibodies:** Elevated levels are seen in auto-immune hepatitis.
- **Iron-TIBC and ferritin level:** Elevated levels are seen in hemo-chromatosis (iron overload); however, elevated iron and ferritin levels are not specific for hemochromatosis. This can also be seen with iron replacement therapy, red blood cell disorders, and significant alcohol consumption, as well as during inflammatory states, including severe Lyme arthritis, hepatitis, other liver diseases, and cancer.
- **Ceruloplasmin levels:** Ceruloplasmin is the major copper-carrying protein in the blood produced in the liver. Low levels of ceruloplasmin are seen in Menkes disease, with high levels of Vitamin C consumption, and in Wilson's disease.
- **Antimitochondrial antibody** (AMA): Elevated levels are seen in primary biliary cirrhosis, a disease in which there is destruction of the small bile ducts that can cause cirrhosis.

• **Hepatitis screen for hepatitis A, B, and C:** Acute hepatitis may present with significantly elevated levels of liver enzymes (AST, ALT), yet chronic hepatitis (B and C) may present with only minimally elevated levels of liver enzymes (transaminases) and be silent causes of liver disease. Hepatitis A usually resolves spontaneously (although rare cases of acute liver failure do exist), but chronic hepatitis B and C can lead to cirrhosis of the liver and liver cancer, and be fatal. Hepatitis sufferers may complain of chronic fatigue, arthralgias, and joint pains, the same symptoms seen in Lyme-MSIDS. These symptoms stem from the virus causing deposition of immune complexes in the joints, arteries, or kidneys, leading to an inflammation in the blood vessels (vasculitis) and in the kidneys (glomerulonephritis). Many chronic hepatitis patients are asymptomatic, and the disease can remain silent for many years, until the liver is severely affected. Many young Americans may have chronic hepatitis C, while Americans of all ages, as well as those of Asian, Indian, and Tibetan descent, often also suffer from chronic hepatitis B. Sexual transmission, maternal-neonatal transmission, IV drug use, body piercing, tattoos, and hemodialysis are associated risk factors. Regular screening of liver functions, viral loads, alpha-fetoprotein levels (an early marker for hepatocellular carcinoma), and imaging studies of the liver are essential in following patients with known hepatitis. Fortunately, some of the newer antiviral combinations for hepatitis B and C are proving to be more effective than prior regimens, and may put the disease into remission.

JIM'S SILENT LIVER DISEASE CONTRIBUTED TO HIS SYMPTOMS

Jim was twenty-one years old and had a past medical history significant for severe depression, anxiety, and mood swings. When he came to see me he also complained of fatigue, migratory joint and muscle pains, headaches, tingling and numbness in the extremities, tremors and neurocognitive deficits, and pronounced difficulties with speech. He told me that he dropped out of college because of the severity of his symptoms. He had a history of several tick bites over the years, and an EM rash. At that time he had received twenty-one days of doxycycline, was pronounced "cured" by his physician, and was told that his ongoing symptoms were due to chronic fatigue syndrome, depression, and fibromyalgia.

His physical examination was essentially unremarkable, except for the tremors and his marked anxiety. His laboratory tests revealed a CDC-positive Lyme IgM Western Blot and prior exposure to *Mycoplasma pneumoniae* and *Chlamydia pneumonia*. He was slightly anemic, and his comprehensive metabolic profile (CMP) was completely normal, including his liver functions. Hormone testing showed normal thyroid functions, and we sent off a salivary DHEA/cortisol test, which returned with a borderline low cortisol in the morning, which may have been responsible in part for his chronic fatigue. We performed a six-hour urine DMSA challenge, which showed an elevated level of mercury (28, normal is less than 3) and an elevated level of lead (36, normal is less than 2). We initially hypothesized that Jim's depression, anxiety, mood swings, tremors, fatigue, and musculoskeletal symptoms were due to his Lyme disease and associated heavy metal burden with borderline adrenal function.

During the first month of treatment, Jim was taking Omnicef, Plaquenil, and Zithromax, as well as nystatin tablets. He had a severe Jarisch-Herxheimer reaction within the first two weeks, and we stopped the antibiotics. Jim was then switched to doxycycline and Plaquenil with meals, but again, within the first two weeks of treatment, we had to stop the antibiotics due to a significant increase in his fatigue and joint pain.

We then performed a new set of routine laboratory tests: His blood counts were normal, but his liver functions had dramatically increased. Although they were normal on his initial screening test, his AST was now 510 and his ALT was 682. These levels were more than ten times normal, and although we occasionally see mild elevations in liver functions with antibiotic therapy, this was an extremely unusual elevation. We therefore sent off blood work for an ANA, AMA, ceruloplasmin, ferritin, alpha-1 antitrypsin level, and screens for hepatitis A, B, and C. These screening tests all came back normal except for the ceruloplasmin. It was low, at 16 mg/dL; normal values are between 20 mg/dL and 40 mg/dL. This suggested Wilson's disease, as the symptoms associated with it were exactly what Jim was experiencing. They were also the same symptoms that we frequently see with Lyme disease and mercury exposure, yet there was one essential difference: Jim's tremors and mood swings were extremely severe. I often see patients with tremors, and I am used to seeing depressed patients with anxiety and mood swings. But there was an extreme nature to Jim's symptoms, and based on his low ceruloplasmin level, I had wondered if he had a copper overload, and if Wilson's disease was responsible for the severity of his complaints on top of neurological Lyme disease with exposure to mercury. The last test confirmed my suspicion.

We sent Jim to a university center that specializes in liver diseases, and referred him to a physician who had extensive experience with Wilson's disease. The results from a liver biopsy showed that his hepatic copper levels were elevated. Jim's Lyme disease and elevated levels of mercury were contributing to his tremors and mood swings, but his elevated levels of copper were responsible for making these symptoms more severe. If he hadn't shown an unusual increase in his liver functions with antibiotic therapy, we would never have screened him for Wilson's disease, and he would never have had the right treatment protocol for his particular issues.

How Can I Improve My Liver Health?

The treatment of elevated liver functions depends on the cause of the elevation. In the case of viral hepatitis, there are newer drug regimens (pegylated interferon and Ribasphere, Baraclude, Viread, Epivir, Hepsera, and Tyzeka) that have helped decrease viral loads and put patients in remission.

For hepatitis C, the treatment has recently evolved from using interferon and a protease inhibitor like Victerilis with ribavirin to newer oral drugs like Harvoni (Simeprevir plus sofosbuvir), and Viekira Pak (ombitasvir/paritaprevir/ritonavir and dasabuvir). Treatment duration is twelve weeks without cirrhosis and twenty-four weeks with cirrhosis. Long-term success rate with these drugs is over 95 percent in treatment of naive patients (without cirrhosis).

For iron and copper overload disorders (hemochromatosis and Wilson's disease), the treatment is to remove the iron (through giving blood regularly, i.e., phlebotomy) and by chelating out the copper (with drugs like Cuprimine).

In lupus and autoimmune diseases, as with an autoimmune hepatitis, steroids and immunosuppressive drugs may be needed (such as Imuran) to decrease signs and symptoms of inflammation. It is important to be sure that there are no underlying infections (i.e., Lyme and associated co-infections), as they may reactivate with immunosuppressive therapy. In endocrine disorders, balancing hormone abnormalities will normalize liver functions, and in bacterial tick-borne diseases causing transaminitis, antibiotic therapy will reduce elevated liver enzymes.

Low-dose naltrexone (LDN) is one newer treatment protocol that also shows promise for those with inflammatory bowel disorders and elevated liver functions.

When the cause of the liver dysfunction has been established and properly treated, other integrative therapies may be useful in decreasing inflammation and supporting liver function. These include antioxidant therapies and supplements that support detoxification reactions. The supplements NAC and alpha-lipoic acid help with the production and regeneration of glutathione, aid in detoxification, and protect the liver from free radical damage. The supplement NAC will also help protect the liver if you are taking large amounts of Tylenol, since cysteine is used in acetaminophen toxicity. Milk thistle (silymarin) is also a useful supplement; extensive scientific research has been done on its liver-protective effects, and we often use broccoli seed extracts, like glucoraphanin, as they have been proven to help the liver detoxify while simultaneously decreasing inflammation. Finally, there are traditional Chinese herbal formulas, such as Hepa #2, by Dr. Zhang. This is useful in lowering liver functions for individuals with chronic liver disease, and we have confirmed the utility of this herbal formulation for our patients with elevated liver functions.

By using the above differential diagnostic categories, and testing and treatment protocols for liver disease, you will be able to move through the complicated maze of possibilities, improve your health, and discover one more clue to your symptoms.

NINETEEN

Lyme and Pain

One of the most disabling symptoms affecting those with Lyme-MSIDS is chronic pain. The pain can be so debilitating that some people lose their ability to function in a meaningful and productive way. Over-the-counter medications such as acetaminophen (Tylenol), ibuprofen (Advil), or naproxen sodium (Naprosyn/Aleve) only provide minimal relief, and many patients take high-dose narcotics to control their pain. These patients often have already seen rheumatologists and may have been told that they suffer from seronegative rheumatoid arthritis or from a nonspecific autoimmune disease. They are then placed on steroids such as prednisone, or disease-modifying antirheumatic drug regimens, such as methotrexate, Arava, or TNF-α blockers such as Enbrel. These agents might give temporary relief but can have significant side effects, such as causing lymphoma and other malignancies, liver toxicity, osteoporosis, and serious infections.

Others turn to pain management specialists, who often prescribe multiple drug regimens of neuroleptic drugs and narcotics, combined with nerve blocks. Despite these physicians' best attempts, the patient may still have pain, and as the narcotics wear off, higher and higher doses are required to control their discomfort, leading to unfortunate and potentially serious painkiller addictions.

WHY AM I IN SO MUCH PAIN?

Lyme disease can cause pain in every part of the body. Although this pain may be limited to one or two areas and be more or less constant, one particular hallmark of tick-borne disease, and particularly *Borrelia burgdorferi*, is pain that comes and goes, and migrates from one area to another. This includes arthritis pain, myalgias (muscle pain), and neuropathic pain (nerve pain), all of which normally do not tend to migrate. In women, pain is also influenced by hormonal cycles, as women usually flare for several days right before, during, and after their menses. We also would suspect a tick-borne disorder when antibiotic use increases pain (from a Jarisch-Herxheimer reaction) or decreases pain. This will occasionally happen in patients treated for an unrelated bacterial infection, such as a sinusitis or urinary tract infection, who are unaware that they have Lyme disease.

If pain is associated with multiple systemic symptoms, especially the ones listed in the HMQ, then it is quite likely that it is caused by Lyme-MSIDS. If you have neck pain or an isolated pain in a joint, you might simply have a herniated disc with neuropathy, or osteoarthritis. But if you have many of the symptoms on the HMQ, one should suspect a tick-borne disorder and order the appropriate tests. This includes testing for co-infections such as Babesia (especially if there are unexplained day and night sweats, chills, flushing, a cough, and shortness of breath) as Babesia increases all of the underlying symptoms of Lyme disease; for Bartonella, a frequent cofactor in neuropathy and encephalopathy; as well as for Mycoplasma and chlamydia, which can increase arthritis pain. Similarly, viruses and yeast may impact pain syndromes, and should be tested for and treated.

Lyme-MSIDS can mimic most common pain syndromes. For example, MSIDS can cause CFS/SEID and fibromyalgia, with widespread pain. It can cause symptoms of common autoimmune diseases such as rheumatoid arthritis, lupus, and MS with associated inflammation. It can present with a varied list of neurological syndromes that cause pain, including headaches and migraines, peripheral neuropathy, neuropathy of the face, dental pain syndromes, trigeminal neuralgia, radiculopathy, associated cranial nerve palsies, and carpal tunnel with ulnar neuropathy. It may present with painful gastrointestinal and genitourinary syndromes, with irritable bowel syndrome, associated inflammatory bowel disease, or interstitial cystitis. We have seen patients with painful gynecological syndromes, including vaginal neuralgia and dysparaneuria (painful intercourse), and painful cardiac presentations, such as resistant chest pain (due to costochondritis, with inflammation in the nerves and cartilage of the chest wall), and pericarditis (inflammation of the sac surrounding the heart). You might have painful inflammatory eye syndromes, such as conjunctivitis, uveitis, retinitis, or optic neuritis. Psychiatric symptoms such as depression and anxiety that result from tick-borne diseases may further increase perception of pain. Gender differences may influence the perception—or at least the report—of pain. A large retrospective study of 72,000 electronic medical records (EMRs) from Stanford University, published in the *Journal of Pain*, showed that women experience pain more intensely than men in virtually every disease category.

You may remember that there are both strains and species of borrelia. Pain syndromes depend on the particular strains and species. Some cause significant pain and others do not. There are approximately one hundred different strains of borrelia in the United States, and three hundred strains worldwide. In Europe, a different species of borrelia, *Borrelia afzelii*, is responsible for the classic purplish skin rash of acrodermatitis chronicum atrophicans (ACA), but another species, *Borrelia garinii*, is responsible for symptoms of Lyme neuroborreliosis with associated neuropathic pain syndromes, like Bannwarth's syndrome. *Borrelia burgdorferi sensu stricto* is the primary form of borrelia found in the United States, and the B31 strain will have different clinical manifestations than European species. In the United States, substrains of outer surface protein C, called RST-1, can cause especially severe pain syndromes, which also depend on the length of the infection and the patient's co-infection status and genetic makeup (HLA status). These cause the release of chemokines and associated cytokines, such as TNF-alpha, IL-1, and IL-6, which increase pain in the muscles, joints, and nerves. Cytokines also have a direct effect on nerve fibers. In the peripheral nervous system, cytokines such as interleukin-1 beta also can cause the release of other inflammatory molecules from the nitric oxide pathway, as well as increase the production of pain-inducing molecules such as bradykinin and/or prostaglandins.

Another possible source of pain arises from the body's production of borrelia-specific antibodies. These may target the 41 kDa flagella and other outer-surface proteins (especially Osp A) in an attempt to disable the bacteria, then cross-react with antigens on the surface of our own nerves and organs, which are structurally similar. This process is called "molecular mimicry," and immune reactions against such shared antigens could play a role in the chronic manifestations of Lyme borreliosis, including pain.

Simultaneously treating the three I's of Lyme disease—infection, inflammation, and immune dysfunction—is often the key to alleviating chronic pain. Blebs, the shed particles containing partial DNA from *Borrelia burgdorferi*, stimulate the immune system, and intracellular borrelia and blebs convert host cells into targets for the immune system, increasing pain. Many co-infections increasing inflammation are also located in the intracellular compartment. Until treatments effectively address the load of intracellular bacteria causing inflammation, pain will often continue.

The nitric oxide (NO) pathway also plays a role in increasing oxidative stress and inflammatory cytokines in Lyme disease, fibromyalgia, environmental illness, and CFS. Diverse stressors, whether viral, bacterial, physical, emotional, or environmental (i.e., exposure to volatile organic solvents or pesticides), can all increase nitric oxide and its oxidant product peroxynitrite, leading to an increase in cytokines and pain syndromes. Finally, inadequate liver detoxification, with inadequate production or overutilization of glutathione, and the subsequent inability to remove neurotoxins and cytokines often seen with Lyme-MSIDS, will also result in pain.

What Are Other Causes of Pain?

Many different medical problems that are listed on the MSIDS map can cause pain, and may be contributing overlapping factors. Apart from the three "I's," each of these different factors can increase free radical production and increase cytokines, and may need to be addressed to achieve adequate pain control. These would include:

- Detoxification problems
- Endocrine abnormalities
- Food allergies and leaky gut
- Imbalances (dysbiosis) in the microbiome of the gut

- Heavy metals and environmental toxins
- Nutritional and enzyme deficiencies
- Other infections, including bacteria, parasites, viruses, and opportunistic infections (Candida)
- Sleep disorders

Psychological disorders may also increase discomfort, as the amygdala is the part of the brain that deals with emotions and pain sensation. When patients suffer from depression and anxiety their pain thresholds can be lowered, leading to increased perception of pain.

BRETT'S PAIN WOULDN'T GO AWAY

Brett was twenty-seven years old with a past medical history significant for kidney stones, hypokalemia (low potassium), low Vitamin D, and hyperlipidemia, but his biggest complaint was his chronic pain. He complained of severe joint and neuropathic pain and was taking MS Contin (morphine sulfate) and Dilaudid. These are high-dose narcotics that were barely addressing his pain. He also had spinal disc problems, which he was told were causing his chronic back pain, and it was keeping him up at night, causing insomnia and depression. He also had been diagnosed with a nonspecific autoimmune disease as well as seronegative rheumatoid arthritis.

Brett had seen over one hundred doctors (you read that number correctly), including eight rheumatologists. He had been on multiple immunosuppressive and biological agents, including prednisone, methotrexate, Enbrel, and Humira. His history included multiple tick bites (five to ten), and he complained of drenching night sweats every night for over a year, severe fatigue, decreased libido, chronic constipation, chest pain, migratory joint pain in the wrists, hands, elbows, shoulders, hips, and ankles, and a slight swelling of the joints. Other symptoms included sore muscles, headaches, facial pain with intermittent Bell's palsy, tingling, numbness, and burning sensations in his arms and legs, floaters in his eyes, and tremors.

His physical examination was unremarkable except for low blood pressure while standing (BP 86/54) with associated dizziness and palpitations (pulse rate: 112 beats per minute), swollen nasal turbinates, and decreased sensation in his hands. Laboratory testing showed a low potassium, low serum zinc, low serum iodine, low RBC magnesium, normal B_{12} and folic acid levels, normal thyroid functions, borderline hypercortisolism, multiple food allergies (IgG positive for milk, soy, wheat, beef, and peanuts), and increased levels of lead and mercury. We determined that part of his autoimmune reaction and neuropathy was connected to antiganglioside antibodies against his nerves. A previous physician had ordered Lyme testing, which revealed a borderline Lyme IgG Western blot and a decreased CD 57 count (an alternative blood test used to help support the clinical diagnosis of Lyme disease and follow the disease's progression, although not specific for borrelia). We then ordered more blood work, which revealed positive titers for *Mycoplasma pneumoniae*, as well as a low-level EBV and HHV-6 titers.

In my clinical judgment, Brett suffered from Lyme disease with co-infections, particularly babesiosis, and POTS/dysautonomia. I started him on Coartem, followed by Omnicef, Plaquenil, Mepron, Zithromax, nystatin, and Serrapeptase. This regimen would address the cell-wall forms, cystic forms, and intracellular location of borrelia as well as treat biofilms and associated parasitic infections. An anti-inflammatory protocol was given, including alpha-lipoic acid, resveratrol, curcumin, and glutathione. He was advised to avoid his allergic foods, and to use EDTA suppositories with DMSA to remove his heavy metals; his mineral deficiencies were addressed by replacing them with a high-potency multimineral supplement that contained calcium, potassium, magnesium, zinc, iodine, and other trace minerals.

Once he started this protocol, his pain and depression initially worsened, but his drenching night sweats became less frequent. After several weeks his incessant joint pain finally decreased to a point where it was tolerable. Cymbalta was added for the depression, fibromyalgia symptoms, and neuropathy, as well as Lyrica for sleep and ongoing neuropathic pain. Florinef was then added for his low blood pressure and autonomic nervous system dysfunction, and Omnicef was rotated to IM Bicillin LA for ongoing severe symptoms.

One month later there was a slight improvement in his pain, and he felt increased energy with the Bicillin injections, but he had a significant relapse of day sweats off the Mepron. Due to the severe pain and neuropathy, I suspected Bartonella, and Factive was prescribed; and cryptolepis for the clinical symptoms of babesiosis.

Once the Bartonella and Babesia were treated, Brett was able to start lowering the doses of the MS Contin and Dilaudid for the first time in years. He reported that he was doing "really well," with a significant decrease in pain while on Factive, but he noticed significant relapses of his pain whenever he was off it. I added minocycline to his regimen, as double and, in some cases, triple and even quadruple intracellular antibiotics are often more effective against resistant intracellular infections (i.e., adding rifampin and Dapsone to a tetracycline and macrolide/or quinolone). Once the minocycline was added, his energy showed further improvement, and the sweats were no longer drenching. We were able to decrease the MS Contin over a two-month period, and he was eventually able to get off all his narcotics. Once his Lyme disease and associated tick-borne infections were properly treated, the pain was much more manageable.

TREATING PAIN RELATED TO MSIDS AND LYME

Some MSIDS patients given oral and IV glutathione will have dramatic decreases in musculoskeletal and arthritic pain, as well as improvements in their headaches, fatigue, and neurocognitive difficulties, within minutes to hours of receiving treatment. In a study I performed in 2004, patients reported improvement in fatigue, joint pain, muscle pain, mood swings, headaches, balance, dizziness, speech problems, and cognitive difficulties within thirty minutes of the administration of glutathione. Glutathione may be acting to metabolize toxins in the short term, and may have an effect on cytokines, prostaglandins, interleukins, oxidative stress, and immune modulation in the long term. We have found detoxification to be crucial in helping patients deal with their chronic resistant pain.

Aside from glutathione, I divide pain treatments into two basic categories. The first would be a pharmaceutical approach, in which we simply treat the symptoms, using medication and minimally invasive techniques, and the second would be an integrative approach, in which we treat the whole person. This would include a body/mind/spiritual approach, using meditation and biofeedback techniques, while addressing biochemical/immunological imbalances, using natural supplements and compounded medications as well as diet and exercise. We always attempt to get to the source of the pain.

Using the Horowitz sixteen-point differential diagnostic map, we have found that a multifaceted approach works best in treating patients with overlapping CFS and FMS. Those who complain of severe headaches, neuralgia, myalgias, and arthritis find that a combination of antibiotics and/ or nutraceuticals and herbs for Lyme disease and co-infections, while detoxifying the body and addressing the multifactorial causes of inflammation, can effectively treat pain. Usually the sickest patients will require a combined approach, using pharmaceuticals and nutraceuticals along with classical pain medications to help relieve their suffering.

Classic Pain Medication Treatments

Multiple treatments from each of the following six categories are often necessary to achieve adequate pain relief:

1. **NSAIDs** (nonsteroidal anti-inflammatory drugs): effective analgesics for muscle pain; includes Motrin, Aleve, Naprosyn, Voltaren, and Zipsor. Contraindications include a history of ulcer disease, bleeding disorders, significant liver and kidney abnormalities, and uncontrolled blood pressure.

2. **Antidepressants:** Some antidepressants are effective in helping to relieve pain. Among the class of SSRIs, which includes Prozac, there are several medications that not only block serotonin uptake in the brain but also block the uptake of another neurotransmitter, norepinephrine. Norepinephrine acts as both a hormone and neurotransmitter, and has an effect on blood pressure and heart rate. Norepinephrine also has an effect on decreasing pain. Those SSRIs (like Cymbalta) that increase serotonin and norepinephrine simultaneously have been proven to be helpful in decreasing both muscular pain and neuropathic pain. Elavil and Pamelor belong to another class of antidepressant medication (tricyclic antidepressants), which have been shown to have an effect on neuropathic pain while also acting as a migraine prophylaxis.

3. **Single-dose Decadron and Neurontin:** Occasionally Lyme patients have to go for surgery from an unrelated illness. Steroids are generally contraindicated in Lyme disease because of their

immune suppressive effects, but a single dose of the steroid Decadron administered with Neurontin has been shown to improve postoperative pain and may be useful. Antibiotics should always be used pre- and post-surgery to prevent a worsening of symptoms. Biofilm busters should also be considered post-op, especially if foreign objects (joint replacements, mesh, implants) are used.

4. **Combination drug regimens:** Lyme-MSIDS patients may have resistant pain that is not controlled with one medication, and combination regimens may improve pain control at lower doses than single analgesics alone. Examples of effective combination drug therapy include using tricyclic antidepressants (Elavil, Pamelor) and/or Neurontin (short- or long-acting forms like Gralise and Horizant can be particularly effective) with or without Cymbalta and/or opioids. This regimen is particularly effective in patients with overlapping migraines and neuropathic pain (burning sensations of the extremities). Combining several neuroleptic drugs together at low doses may be efficacious, and oftentimes allows us to avoid narcotic use.

5. **IVIG:** This is the treatment of choice for pain secondary to small-fiber neuropathy and chronic inflammatory demyelinating polyneuropathy (CIDP), which is an immune-mediated inflammatory disorder of the peripheral nervous system seen with Lyme disease. We use IVIG for patients with significant immunoglobulin deficiencies, for autoimmune encephalitis (often with positive autoimmune markers on the Cunningham panel), as well as for neuropathic pain that has persisted in patients with Lyme-MSIDS. IVIG is used for patients with resistant neuropathy despite treating borrelia and co-infections such as Bartonella, and despite detoxing heavy metals such as mercury, lead, and arsenic, which can both affect nerve function and cause neuropathy.

6. **Nondestructive, minimally invasive techniques for refractory pain:** electronic stimulators, pulsed radiofrequency, and Botox injections. Electronic stimulators (peripheral, spinal, and motor cortex) can improve difficult-to-manage chronic pain syndromes, pulsed radiofrequency can decrease pain without tissue damage, and Botox may be able to decrease targeted neuropathic pain.

Botox can help alleviate neuropathic pain by blocking the release of pain mediators (glutamate, substance P) from peripheral nerve terminals and spinal cord neurons, decreasing local inflammation around nerves, and decreasing sympathetic activity.

Integrative Treatments

1. **Low-dose naltrexone (LDN):** We have found LDN to be an extremely useful and effective medication in patients with resistant pain, and it should be routinely considered in patients with Lyme-MSIDS with overlapping pain syndromes, not on long-acting narcotics. LDN has been studied for treating MS and fibromyalgia. A study published in 2010 in *Online Annals of Neurology* showed that LDN was well tolerated, and it significantly improved mental health quality-of-life indicators. These studies have important implications for those with MSIDS, because the same cytokines seen in Lyme disease, FM, and CFS that increase inflammation and pain are also found in those with inflammation from Crohn's disease and MS. LDN helped decrease pain and inflammation in each of these diverse groups. Mechanisms of action of LDN include decreasing glial cell activation in the brain (glial cells release pro-inflammatory cytokines), blocking NFKappa-B and production of IL-6 and TNF-alpha, modulating T and B lymphocyte production, and shifting immune responses from TH2 (making antibodies) to TH1 (helping to fight intracellular infections).

   I performed a study of LDN with my patients, starting in 2009, and it is continuing to date. Those with CFS- and fibromyalgia-type symptoms, who had been diagnosed with Lyme and co-infections and are not on long-acting narcotics, are given LDN at gradually increasing doses. Over one thousand patients have participated in our clinical study. The results have shown that approximately 75 percent of patients with Lyme-MSIDS improved their FM and CFS symptoms, including fatigue, myalgias, and arthralgias. LDN was well tolerated without any significant side effects, although a small percentage

(10 percent to 20 percent) had to decrease the dosage or stop the drug due to insomnia. Those who cannot tolerate LDN at bedtime can take it upon awakening in the morning on an empty stomach.

2. **Antioxidant therapies:** Pharmaceuticals such as glutathione, and nutraceuticals such as alpha-lipoic acid, NAC, glycine, omega-3 fatty acids, sulforaphane, resveratrol, and curcumin. NAC, glycine, and alpha-lipoic acid all help augment the production of glutathione, which has been shown to be clinically beneficial in decreasing pain, fatigue, and brain fog in the resistant Lyme patient. Antioxidant therapies may be helpful, especially for those with overstimulated immune systems producing large numbers of inflammatory cytokines and prostaglandins. These supplements lower oxidative stress, which subsequently decreases the stimulation of NFKappaB, thereby turning off the switch that is responsible for the production of inflammatory cytokines. In our medical practice, we combine the antioxidants mentioned above to achieve a synergistic effect, especially if lipid peroxide levels are elevated (a biomarker of oxidative stress) or if there is resistant pain. In our study on LDN, we often combined LDN with antioxidants such as alpha-lipoic acid, glutathione, resveratrol, and curcumin to reduce free radicals and inflammation, which increase pain, as well as using supplements to support detoxification and removal of inflammatory cytokines.

3. **Angiotensin receptor blockers (ARBs):** Angiotensin II is a hormone that regulates vascular tone, stimulates the release of proinflammatory cytokines, activates NFKappaB, and increases oxidative stress, thus functioning as an inflammatory molecule. ARBs are known to decrease levels of TNF-alpha, and ARBs such as Benicar may be useful in certain cases of persistent inflammation, especially when associated with uncontrolled hypertension. These medications are often associated with the Marshall protocol for treating Lyme disease, which incorporates ARBs and lowering Vitamin D levels as a means of controlling inflammation. Some now believe that low 25(OH) Vitamin D levels is a consequence of chronic inflammation

rather than the cause. Research points to a bacterial etiology which results in high 1,25(OH) Vitamin D and low 25(OH)D levels, and that eradicating persistent intracellular pathogens corrects dysregulated Vitamin D metabolism and resolves inflammatory symptoms. The Marshall protocol is occasionally useful for those with ongoing, severe Jarisch-Herxheimer reactions who cannot tolerate intracellular antibiotics such as tetracyclines and macrolides.

Several of our patients have had a positive response to ARBs, but I have been hesitant to use the high doses recommended in the Marshall protocol because of concerns about lowering blood pressure significantly. I prefer to use other methods, such as LDN and antioxidants, to decrease inflammatory cytokines. Based on recent scientific evidence that Vitamin D can help to decrease morbidity and mortality, and that the vast majority of our patients are Vitamin D deficient and can tolerate Vitamin D supplementation, I believe that the benefit outweighs the risk of using it in the MSIDS population. Using ARBs and lowering Vitamin D would only be a reasonable intervention for those with inflammation who are unresponsive to other treatment protocols.

4. **Changing your diet:** Anti-inflammatory diets consist of increasing the amounts of omega-3 (fish) and omega-9 fatty acids (extra-virgin olive oil) while decreasing omega-6 fatty acids (meat, eggs, dairy) and eating healthy fruits and vegetables (a Mediterranean style diet) and/or following a Paleo diet. Both have been shown to help lower inflammation. When the ratio of omega-3 to omega-6 fatty acids is out of balance, this contributes to inflammation, thus increasing pain. Levels of fatty acids can be tested through some local laboratories, as well as specialized functional medicine laboratories such as Genova or Kennedy-Kreiger. If the ratios are too high toward the omega-6 side, and there is evidence of inflammation, we recommend a diet change and adding nutritional supplements, such as high doses of omega-3 fatty acids in the form of mercury-free fish oils that are also high in DHA.

Anti-inflammatory diets are important in both chronic

disease prevention and in those with active Lyme-MSIDS. Mediterranean-style menus incorporate the use of increased fresh fruits and vegetables (preferably low carb), olive oil, decreased consumption of red meat, eggs, and dairy, and eating fish high in omega-3 fatty acids. This is typically combined with the occasional consumption of red wine (for increasing resveratrol) and avoiding simple sugars, although I do not recommend drinking alcohol to my MSIDS patients while they are being treated with antibiotics, since most people with tick-borne diseases tend to feel worse after drinking (especially if they are on Flagyl or Tindamax). Due to the high levels of mercury often found in seafood, I recommend wild organic salmon and limiting consumption of farm-raised fish (especially in pregnant women) unless you know how they are raised, as well as avoiding eating raw fish or sushi, due to the possibility of parasites. Eating smaller fish is also advisable, since larger fish, such as tuna, tilefish, and swordfish, accumulate more mercury (they are higher up in the food chain). A 2016 study in *JAMA* showed that increased fish consumption decreased the incidence of Alzheimer's disease among apolipoprotein E (APOE ε4) carriers, and the Mediterranean diet has also been shown to increase telomere length of chromosomes, associated with longevity.

A Paleo diet has had some provocative results with chronically ill patients. The diet consists of eating lean meat, fish, low-carb fruits such as berries, vegetables, nuts, and healthy fats, while avoiding high-carb foods, grains, dairy, and salt. This type of diet may be warranted in people with resistant fatigue, joint and muscle pain, headaches, dizziness, palpitations, mood swings, and insomnia for whom other treatment and dietary interventions have failed. These symptoms overlap those of Lyme-MSIDS, and patients report that their Lyme disease symptoms are exacerbated when their blood sugars swing toward the low side. The Paleo diet helps stabilize hypoglycemia, and it can also be beneficial for those patients with overlapping food allergies and food sensitivities to gluten and grains, which may account for its clinical effect. Avoiding gluten may be indicated for those who complain of resistant fatigue, myalgias, arthralgias, headaches, and gastrointestinal complaints. Individuals who do not have true celiac disease but are still sensitive to grains also report that they feel much better avoiding these foods. Similarly, those who are sensitive to certain histamine containing/releasing foods or have a mast cell disorder feel much better on a histamine-free diet, which helps to decrease fatigue, headaches, and pain, apart from decreasing allergic manifestations (wheezing, itching, sneezing, urticaria/hives).

5. **Stress-reduction techniques:** Meditation, yoga, and tai chi can be helpful, since repeated episodes of acute or chronic psychological stress can induce an acute phase response and subsequently a chronic inflammatory process. The practices of mindfulness meditation (Kabat-Zinn), calm abiding meditation, or other stress-reduction techniques provide a way to better cope with our illness, but also decrease stress as another factor driving the inflammatory response. These techniques are discussed in more detail in Chapter 21.

6. **Treatments for Jarisch-Herxheimer reactions:** This would include the five-pronged approach laid out in Chapter 3, and using methods described above to decrease the levels of cytokines.

TWENTY

Lyme and Exercise

The most basic component of our overall health lies in our genetic code: our DNA. Just as we know that we inherit certain physical characteristics and social/emotional traits from our parents, we also inherit their health profile. This is why doctors have been taught to take a comprehensive family history during an initial consultation.

However, we now know that these genes do not always predict our destiny. In many instances environment and lifestyle choices can affect the way genes are expressed. Instead of resigning yourself to the fact that you will have a chronic disease because one or both of your parents experienced the same illness, we have come to understand that you can prevent this scenario by taking better care of your overall health before symptoms present. This involves changing your diet and getting enough exercise. These simple steps not only make you feel better, but they actually change the structure and function of your DNA. The science that backs up this theory is known as *epigenetics*.

WHY SHOULD I EXERCISE?

We have all heard that exercise is important, but did you know that inactivity accounts for 5 percent of global mortality, and is a greater health risk than being overweight or obese? Patients with Lyme disease, fibromyalgia, and CFS/SEID find that their fatigue and pain syndromes improve with increased exercise, independent of other changes in their medical regimens. By losing weight and exercising, we are helping to decrease inflammation and increase detoxification, which are of paramount importance in MSIDS. You may feel much better, both physically and mentally, once you have adopted a healthy lifestyle program.

Scientists have found that short bursts of high-intensity exercise, called high-intensity interval training (HIIT), interspersed with regular exercise have an even greater cardiovascular benefit. It positively affects not only traditional cardiovascular risk factors but also further decreases oxidative stress and inflammation while improving insulin sensitivity, which are all necessary for improved health in those with Lyme-MSIDS. High-intensity interval training may also help brain health by increasing production of an important hormone, known as brain-derived neurotropic factor (BDNF), which helps with the growth and differentiation of neurons and synapses in the memory centers of our brain (hippocampus).

Starting with a gentle exercise program and working up to more vigorous exercise over time (at least four hours a week) is ideal, but any form of daily movement can literally add years to your life. Vigorous walking for at least twenty minutes per day may positively influence many chronic health conditions, ranging from diabetes to cancer. Studies have shown that those who are able to adhere to the American Heart Association's seven ideal cardiovascular health components not only reduced the incidence of cardiovascular disease but even lowered the incidence of several major types of cancer. These include:

1. Maintaining a body mass index (BMI) below 25 (visit http://www.nhlbi.nih.gov for more information and to access a BMI scale)
2. Refraining from smoking
3. Maintaining an untreated total cholesterol below 200 mg/dl
4. Maintaining an untreated blood pressure below 120/80 mm Hg
5. Maintaining an untreated fasting blood glucose below 100 mg/dl
6. Performing at least 150 minutes per week of moderate exercise, or 75 minutes per week of vigorous physical activity. Moderate exercise would include fast walking, a slow jog, and slow bicycling (an activity during which you can still carry on a conversation),

and vigorous physical activity would include high-intensity aerobics (running, cycling, swimming, elliptical training, Stair-Master, kickboxing, Zumba, and team sports) at the level of activity that precludes talking because of the increased intensity

7. Following a healthy diet, as outlined in this book

MSIDS AND EXERCISE

I have seen patients significantly improve their symptoms and recover their health once they begin to exercise. Aerobic exercise has been shown to be effective in reducing fatigue among adults with chronic autoimmune conditions as well as those with depression, cancer, multiple sclerosis, and chronic fatigue syndrome. Lack of exercise contributes to obesity and presents a significant health challenge to those with arthritis or joint pain (seen in Lyme disease) who are deconditioned. The majority of my patients have been ill for an extended period of time. Some are bedbound or are forced to use wheelchairs, and have lost a significant amount of muscle tone. Others continue to suffer from chronic fatigue, dizziness, muscle pains, joint pains, and weakness of the lower extremities that make starting an exercise program difficult. While we can address and treat their symptoms based on the differential diagnoses on the MSIDS map, none of these measures will address the severe deconditioning that can take place. This is why physical therapy and progressive reconditioning with stretching are often essential to get Lyme sufferers back to an optimal level of functioning.

In a case report that was published in the journal *Physical Therapy*, Myriam M. C. Moser, PT, DPT, profiled a typical scenario that we see in our medical office. A fourteen-year-old girl had been infected with Lyme disease one year before receiving appropriate treatment. This young girl had received antibiotic therapy for Lyme disease but still had impaired functional mobility in the activities of daily living. It wasn't until she participated in a combination of therapeutic exercise and a home exercise program that her energy, strength, and range of motion deficits improved.

Creating a Lasting Exercise Program

The ideal exercise program for people with Lyme disease is one that can be built up slowly, gradually increasing levels of exertion. This will ensure that you can stick with the program, and that you won't overdo it early on in therapy and subsequently feel worse.

Patients with Lyme and non-Lyme-MSIDS often tell me that as they begin to feel better and have good days, they tend to overdo their exercise and then crash, ending up in bed for days. They ignored the signals that they were pushing too hard. This can be due to impaired adrenal function, combined with mitochondrial dysfunction, dysautonomia, as well as deconditioning. This is why I believe that a graded exercise program that improves stamina offers the best results for relieving symptoms and improving health, while making sure that you have addressed all overlapping abnormalities on the sixteen-point MSIDS map. When you are healthier and able to do more, increasing the number of hours of exercise and intensity will be possible.

Supervised exercise is advised if you have been ill for a long time and are deconditioned. I strongly recommend that you see your doctor before you start any exercise program, and then begin with a gentle whole-body stretching and conditioning routine. Yoga stretches with an instructor are a good place to start. Never push beyond your body's level of comfort. Slow and gentle is always preferable. As you improve over time, you can lengthen both your yoga routine and exercise practice.

Each week, try and gradually increase the level of exercise, but do it in a systematic fashion, keeping a diary of your progress. Try and work up to at least twenty-five minutes a day, as this will ensure that you get all of the cardiovascular health benefits. Water-based exercise is also a good choice if you have a chronic illness, as you can exercise longer in water than on land without increased effort, or joint or muscle pain, but with all of the cardiovascular benefits.

As you become stronger over time, endurance training, resistance and weight training, and combined training may then be used with HIIT. Strength training with weights has been shown to be beneficial in relieving fatigue, increasing muscle strength and endurance, and improving mood. If you are new to working with weights, I strongly recommend that you work with a personal trainer to make sure you are performing the exercises correctly, and therefore averting injury.

Nutritional Support Can Facilitate Exercise

Many nutritional supplements are useful to help with fatigue and deconditioning, and research has shown that they are the same ones we frequently use with our MSIDS patients. For example, a statistically significant reduction in fatigue of deconditioned patients was achieved with the use of acetyl-L-carnitine, which I commonly prescribe. L-carnitine helps to shuttle fatty acids into the mitochondria as an energy source, and they may be useful if you are deconditioned and too weak to exercise. In a randomized, double-blind, crossover trial published in the *Journal of the Neurological Sciences*, researchers compared the effects of acetyl-L-carnitine and prescription amantadine for the treatment of fatigue in multiple sclerosis. They found that acetyl-L-carnitine was superior to, and better tolerated, than amantadine, which is usually a first-line pharmacological treatment for MS fatigue. L-carnitine should therefore routinely be considered for those with Lyme-MSIDS who are fatigued and don't have adequate energy to participate in a reconditioning program, as well as using mitochondrial support supplements, like NT factors, CoQ-10, resveratrol, and alpha-lipoic acid. Nutritional supplements like biotin also helped disability in MS, as researchers found that 300 mg/day helped activate acetyl-CoA in the Krebs cycle used to make energy while increasing myelin production.

Fish oil has long been shown to help decrease inflammation, primarily through decreasing the production of inflammatory prostaglandins. In a study of patients with rheumatoid arthritis, the ones consuming fish oil were able to exercise over two hours longer before fatigue onset compared to a placebo group. Similarly, antioxidants such as Vitamins C and E, combined with exercise, have been shown to be superior to exercise alone in patients with fibromyalgia. In this study, lipid peroxide levels (a marker for oxidative stress) were lower, and reduced glutathione levels were higher in the vitamin-supplemented group who exercised. As we have previously discussed, glutathione can help detoxify chemicals and modulate prostaglandins and cytokines, which subsequently may have an effect on decreasing fatigue and pain. This explains why glutathione is often helpful in patients in a medically supervised exercise program in which pain and fatigue limit their ability to fully participate in physical therapy.

THE BENEFITS OF MASSAGE

Medical massage and whole-body vibration (using electric vibrators over the major muscle groups) should also be considered if your pain interferes with your ability to participate in graded exercise therapy. In a 2008 study published in the *Journal of Alternative and Complementary Medicine*, researchers recorded the effectiveness of a six-week traditional exercise program, with or without supplementary whole-body vibration therapy. They found that pain and fatigue scores were significantly reduced from the baseline of the exercise and vibration group, but not of the control group or in the group with exercise alone.

Medical massage therapy is another option to improve outcomes during physical therapy and rehabilitation, especially when pain and stiffness interferes with participation in a physical therapy program. Massage has been shown to decrease inflammation and promote mitochondrial biogenesis, two of the most important factors necessary for reducing fatigue and pain for patients with Lyme-MSIDS.

Although we may address all of the other fifteen points on the MSIDS map and improve our health, without putting a proper exercise and progressive reconditioning program in place, those who have been chronically ill will have a much more difficult time maintaining their gains.

TWENTY-ONE

Meditation and the MSIDS Model

Over the years I have found that the pain and suffering associated with Lyme-MSIDS not only manifests as physical symptoms but also has a strong emotional component. The vast majority of my patients share their emotional life with me, and their experiences range from mild sadness to severe depression, with elements of anxiety, shame, anger, guilt, fear, and grief. Sometimes these emotions are directly related to their physical symptoms and coping with an ongoing illness. However, some experience post-traumatic stress disorder that comes from issues completely unrelated to their Lyme disease. This can often include emotional, physical, and sexual abuse. These patients are the most challenging to treat. There is evidence that early trauma can damage the immune system, and it makes these individuals, once infected, more vulnerable to the worst ravages of the disease. However, I know that once they have gathered the courage to go into their own pain and suffering and transform it, they will have an easier time healing. I have seen this happen over and over again.

When patients tell me about their migraines, irritable bowel syndrome, and asthma, I know it is possible that some underlying emotional wound might be contributing to the illness. This phenomenon has been described in detail in the scientific literature. I'm not saying that migraines can't be triggered by food allergies, lack of sleep, stress, hypoglycemia, nutritional deficiencies, and Lyme disease with co-infections. Yet my clinical experience has convinced me that we are carrying around our emotions within our bodies, and that they have a profound effect on our health. Books such as Bruce H. Lipton's *The Biology of Belief* and Candace Pert's *Molecules of Emotion* discuss studies on psychoneuroimmunology, the complex interaction between psychosocial factors such as stress and trauma and the nervous, cardiovascular, endocrine, and immune systems.

We know that the immune system can be influenced by the outside world. For example, high levels of the stress hormone cortisol can trigger cell death of white blood cells and other changes in inflammatory processes during traumatic experiences. In this way the mind and body work as one. Psychiatric medications can be helpful with symptom relief, but they do not address deeper emotional wounds and the way they affect our immune system. Some doctors trained in integrative medicine have devoted their lives to understanding mind-body interactions at an even deeper level to help their patients with emotional trauma, and have combined Western and Eastern traditions to help find new solutions. Working within the framework of the Chinese, Tibetan, and Ayurvedic systems of medicine, these doctors work to balance and strengthen the subtle energy channels in the body (known as the energy meridians in Chinese medicine), which, when out of balance, lead to diseases of the body and mind.

While there is no one right way to resolve an illness, a multidisciplinary approach to clear emotional issues and past trauma is often helpful. Talk therapy and cognitive-behavioral therapy can be beneficial, and techniques such as EMDR (eye movement desensitization and reprocessing), neurofeedback (EEG biofeedback), and hands-on bodywork (i.e., Rosen Method Bodywork) can also help in those cases of deep trauma associated with grief. Working with the mind and learning to find peace in the midst of pain and suffering is essential when dealing with significant illness.

This is also where the practice of meditation can be of immense benefit. Meditation and stress reduction techniques are another way to improve our physical and mental health, and optimally would be used in conjunction with a focused diet and exercise plan.

MEDITATIONS TO CALM THE MIND
AND HEAL THE BODY

I have been blessed by having the opportunity to study for more than thirty years with meditation masters of the Kagyu school of Tibetan Buddhism. They have passed down an unbroken lineage of teachings from twenty-five hundred years ago that is still accessible and fresh today. These teachings allow us to develop greater loving kindness and compassion that can help deepen a person's faith and devotion, irrespective of their own spiritual path. That is because these teachings transcend religious beliefs, as they deal with the direct experience of the mind itself, and allow one to experience a deep peace and joy. As we learn to calm our mind and listen to the body, the body will speak its truth, allowing our innate potential to surface. Ultimately, this will have a healing effect.

Meditation has been proven to have scientific health benefits that can assist us in our healing and in maintaining our well-being. Meditation may be one way to mute the impact of stressful events on our lives and give us a chance to experience deep relaxation. It is like taking a minivacation in the midst of a busy life.

The health benefits of meditation were first studied by Dr. Herbert Benson at Harvard, when he studied the relaxation response. He found numerous beneficial effects of meditation on our physiology, including decreased sympathetic nervous system activity with a decrease in our heart rate, respiratory rate, and cortisol levels as well as decreased oxygen consumption and decreased blood lactate levels, implying better metabolic activity, with an increase in alpha and theta waves on the EEG (deeper, calmer states of consciousness), with hemispheric symmetry (symmetric brain-wave patterns in both the right and left brain). As we have seen, patients with Lyme-MSIDS often have problems with their autonomic and endocrine systems, with abnormal levels of norepinephrine and cortisol secretion. These patients are often anxious about their illnesses, and have associated significant neurocognitive difficulties. A review of the medical literature published in *JAMA* in 2014 showed that mindfulness-based meditation techniques improved anxiety, depression, and pain. By meditating we can help balance these abnormalities and teach the mind to be clear and rest in a relaxed state.

Another 2008 study, published in the *Journal of Personality and Social*

Psychology, found that the practice of loving-kindness meditation produced increases in daily experiences of positive emotions, which over time produced increases in a wide range of personal resources (e.g., increased mindfulness, purpose in life, and social support). In turn, these increments predicted increased life satisfaction and reduced depressive and physical symptoms. Similar studies verified earlier work, in which mindfulness-based stress meditation has been found to have numerous health benefits, including a decrease in IBS symptoms with lower anxiety levels; increased grey matter density levels of the brain in areas of learning and memory with increased BDNF and neuroplasticity; increased telomere length and telomerase activity, associated with longevity, as well as lower inflammatory cytokine levels, an important effect for those suffering from the "sickness syndrome" in MSIDS. Lastly, meditation helps patients better cope with their illness.

A simple meditation practice has three parts. The first part is the motivation behind meditation, the second is the meditation practice itself, and the third involves a dedication of merit after completing the practice. By following this three-step process, you will learn to access the deeper states of meditation by calming the mind and then examining the nature of what arises in that state.

The motivation behind the meditation teaches us that while we want to find peace and happiness and relieve our own suffering, others are also suffering. If we develop a broader motivation of loving-kindness and compassion for others, then, according to my teachers, the meditation practice will bear the greatest fruit. Love is wanting others to be happy, and compassion is wanting others to be free from suffering. Loving-kindness and compassion are the highest level of motivation, and they prepare the ground for a successful practice.

The meditation practice is also divided into three parts. The first part is calm abiding meditation, the second part is insight meditation, and the third part is Mahamudra meditation, which integrates calm abiding and insight meditation.

Before You Begin

You can start to practice meditation in short, five-minute sessions and eventually expand this to a half hour per day. All you need is a space where you can be quiet and alone.

Your physical posture is important when meditating. This allows the proper flow of energy to take place during the practice so that we do not fall asleep or become too agitated. Be free and easy and deeply relaxed with the posture! Do not force it, and do not hold the body too tightly or too loosely. Simply be mindful of your body and gently try and keep the following seven essential points in mind while performing the different meditation exercises:

1. Sit cross-legged on a cushion (sattva posture), or if you are an experienced meditator or have experience doing yoga, you can sit in a full lotus posture (vajra posture). Never force the position. If either of those are too difficult, simply sit in a chair.
2. Position your arms and hands so that the hands are folded on the lap with the right hand resting in the left hand ("gesture of equanimity"), or the hands are placed on the knees, the fingers extended toward the ground ("the gesture of ease").
3. Sit with your back straight and upright in either a chair or cushion. This allows the energies in the subtle channels to flow more freely and straight, allowing the mind and attention to remain at ease.
4. Extend the shoulders and elbows until they are straight.
5. Slightly tilt the neck, and tuck the chin in slightly toward the chest.
6. Connect the tip of the tongue to the palate. This helps stop the flow of excessive saliva.
7. Keep your eyes open, gazing toward the tip of the nose (forty-five degrees downward).

THE FIRST MEDITATION:
CALM ABIDING MEDITATION

In a seated posture, you will perform the following meditation for five minutes, three times a day. Over time, you can combine these sessions into one longer session, working your way to a total length of one thirty-minute session once a day. If you are new to a meditation practice, work with this exercise until you are not distracted by your own thoughts and feelings. When this occurs, you will know that you are ready to move to the next stage of insight meditation.

Choose a physical object as a mental support, such as a small pebble, flower, picture, or statue, or you can focus on your breath. The technique is simply to gently place your awareness on the object. Don't examine the object and mentally discuss its qualities, just use the object as a way of anchoring your attention. Don't follow thoughts of the past (the past is gone), don't follow thoughts of the future (where fear lies), and don't follow thoughts of the present (which are gone the moment you notice them). Just place enough attention on the object to anchor the mind and not be distracted. Constant mindfulness and awareness are necessary. If you lose your mindfulness and your attention wanders off of the object of meditation, as it is likely to do, once you notice that you have been distracted, bring your attention back to the object.

If you choose to focus on your breath, count your breath twenty-one times, where a single inhalation and exhalation are counted as one breath. If you make it to twenty-one without being distracted, start over again. If you notice that you have forgotten what number you are on, or are no longer watching the breath, start counting again from the beginning. This method allows us to track our progress, and see how far we can get before we are distracted.

Obstacles to Overcome

Two main obstacles frequently arise in meditation, both of which cause distraction: drowsiness and agitation. If you become drowsy, straighten your posture and raise your gaze. If this does not work, imagine a white lotus at the level of your heart with a small bright sphere the size of the pea that sits in the center of the lotus. This pea is white on the outside and red on the inside and represents your mind and awareness. It is the nature of light and should not to be visualized as a solid object. With a forceful exhale, imagine shooting this small sphere up through the top of your head into space. Continue to visualize this bright white sphere in space above your head until the drowsiness resolves.

The second obstacle to meditation is agitation: When you try to settle your mind, it gets caught up in thoughts. Remedies include cutting thoughts at their root: Take the attitude from the beginning that you are not going to get involved in any thoughts whatsoever during the meditation, no matter how interesting. If you become too agitated, relax your posture and lower your gaze, and if this is ineffective, imagine a four-petalled black lotus upside down at the level of the heart (also of the nature of light) with a dark pea-sized sphere of light in its center. Imagine this sphere slowly traveling down through the body into the earth. Continue to visualize this heavy and dark sphere non-distractedly until the agitation resolves.

INSIGHT MEDITATION

Even when we are feeling well, human nature has us experience the world in terms of opposites: good/bad, happy/sad, man/woman, life/death. Insight meditation allows us to realize that the ultimate nature of consciousness is a more unified state of perception instead of a dualistic one. This helps us break the connection between pain and suffering.

During this meditation you will be looking directly at the mind to see the nature of thoughts and emotions, and the nature of mind itself. You will not focus on the content of thoughts, whether they are good or bad, virtuous or not. Instead, you will simply ask yourself the following questions and look at the mind to directly see the answers, rather than taking an intellectual or conceptual approach to them. This process is creating a direct experience of the answer, not an intellectual approach to answering it. Don't worry if this seems complicated: You have to sit down and do it to see what your direct experience is.

These instructions are particularly helpful for people who suffer with strong emotions, especially great anxiety and fear regarding their illness. Instead of running from the fear, we learn to relax our minds and turn toward it, looking at its essential nature. This was eloquently stated by the meditation master, Mingyur Rinpoche: "At any given moment you can choose to follow the chain of thoughts, emotions, and sensations that reinforce the perception of yourself as vulnerable and limited. Or you can remember that your true nature is pure, unconditioned, and incapable of being harmed." We can then use meditation as a way to help us transform our fear about our illness. Once we are able to relax and see the deeper truth of our experience, it cannot harm us in the same way.

Focus on one question for each session during insight meditation. You can break up each session into several parts and focus on each question individually for several minutes, until you are ready to move on to the next. Once you have practiced calm abiding meditation for several minutes, and your mind is calm and not distracted, ask yourself the following questions during the practice of insight meditation:

- Where does the mind come from, where does it reside, and where does it go?
- Where do thoughts come from, reside, and go?
- Where do emotions come from, reside, and go?
- Look at the mind when it is still, and look at the mind when it is in motion. Is there a difference?
- Look at the essence of the one who is meditating. Who is meditating?
- Does the "I" that is experiencing suffering have a color or form? Does the mind experiencing suffering have a color or form?
- Where does fear come from, reside, or go? Does it have a color or form?

After you have asked these questions, and directly looked and seen whatever you have seen, rest naturally and at ease in the essence of the mind (the inseparable unity of clarity and emptiness). Do this non-distractedly, without effort, and without grasping on to concepts. Non-distraction, non-meditation (meditation without effort), and non-conception (not grasping on to concepts) are the three essential points to this third and final stage of Mahamudra meditation.

WORKING WITH THE MIND IN POST-MEDITATION

Once you get up from your meditation cushion, try and maintain the mindfulness and awareness that was developed during meditation. To enhance the mind that has been stabilized, we need to apply "watchfulness," which is being aware of what the mind is doing. Throughout the day, recognize what thoughts are present. If virtuous thoughts arise, recognize them as positive. If nonvirtuous thoughts arise, recognize them as being negative. By doing this we are sure to progress on the path, and we will not find ourselves easily distracted by the sounds and activities that can disturb our minds.

At the end of your practice, take a few moments to dedicate the merit of the practice for the sake of all sentient beings limitlessly through time and space. Finish the meditation by reciting a four-line prayer that encapsulates the essential meaning of this meditation, known as the Four Immeasurables. Repeat this calmly at the end of each session:

May all beings have happiness and the causes of happiness.
May all beings be free from suffering and the causes of suffering.
May all beings know the great bliss which is free from all suffering.
May all beings know the great equanimity which is free from
　　attachment and aversion.

FINAL THOUGHTS

Restoring health takes work, and perseverance, but you have already taken the first important step. You can now continue on your journey with the confidence of knowing exactly how you can, and will, feel better. As you work through the differential diagnostic map, implementing the seven-point Action Plan strategies discussed in this book, you'll notice your overall health will improve as well as your specific symptoms. You may notice that your energy improves, your joint and muscle pain is better, that your brain fog has lifted, and that you no longer have difficulty concentrating. Your sleep may improve, and at the same time, you might find that your mood is better. People may start telling you that you look well.

Share this book with your doctor. Review together the extensive scientific references on the new cutting-edge diagnostic and treatment regimens that are now available, so that you can work in a healing partnership. If your physician is not open to this information, you may find that doctors trained in integrative medicine are more familiar with some of these concepts, and can be part of your medical team. The biggest difference between the MSIDS model and the standard medical approach to chronic illness is a new emphasis on several distinct aspects of diagnosis and treatment: the MSIDS model postulates that the rising incidence of chronic illnesses are due to multiple overlapping causes that increase inflammation. These factors, in combination, contribute to mitochondrial dysfunction and cellular damage. When we treat all of the sources of inflammation and repair the damage to the body, we give ourselves the best chance to fully recover. I wish you peace, joy, love, and healing as you proceed on this journey to better health.

Appendix A

Medications, Dosages, and Common Side Effects

There may be additional side effects of the medications/antibiotics/herbal protocols described below. Please consult your healthcare provider and the *Physician's Desk Reference* for a full listing of potential side effects.

A complete blood count (CBC) and biochemistry profile that follows electrolytes, kidney and liver functions are advisable every four weeks (occasionally every six to eight weeks if prior blood testing is stable) for most antibiotics (more often for IV medications and Dapsone/PZA).

General Antibiotic Guidelines

Take antibiotics with a full glass of water immediately after a meal to minimize GI upset, unless otherwise specified. Do not take multimineral supplements or antacids with antibiotics or thyroid medications (wait at least one to two hours before or after), as they may interfere with their absorption.

If you are taking multiple antibiotics and you have GI discomfort, make sure that you take antibiotics on a full stomach. H2 blockers like Zantac (over the counter) 75–150 mg twice a day, with supplements that protect the stomach (i.e., glutamine, aloe vera, DGL) with ginger capsules may also be helpful for nausea. If you are using NSAIDs (Motrin, Naprosyn, Voltaren), then misoprostol (Cytotec) 200 mcg twice a day may be necessary for GI protection (if you are not pregnant).

All antibiotics may decrease the efficacy of birth control pills. Consider using additional protection (i.e., condoms) while taking antibiotics.

Probiotics and Prebiotics

Antibiotics upset the balance of microflora in your intestinal tract, which are essential for proper digestion and detoxification. Replacing the good bacteria is essential and not optional. Take probiotics at least one hour before or after taking antibiotics, but if this routine becomes too complicated and you are missing doses, a simple and effective regimen is to take the probiotics first thing in the morning and again when you go to bed at night. If you take antibiotics with breakfast and dinner, an alternative schedule is to take probiotics before lunch and bedtime.

We recommend taking at least three different probiotics simultaneously twice a day if your bowels are normal. A third dose or additional probiotics and/or a prebiotic (like Trufiber, Master Supplements) may be necessary if the bowels become loose. Extremely loose stools or diarrhea require temporarily stopping antibiotics, increasing probiotics, and/or checking for *Clostridium difficile* toxin A and B (and PCRs) in the stool by a local laboratory. It is important to contact your healthcare provider if significant loose stools or diarrhea occur despite being on high-dose probiotics.

The regimen I usually prescribe includes:

- Theralac 1, 2x/day (Master supplements)
- *Saccharomyces boulardii* 1, 2x/day
- Ultraflora DF 1, 2x/day (Metagenics) or Probiomax 1, 2x/day (Xymogen) and/or Orthobiotic 1, 2x/day (Orthomolecular products) and/or VSL#3 (regular or DS) if necessary for a total dosage of over 200 billion CFUs/day.

Biofilm Busters/Candida

The following biofilm busters are recommended with antibiotic and herbal protocols. Slowly increase the dose of biofilm busters if you have a history of Herxheimer reactions, and lower the dose of monolaurin if stools become too loose. Follow a strict yeast-free, sugar-free diet. Some biofilm busters like monolaurin and herbal protocols like Biocidin (Bio-Botanical Research) also help to decrease yeast overgrowth and treat imbalances in gut flora.

- Serrapeptase (Nutramedix, 1–2 capsules twice a day on an empty stomach)
- Stevia (Nutramedix, slowly working up to a minimum of 15 drops twice a day)
- monolaurin (Lauricidin) one scoop, 1–2 times per day
- nystatin 500,000 units, two tablets twice a day with antibiotics and healthy probiotics to decrease yeast overgrowth in the intestine
- Biocidin and supplements like berberine, garlic, oregano oil, and Pau D'Arco bark extract may also be helpful to decrease Candida overgrowth

Herxheimer Reactions

If you are Herxing, take Alka-Seltzer Gold (2) or a comparable product with sodium bicarbonate with up to 2,000 mg of liposomal glutathione (i.e., 6–8 Essential Pro, Wellness Pharmacy). This can be repeated up to three times a day if necessary. Consider alkalizing with Lemon-Lime Therapy: 1–2 fresh lemons or limes squeezed in water, taken over ½ hour. Sip through a straw and brush your teeth afterward to protect the enamel of your teeth.

If Herxheimer reactions (JH reactions) improve with the above protocol, consider an alkaline diet and Lemon-Lime Therapy as needed with intermittent use of liposomal glutathione. Other regimens that may help with Herxheimer reactions are included in the list below. Some of these agents are also used if there is associated mold toxicity or chemical sensitivity with environmental illness (EI):

- Burbur and/or parsley (Nutramedix) 10 drops in water every 10 minutes (up to 6 times per hour), for one hour for JH flares; three times a day for detoxification support
- drainage remedies (i.e., Pekana drainage, 15 drops of Itires, Renelix, and Apo-HEPAT, three times per day)
- binding agents (i.e., clay, charcoal, cholestyramine, Welchol). Binding agents need to be taken at least 2 hours before or after medication and supplements, and may cause constipation requiring increased doses of magnesium. Binding agents can also affect drug levels of your medications and can require extra multivitamin/minerals supplementation, as they can deplete the body of minerals and/or fat-soluble vitamins. Specific binding agents include:

- Byron White Detox 2 (⅛ to ¼ tsp/day)
- GI Detox (one capsule/day, with or without the Biocidin protocol)
- Intestinal Drawing Formula (one tsp/day)
- Questran (cholestyramine) one packet or scoop/day, working up the dose as tolerated (many individuals have difficulty increasing past twice a day due to medication schedules and GI upset)
- WelChol (colesevelam) 625 mg, 3 PO QD or BID

Other regimens that can be helpful with Herxheimer reactions include medications and/or supplements that decrease inflammation. These include:

- broccoli seed extract (Glucoraphanin), i.e., Oncoplex ES (Xymogen), one capsule QD or BID
- curcurmin (between 2 and 6 grams/day), i.e., CurcuPlex-95 (Xymogen), one capsule PO BID
- green tea extract
- resveratrol
- omega-3 fatty acids and their derivatives (i.e., Omega Genics SPM Active, Metagenics two PO QD; Xymogen Omega Pure/MonoPure/Krill oil with astaxanthin two PO QD)
- low-dose naltrexone (LDN), which can be obtained through a compounding pharmacy, is also effective in helping to decrease inflammation in the majority of patients. Doses start at 2 mg at bedtime, increasing to 3 mg after one month, working up to 4.5 mg HS. Patients on long-acting narcotics should not take LDN, as it interferes with their action and may cause withdrawal symptoms. If any insomnia should result from using LDN, then take it first thing upon awakening in the morning

If Herxheimer reactions persist despite the above protocols, speak to your healthcare provider about changing your antibiotic and/or herbal regimen.

Routes of Antibiotic Administration

Oral: PO QD (1x/day), BID (2x/day), TID (3x/day), QID (4x/day), QOD (every other day)
Q 6, Q 8, Q 12, Q 24 hours: refers to dosing every 6, 8, 12, or 24 hours respectively

IM: intramuscular
IV: intravenous
PR: rectal
PRN: as needed

Commonly Used Antibiotic Dosing for Lyme Disease
AMOXICILLIN

Dosages range according to body weight and if there are central nervous system symptoms (stiff neck, headache, light and sound sensitivity, dizziness, memory/concentration problems, Bell's Palsy, increased or new neuropsychiatric symptoms). Take the oral medications below with meals:

- Amoxicillin: 500 mg or 875 mg, PO BID. Total dosage may go up to 6,000 mg per/day for CNS Lyme, i.e., 875 mg, three PO BID. Check peak levels of Amoxicillin one hour after administration, which should be between 12–15 mcg/mL for adequate CNS penetration
- Augmentin: 875 mg/125 mg, PO BID or 1,000/62.5 mg XR, 1–2 PO BID

- Probenecid: 500 mg, 1 PO BID-TID. This raises the levels of penicillins and cephalo-sporins, allowing lower doses of these antibiotics to be used, and/or helping to raise penicillin levels for CNS Lyme. It can also be used with long-acting Bicillin injections (as can long-acting penicillins like Moxatag or Augmentin, therefore requiring less IM injections), but should be avoided with a history of sulfa sensitivity, kidney stones, acute gout, or renal impairment
- Amoxicillin ER: 267 mg, 3 PO QD (compounded)
- Moxatag: 775 mg, 1 QD (availability is limited)

CEPHALOSPORINS

Penicillins and cephalosporins are considered safe in pregnancy. Speak to your healthcare provider about their use if you are pregnant or plan on becoming pregnant.

- Ceftin (cefuroxime axetil): 500–1,000 mg PO BID
- Omnicef (cefdinir): 300–600 mg, PO BID (higher doses are used for resistant CNS symptoms)
- Omnicef: 125–250 mg/5ml, one tsp PO BID (pediatric)
- Probenecid: 500 mg, 1 PO BID (helps raise levels of cephalosporins, same contraindi-cations as listed above for penicillins). Generally reserved for adult use.
- Cedax (ceftibuten): 400 mg, 1 PO QD or BID (q 12 hours)
- Suprax (Cefixime): 400 mg, 1 PO QD or BID (q 12 hours)

FLAGYL AND TINDAMAX

Take these with meals. Intravenous formulations are available if GI intolerant. Interaction between alcohol and these medications may cause severe nausea and vomiting, so decrease herbal alcohol-based tinctures if nausea occurs as well as refrain from all alcohol, including cough syrup with alcohol, mouthwash, and perfumes/colognes containing alcohol. Flagyl and Tin-damax can cause neuropathy or increase prior Lyme neuropathy (it can also help), so take a multi-vitamin with a B-complex, or Methylprotect (Xymogen, 1x/day) and/or Vitamin B_6 100 mg per day, 1 hour before or after taking Flagyl or Tindamax. If there is any increase in tingling and numbness, stop the medication and speak to your provider.

If you weigh:

- <120 lbs.=250 mg, PO TID
- 121–150 lbs.=500 mg, PO BID
- >150 lbs.=500 mg, PO TID (can also be taken, 2 PO in the A.M., one in the P.M.)
- Flagyl ER 750 mg, 1 PO QD-BID (an extended release Flagyl is available for GI intolerance)

PLAQUENIL

Before starting Plaquenil, inform your healthcare provider if you have a history of eye prob-lems (i.e., visual field or retinal problems). Stop if you develop visual field or color vision prob-lems while on the medication, and contact your healthcare provider. Get an eye exam every six months to yearly. Most ophthalmologists only require yearly exams on Plaquenil, as retinal prob-lems are rare with proper use. Plaquenil should be used with caution in pediatric patients, or if there is psoriasis or porphyria. If taking Depen as part of chelation therapy, do not take Plaque-nil during the two days per week taking Depen.

- 200 mg, 1 PO BID. Can be taken at the same time as antibiotics and nystatin.

RIFAMPIN

Rifampin is usually prescribed on an empty stomach. It is classically used for infections like tuberculosis and leprosy, but is very useful for other intracellular infections such as Lyme, Ehrlichia, Bartonella, Q fever, and Brucella, especially when there is associated neuropathy. Inform your healthcare provider if you are taking other medications, as it can affect other drug levels (i.e., like thyroid and sex hormones, psychiatric medications, seizure medications, etc.) and may require extra monitoring of drug levels. An expected side effect of rifampin is that your urine and tears may turn orange, and it may stain contact lenses. Do not take multimineral supplements or antacids 1–2 hours before or after antibiotics.

- 300 mg, 1 PO BID or 300 mg, 2 PO QD. IV dosing is available for GI intolerance (10 mg/kg IV QD)
- 300 mg, 2 PO BID: higher dose rifampin can be pulsed one to several times per week (QOD) in severe, resistant intracellular infections, or when needing to decrease regular rifampin use secondary to adverse drug-to-drug interactions. Follow LFTs regularly. High-dose pulsed rifampin in combination with Dapsone and other intracellular antibiotics like doxycycline has been effective in some resistant patients (they had JH flares and then improved). Long-term clinical outcome data on pulsed therapy is unavailable. Recent culture studies showed that rifampin is effective alone and in combination with other intracellular antibiotics in reducing biofilms.
- 150 mg, PO BID (for lower body weights, younger age, decreased renal function, intolerance)

TETRACYCLINES

Do not lie down immediately after taking tetracyclines (it can cause esophagitis). Do not eat dairy products or take minerals and antacids within 1 hour before or after taking tetracyclines, as it can interfere with absorption. Strict sun avoidance is necessary, as tetracyclines can cause photosensitive reactions and sunburn. Wear a >35 SPF (60 SPF or higher is recommended) on all exposed areas (face, lips, hands, etc.). Wear sunblock even when driving in the car, placing it on hands, face, and any exposed areas. Tetracyclines may cause loose stools. See your doctor if loose stools persist more than once a week or if any watery stools occur (this may require stopping all of your antibiotics and increasing beneficial probiotics). Tetracyclines can stain teeth in children less than 8 years old, before adult teeth have come in, but may be used for short courses (7–10 days) in life-threatening infections such as Rocky Mountain spotted fever/Ehrlichia/Anaplasma according to recent CDC guidelines. Speak to your pediatrician about risks/benefits. A rare side effect of tetracyclines is pseudotumor cerebri (increased intracranial pressure), causing headaches with nausea/vomiting and/or papilledema with swelling of the optic nerve. Any of these symptoms should be evaluated by your healthcare practitioner/ophthalmologist. This medication group is contraindicated in pregnancy.

- Doxycycline (generic): 100 mg, PO BID (children, lower body weight), up to 2 PO BID with meals (total of 400 mg/day). If there is no GI intolerance, 2 PO BID is a preferable starting dose. If there is significant stomach upset using 1, 2x/day, try brand Monodox, and/or do not increase to the higher dosage until well tolerated. Long-acting forms of doxycycline (i.e., Doryx, LA doxycycline) may be more efficacious with less GI side effects.
- Tetracycline HCL: 500 mg, PO BID-TID-QID. This is usually taken on an empty stomach.

- Minocin (minocycline): 50 mg or 100 mg, PO BID. Lower doses may be used in combination therapy with other tetracyclines like doxycycline if there are side effects or flares. Lower the dose if there is any dizziness (100 mg PO BID is usually well tolerated). Same contraindications as doxycycline exist, as well as the possibility of rare cases of hyperpigmentation, where the medication should be discontinued.
- Doryx: 150 mg, 1 PO QD-BID. Can be used in combination with other tetracyclines (doxycycline, minocycline) to get to 400 mg/day for increased CNS penetration.
- Long-Acting doxycycline (GenRx): 150 mg, PO QD-BID. This may be added to other forms of doxycycline to increase levels and for improved GI tolerance.
- Long-Acting Minocin (Gen Rx): 90 mg, 1–2x/day. This may be added to other forms of minocycline and/or doxycycline to increase drug levels.

MACROLIDES

Your doctor may require that you have an EKG while on this treatment to monitor your QT interval. Give your provider a complete list of medications you are taking to check for potential interactions. If you experience new or increased ringing in the ears or hearing problems, call your doctor. Zithromax may be used in pregnancy (Biaxin has potential risks), and has less potential drug interactions.

- Zithromax: 100, 200 mg/5mL, 1–2 tsp. PO QD with meals (i.e., pediatric dosing). The starting dose is 10 mg/kg on day 1, followed by 5 mg/kg, PO QD.
- Zithromax: 250 mg, 1 PO BID with meals (adults), or 500–600 mg, 1 PO QD.
- Biaxin: 500 mg, 1 PO BID with meals. If you are taking a statin (Mevacor, Zocor, Pravachol, Lipitor, or Lescol), a possible interaction exists; inform your healthcare provider. If any significant and persistent new muscle pain occurs on a statin, inform your healthcare provider, and your provider may need to check a blood test (i.e., CPK). Biaxin may cause an abnormal taste in your mouth. This is normal, and can be minimized by taking Biaxin with a small amount of cranberry juice diluted in water.
- Biaxin XL: 500 mg, 2 PO QD or 1 PO BID. The long-acting form of Biaxin has less side effects and may be more efficacious in some individuals.
- Roxithromycin: 150 mg, 1 PO BID, or 2 PO QD (300 mg/day). This medication must be compounded in the United States but is regularly available in Europe.

SEPTRA DS/BACTRIM DS

Inform your healthcare provider if you have had any prior reactions (i.e., rash) to sulfa drugs. If you are unsure about a sensitivity to sulfa drugs, speak to your healthcare provider about premedicating with an H1 (Benadryl, Zyrtec) and H2 blocker (Zantac) before use. This is a sunsensitive drug. Please wear >35 SPF. A 50–60 SPF or higher is recommended.

- 1 PO BID with meals
- Do not mix with other sulfa drugs like Dapsone

QUINOLONES

You may be asked to have an EKG while on this treatment to monitor your QT interval. Do not take if less than eighteen years old, unless advised by your provider. There are occasional reports of tendon problems (tendonitis/rupture) with this class of antibiotics. Tell your healthcare provider if you presently suffer from tendonitis, or have had a history of tendonitis in the past. If you experience unusual tendon pain, worsening of symptoms, or new musculoskeletal symptoms, stop the medication, rest and refrain from exercise, and contact your doctor. Do not overexert with exercises that may strain tendons while taking these medications. Do not take concurrently with milk or yogurt alone, since absorption of antibiotics may be significantly reduced. Dietary calcium as part of a meal, however, does not significantly affect absorption. We recommend magnesium supplements (1 hour before or after antibiotics) and alpha-lipoic acid 2x/day while on quinolones to help decrease muscle spasm and oxidative stress/inflammation, which may adversely affect the tendons. May cause loose stools. Call your doctor if loose stools persist more than once a week, or if any watery stools occur, which require stopping antibiotics.

Caffeinated beverages should not be consumed while on Avelox or Cipro as they may cause a jittery, nervous feeling. These are sun-sensitive drugs. Wear >35 SPF. A 50–60 SPF or higher is recommended. Do not mix quinolones with macrolides (Zithromax/Biaxin), Diflucan, Larium, certain PPIs, or other medications that may increase QT intervals. If these medications must be used together, consider obtaining an EKG, especially if elderly, and/or cardiovascular risk factors exist.

- Cipro: 500 mg, 1 PO BID with meals
- Cipro XR: 500 mg up to 1,000 mg, 1 PO QD
- Levaquin: 500 mg, 1 PO QD (Lyme, co-infections); 750 mg dosing is usually used for pneumonia, pyelonephritis, and/or severe skin reactions. IV dosing is available for quinolones if there is GI intolerance
- Avelox: 400 mg, 1 PO QD
- Factive: 320 mg, 1 PO QD (availability may be limited)

Intramuscular and IV Medications
BICILLIN

Bicillin is an effective option for treating Lyme disease for those who cannot tolerate oral medications, have failed oral medications, or wish to provide 24-hour coverage with a penicillin during pregnancy. It can be supplemented with oral penicillins and/or probenecid (if not pregnant, sulfa sensitive, with a history of kidney stones, acute gout, or renal impairment) to increase levels for higher CNS penetration. Warm the medication by taking it out of the refrigerator one hour prior to use. Have a CBC and CMP done monthly, as with most antibiotic protocols, unless otherwise specified by your provider.

- Bicillin LA Injections: 1.2 million units, one injection 2x/week (i.e. Mondays and Thursdays), or 3–4x/week. An injection can also be placed in each buttock one to two days/week, for a total of 2.4 to 4.8 million U/week to decrease trips to your provider. Higher doses of Bicillin are often more effective than lower doses, but a long-acting oral penicillin and/or a penicillin with probenecid may also be added to increase blood levels and avoid an increase in the number of injections.
- 2.4 million units per injection 1x/week or 2x/week (these are larger shots with bigger needles, and therefore not usually used as often).
- To minimize the discomfort of the injection, use Xylocaine Topical Ointment 5 percent or EMLA cream on the anticipated injection site 1 hour before. You can also bring a cold pack and numb the area before your injection. The use of a hot bath or hot tub after the injection will also help decrease discomfort. Tylenol or ibuprofen is OK half an hour before the injection or as needed afterward (if there are no contraindications). After the injection, massage the injection site for 3–5 minutes to ensure antibiotic dispersion.

IV ROCEPHIN

Rocephin is used for those with resistant Lyme symptoms and/or severe neurological problems (i.e., Bell's palsy, optic neuritis, meningitis, resistant neurocognitive deficits). Rocephin may cause gallbladder problems; inform your provider if you have ever had gallbladder issues. An ultrasound of the gallbladder may be necessary before and/or during treatment. Inform your healthcare provider if you experience right upper abdominal pain with nausea, vomiting, or jaundice. Perform a CBC and CMP at least every 2 weeks while on IV therapy.

- 2g IV QD, 4–7 days per week. Some healthcare providers have seen benefits using higher doses, i.e., 2 grams IV Q 12, 4 days in a row/week, or 2 grams pulsed three days per week (Monday, Wednesday, Saturday) when combined with a cystic drug (like Tindamax) and intracellular drugs (like Minocin, or Zithromax alone, or used in combination therapy with other intracellular drugs like Dapsone). Pulsed therapy may keep down potential side effects.
- To protect the gallbladder, start Actigall 300 mg, 1 PO BID, and consider pulsed therapy. Long-term clinical outcome data on pulsed therapy is unavailable.

IV VANCOMYCIN

Vancomycin can be effective in some patients who are allergic or failed other IV medications. This drug can however cause "red man syndrome"—a rash that is not a true allergic reaction, but due to mast cell degranulation causing a red rash/flushing in the face, neck, and torso—and hypotension if given too rapidly. It should be administered as a diluted solution in a slow IV drip over one hour or longer. Premedication with antihistamines (H1 and H2 blockers) will decrease the possibility of a reaction. A trough level should be done after the fourth dose, and the dose is then adjusted based on serum levels. A trough level greater than 10 mcg/ml is necessary, and higher levels (15–20 mcg/ml) are used for life-threatening infections. Toxic levels greater than 20 mcg/ml require decreasing the dose. Renal impairment also requires lower starting doses. Tell your provider if you experience any changes in hearing or have significant ringing in the ears before starting vancomycin. Follow a CBC and CMP with renal and liver functions during treatment (every week initially).

- Dosing is based on body weight. For patients over sixteen years old, an average starting dose is 1,000 mg IV Q 12 hours.
- Take 25–50 mg of Benadryl orally 1 hour before administration to prevent a rash. Zyrtec (10 mg), Claritin (10 mg), or Allegra (180 mg) with Zantac 75–150 mg 2x/day before administration, with or without Benadryl, may decrease the incidence of a rash.

IV TEFLARO

This is a fifth-generation cephalosporin without the potential gallbladder complications seen with Rocephin. It can be used for Lyme patients with a history of gallbladder disease if an IV cephalosporin is required (long-term outcome data is unavailable). The same precautions otherwise apply as with IV Rocephin.

- 600 mg IV Q 12 hours, infused over 1 hour.

IV CLINDAMYCIN

IV clindamycin can be effective in babesiosis when oral regimens (including PO Clindamycin) are insufficient. Take high-dose probiotics while on Clindamycin, as there is a risk of C. difficile.

- 600 mg IV q 12 hours, 600 mg IV q 8 hours, 900 mg IV q 12 hours.

IV DAPTOMYCIN

Clinical studies still need to be performed to evaluate the efficacy of this combination of a persister drug (daptomycin) with an active drug (cefuroxime) and doxycycline, and it is therefore not recommended for regular use at this time. Severe Herxheimer reactions may result from use, as with other medications. Caution is needed in the elderly with renal impairment. Muscle pain (myalgias), and rhabdomyolysis are possible side effects; regular blood work with a CBC, CMP, and CPK levels is necessary.

- 4 mg/kg to 6 mg/kg IV every 24 hours.

OTHER IV MEDICATIONS:

- **IV doxycycline**: can be used for those with Lyme and intracellular infections who are intolerant of oral preparations, but it must be given through a PICC line (not a mid-line or peripheral line) as the drug can irritate the veins and cause phlebitis. A dose of 100 to 200 mg, IV Q 12 is used based on severity of symptoms and body weight. The same precautions as oral doxycycline are applicable.
- **IV Primaxin**: 500 mg, IV Q6. This is a less commonly used drug regimen for Lyme due to the inconvenience of the dosing regimen.
- **IV gentamycin**: usually reserved for severe gram-negative tick-borne infections such as tularemia and Brucella. Average dosage is 5 mg/kg/day in three divided doses and peak and trough levels are necessary to avoid side effects, which include neurotoxicity (vertigo, numbness/tingling), ototoxicity (hearing loss), and nephrotoxicity (renal impairment). Renal function must be followed carefully since side effects are increased if there is renal impairment.

Co-infection Treatment Dosages

TREATING BABESIA

Clindamycin

- 300 mg, 2 PO BID-TID with meals
- Clindamycin can be mixed with a macrolide (Zithromax, Biaxin) and Bactrim DS for greater efficacy, as well as Mepron (1–2 tsp, twice a day with a high-fat meal) or Malarone (1–2 tablets, PO BID).
- Antimalarial herbal protocols (listed below) may also be added for increased efficacy if there are ongoing malarial symptoms (sweats, chills, flushing, an unexplained cough, and "air hunger") despite use of classical medications.

Quinine:

- 325 mg, 2 PO TID: This is usually mixed with clindamycin, and reserved for resistant Babesia cases who have failed Clindamycin with Mepron and Zithromax. Side effects include ringing in the ears, nausea, vomiting, and rashes. May cause QT prolongation.

Mepron:

Mepron absorbs better with fat, therefore take with a high-fat meal that includes milk, salad dressings with oil, cheese, almond butter or other nut butters, avocados, olive oil, etc. (assuming there are no food sensitivities). Do not take any supplements with enzyme CoQ10, as it will interfere with the action of Mepron. Inform your healthcare provider if you are taking Mepron and rifampin together because rifampin will lower the levels of atovaquone in the body. Contact your doctor if you have loose stools or diarrhea.

- 750 mg / 5 cc, 1–2 tsp PO BID. There is Mepron resistance in the United States, so 2 tsp twice a day is required if Babesia symptoms are severe and persist (day and night sweats, chills, flushing, an unexplained cough, and "air hunger").

Malarone:

Malarone absorbs better with fat, therefore take with a high-fat meal that includes milk, salad dressings with oil, cheese, almond butter or other nut butters, avocados, olive oil, etc. (assuming there are no food sensitivities). Do not take any supplements with enzyme CoQ10, as it will interfere with the action of Malarone. Inform your healthcare provider if you are taking Malarone and rifampin together because rifampin will lower the levels of Malarone in the body. Contact your doctor if you have loose stools or diarrhea. Certain SSRIs and antifungal medications may decrease Malarone levels; inform your provider if you are on them.

- 100/250 mg tablets (adult), or 62.5/25 mg tablets (pediatric). Start with 4 tablets/day × 3 days (loading dose), then 1–2 tablet(s) PO QD or BID thereafter. As with Mepron, higher doses of Malarone are often required in resistant babesiosis.

Coartem:

Stop any medications that may affect your QT interval at least 3 days before and 3 days after Coartem (unless on drugs with an even longer half-life, which may require stopping even further in advance). Medications that may affect the QT interval includes Diflucan, other antifungal medication (Sporanox), macrolides, quinolones, certain SSRIs, certain psychiatric medications (trazodone), PPIs, and Elavil. Antimalarial supplements (Artemisia, NEEM, cryptolepis, A-Bab, and Bab 2) should also be stopped several days before and after using Coartem.

- 4 tablets PO BID × 3 days. Coartem can be used alone or with Daraprim 25 mg, 2 PO QD × 3 days in severely ill patients, and/or in combination with Clindamycin, or other medications like doxycycline for resistant babesiosis. One course of Coartem is usually inadequate to "cure" Babesia, and once-a-month pulses of Coartem may be necessary in a comprehensive antiparasitic protocol to lower the load of the parasites.
- Day 1: take at 7:00 A.M. and 3:00 P.M. (8 hours apart)
- Day 2 and 3: take at 7:00 A.M. and 7:00 P.M. (12 hours apart)

Alinia

Alinia is primarily used for clearing intestinal parasites like Entamoeba histolytica, Giardia, and cryptosporidium, but may also be used for bacteria like Clostridium difficile and viruses like norovirus (causing diarrhea), as well as SIBO. It also appears to clinically have some efficacy against babesiosis. Since Babesia suppresses the immune system's ability to clear other parasites, it can be considered as part of a comprehensive antiparasitic protocol. Side effects include abdominal pain and nausea. Usual dosing:

- 500 mg, PO Q12 for 3–5 days.

Other Anti-Parasitic Protocols for Associated Intestinal Parasites

ALBENZA (ALBENDAZOLE): 200 mg, average dose is 2 PO BID (total dose 800 mg/day) with food. Length of treatment depends on the parasite. See the PDR.
- Addresses neurocysticercosis, hydatid disease (tapeworms like echinococcus), hookworm, pinworm, ascariasis (roundworm), whipworm, and larva migrans (cutaneous).

- Side effects include abdominal pain, nausea, vomiting, and headaches. Consult the PDR for full listing of potential side effects.

BILTRICIDE (PRAZIQUANTEL): average dose 600 mg, two PO TID X 2 days.
- Addresses intestinal parasites, including schistosomiasis, liver flukes, tapeworms, and cysticercosis.
- Do not take with grapefruit juice, as it may interfere with absorption.
- Side effects include GI symptoms (abdominal pain, nausea, vomiting). Check the PDR for a full listing of potential side effects for all intestinal parasitic medications.

IVERMECTIN: 0.2 mg/kg PO 1x
- Addresses strongyloidiasis, onchocerciasis.
- Can be pulsed for ongoing symptoms.

PIN-X (PYRANTEL PAMOATE): chewable tablets or liquid preparations, dose according to body weight.
- Addresses pinworm infections
- <37 lbs.=½ tab PO x1, or oral suspension, 2.5 ml PO x 1
- 38–62 lbs.=1 tab PO x 1, or oral suspension, 5 ml PO x 1
- 63–87 lbs.=1.5 tabs PO x 1, or oral suspension, 7.5 ml PO x 1
- 88–112 lbs.=2 tabs PO x 1, or oral suspension, 10 ml PO x 1
- 113–137 lbs.=2.5 tabs PO x 1, or oral suspension, 12.5 ml PO x 1
- 138–162 lbs.=3 tabs PO x 1, or oral suspension, 15 ml PO x 1
- 163–187 lbs.=3.5 tabs PO x 1, or oral suspension, 17.5 ml PO x 1
- >187 lbs.=4 tabs PO x 1, or oral suspension, 20 ml PO x 1

ANTIMALARIAL HERBAL PROTOCOLS USED TO TREAT BABESIA AND OTHER CO-INFECTIONS:
- Alcohol-Free Cryptolepis: 1 tsp three times a day (order through Infuserve @ 1-800-886-9222) or
- Cryptoplus (Researched Nutritionals): Start with ½ tsp twice a day and work up to 1 tsp three times a day as tolerated. Herxheimer reactions are common, so dosing must gradually increase based on tolerance.
- NEEM: 30 drops 3–4 times per day (order through Greenwood Herbals: 207-793-3553)
- Liposomal Artemisia: 2x/day. Order through a compounding pharmacy.
- A-Bab (Byron White): Work up to 15 drops 2x/day. This also contains Samento to treat Lyme, and may cause Herxheimer reactions. Gradually increase the dose based on tolerance.
- MC Bab 1,2,3 (Beyond Balance): 15–18 drops PO BID.
- Sida Acuta: An herbal protocol recommended by Steven Buhner, which has shown some clinical efficacy against Babesia. It can be used alone or blended with *Alchornea cordifolia* and *Cryptolepis sanguinolenta*: ¼ tsp (up to ½ tsp) of each 3x/day (i.e., CSA formula). These tinctures can be purchased from woodlandessence.com.
- Artemisia: 3x/day, 15 to 30 minutes before meals. Artemisia has been recommended by the World Health Organization to be used in conjunction with antimalarial treatment to improve the effectiveness of the medications. Artemisia is also known as "wormwood" and is an herb used in many parts of the world to treat parasites such as Babesia and malaria. We do not generally use Artemisia longer than several months at a time. Inform your provider the length of time you have been on it and whether

you are still having Babesia symptoms. Artemisia should be not be used during pregnancy. Although Artemisia can be helpful, we do see Artemisia resistance, requiring
the use of combinations of the above herbal protocols to increase efficacy.

Dapsone: For Treating Lyme and Associated Co-Infections (i.e., Babesia):

Dapsone has good antimalarial activity and was effective in decreasing Babesia symptoms
in our published retrospective study when used at full dose (100 mg) with Malarone (4 per day)
and antimalarial herbs. Consider Dapsone if you have ongoing symptoms of Babesia and have
failed other antiparasitic protocols, if you are not sulfa sensitive. Coartem may temporarily decrease Dapsone levels. The higher the dose, the greater the efficacy (and side effects) in our clinical studies. The efficacy appears to be increased using rifampin and other intracellular
medications simultaneously (i.e., rifampin with tetracyclines, macrolides, and/or quinolones).
Choose the intracellular drugs to mix with Dapsone based on the individual's co-infections,
prior response, side effects, and/or Herxheimer reactions. Consult the PDR for a full listing of
potential side effects.

- Dosing ranges from 25 mg, 1 PO QOD, up to 100 mg, PO QD. For those who are sulfa
  sensitive or have a history of severe Herxheimer reactions, start at the lowest dose, of
  25 mg, PO QOD, and gradually increase (in one or two weeks) to 25 mg/day. Then
  increase to 50 mg, PO QD after several more weeks (if tolerated), which can be done
  by alternating doses of 25 mg/50 mg, QOD. Doses can then be increased in the following manner: 50 mg/75 mg, QOD x several weeks, then 75 mg, PO QD, until reaching
  the maximum dose of 100 mg, PO QD.
- For those who are not sulfa sensitive, without severe Herxheimer reactions, you can
  start at a higher dose, i.e., 50 mg, PO QD, working up gradually over several weeks or
  a month to 100 mg/day. Lower the dose if there are severe Herxheimer reactions or
  other side effects (see below). Occasionally taking a few days off Dapsone and restart-
  ing at the same dose will help to minimize side effects.
- Consider using an H1 and H2 blocker (Zyrtec and Zantac) twice a day if there is a history of a mild sulfa sensitivity.
- Dapsone causes a folic acid–induced anemia, and women who are iron deficient, or
  are prone to heavy menstrual bleeding, should take adequate iron (i.e., 325 mg iron,
  PO QD or BID) while on Dapsone and correct an iron deficiency anemia before using
  the drug. If sustained heavy menstrual bleeding occurs, or there is loss of blood from
  a procedure, gastroenteritis, etc., stop the Dapsone immediately, double up on your
  folic acid and iron supplementation, and contact your healthcare provider for further instructions. While on Dapsone, take several folic acid supplements to help decrease anemia. These include: MTHF-ES (5 mg) 1–2 PO BID (Xymogen); Leucovorin
  15 mg, 1–2 PO QD BID; Leucovorin 25 mg, PO QD-BID; Folafy ER 15 mg, 1–2 PO
  QD-BID (Xymogen), and/or Deplin 15mg once a day. A total dose of 30–45 mg of folic
  acid QD is recommended (rarely higher doses are required, i.e. 60 mg/day) for the
  majority of individuals to prevent more than a 3-gram drop in hemoglobin. The hemoglobin and hematocrit will usually return to normal within several weeks off the
  drug, if adequate folic acid supplementation is continued after using Dapsone. If you
  have a history of being sensitive to high doses of methylation support (methyl B_{12} or
  methyl folate), which cause symptoms such as irritability and/or agitation, inform
  your provider. Other forms of folic acid can be used.
- In rare cases other side effects include neuropathy (although most patients' neuropathies
  improve on Dapsone), methemoglobinemia (blue hands and lips, shortness of breath,

and/or increased underlying symptoms like fatigue and headache), and Herxheimer reactions requiring extra detox support +/– adjusting medication dosage. We suggest using NAC, 600 mg, two capsules twice a day (Xymogen), alpha-lipoic acid twice a day (i.e., ALAMAX, Xymogen) as well as liposomal glutathione (i.e., Essential Pro, Wellness Pharmacy), two capsules (500 mg) twice a day to support detoxification pathways and help minimize the possibility of methemoglobinemia (glutathione has been shown to be helpful). Follow a CBC, CMP, and methemoglobin levels regularly (q 2 weeks initially), then q 3–4 weeks if stable.

- If methemoglobin levels significantly rise on Dapsone (they should be checked intermittently, especially on doses of 50 mg or higher), i.e., levels in the range of 5%-8%, and you are mildly symptomatic with fatigue, shortness of breath, and/or blue hands/lips, stop Dapsone, increase methyl folate and glutathione and contact your healthcare provider. Levels will usually rapidly return to normal once the drug is stopped, with extra antioxidant and folate support. Levels below 5% do not usually cause significant symptoms. Significant methemoglobin levels (over 8%-10%) in symptomatic individuals (i.e., significant blue hands, blue lips, fatigue, headaches, and/or shortness of breath) may require going to the emergency room for oxygen and an injection of methylene blue if symptoms do not rapidly resolve with stopping Dapsone, increasing folic acid and glutathione. Methylene blue is given as a 1% solution (10 mg/ml) 1–2 mg/kg IV, over 5 minutes, and can be repeated in 1 hour. It is usually immediately effective in relieving symptoms and reversing the oxidized hemoglobin causing methemoglobinemia.

- G6PD deficiency may predispose to hemolytic anemia on Dapsone, so if you are of Mediterranean or African origin, inform your healthcare provider so you can be tested. We have had several individuals who were Coombs positive on Dapsone, but have not yet seen a case of hemolysis (just folic acid–induced anemia, which is to be expected on the medication). Follow labs post treatment.

Pyrazinamide (PZA)

This is an experimental protocol for treating Lyme and certain co-infections, like Bartonella. Speak with your healthcare provider about the risks and benefits. Pyrazinamide (PZA) is a powerful mycobacterium drug with potential liver toxicity, and should only be considered in combination with rifampin and other intracellular antibiotics, in severely ill patients with a poor quality of life who have failed traditional antibiotic protocols, with evidence of one or multiple resistant intracellular infections. We have seen significant positive responses to PZA, but it can also cause severe Herxheimer reactions. Tell your provider if you have ever had any significant elevation of liver functions on prior medications, or have a history of liver disease. Consult the PDR for a full listing of potential side effects.

- PZA is usually used for 2 months in initial mycobacterial drug therapy, in combination with rifampin and other intracellular medications
- Dosing: Pyrazinamide 500 mg, two to four tablets once per day, based on body weight:
- 40–55 kg: 1,000 mg PO QD
- 56–75 kg: 1,500 mg PO QD
- 76–90 kg: 2,000 mg PO QD
- Follow LFTs Q week initially during therapy (with a CBC, CMP)
- Use the following liver-support protocol while taking pyrazinamide:
  - NAC, 1–2 PO BID
  - ALAMAX, 1–2 PO BID (following liver functions)
- DIM, 1 PO QD

- Oncoplex ES (Xymogen), one PO BID
- Hepa #2 (TCM, Dr. Zhang), two PO BID
- MedCaps DPO (Xymogen), one to two PO BID
- Glutathione (Essential Pro, Wellness Pharmacy), one to two capsules, PO BID

TREATING TULAREMIA/BRUCELLA

- IV/PO doxycycline (200 mg to 400 mg per day), quinolones, such as IV/PO Cipro (dosage based on body weight), with other quinolones like Levaquin, IM/IV streptomycin (1 gram Q 12 x ten days in adults, lower dosing in children, i.e., 20 to 40 mg/kg day in divided doses), IV gentamycin (5 mg/kg per day in three divided doses). Chloramphenicol can be considered in treatment-resistant cases (50 mg/kg per day, up to 100 mg/kg per day in four divided doses). Combination therapy is often required.
- One regimen proven to be effective in an immunosuppressed patient with relapsing tularemia that we published in the medical literature was doxycycline 100 mg PO BID, rifampin 300 mg, PO BID, Avelox 400 mg, PO QD, and Dapsone 100 mg, PO QD. This regimen requires further scientific study regarding long-term efficacy.

MSIDS Treatment Dosages

TREATING IMMUNE DYSFUNCTION

Plaquenil (hydroxychloroquine) 200 mg, PO BID is a commonly used medication to modulate an overstimulated immune system, except in patients with psoriasis or porphyria, where the drug must be used with caution. Yearly eye exams are recommended.

INFLAMMATION

Immune dysfunction with associated inflammation: Consider immune modulators (Plaquenil, DMARDs), drugs with anti-inflammatory effects (macrolides, tetracyclines), IVIG for decreased immunoglobulin levels (CVID), and/or autoimmune encephalopathy/neuropathy (CIDP and small fiber neuropathy). Common brands of IVIG include Gamunex-C, Gammagard and Privigen, usually administered at 400 mg/kg, q 3–4 weeks. Dosing and administration varies based on the condition, i.e., some patients with severe flulike symptoms from cytokine release may feel better with lower q 2 week dosing vs. higher doses q 3–4 weeks. Oftentimes Tylenol and Benadryl are administered beforehand to decrease systemic reactions. Occasionally steroids are also administered before the first dose, and/or for severe reactions. This should be done with caution in patients with active Lyme disease, as steroids may cause a relapse of symptoms. Hizentra, subcutaneous immunoglobulin therapy administered weekly, is an option for those who have CVID and do not require IVIG. Speak to your neurologist or immunologist regarding immunoglobulin therapy dosing and administration.

Properly treating Lyme disease and associated co-infections and lowering down the total load of organisms in the body is essential in order to significantly decrease inflammation and control symptom flares. This can be accomplished with the antibiotics and classical therapies discussed above, as well as integrative therapies that focus on the down-regulation of the nitric oxide pathway to help decrease inflammatory cytokines, prostaglandins, and leukotrienes. This would include using protocols discussed under treating Herxheimer reactions, i.e., similar dosing for LDN, curcurmin, resveratrol, green tea extract and broccoli seed extract, glutathione precursors (NAC, alpha-lipoic acid), and liposomal glutathione. Other protocols include:

- CoQ10 (100 mg–200 mg/day starting dose) if not on Mepron or Malarone
- B vitamins (especially oral B_1, B_2, B_6, methyl B_{12}), and subcutaneous injections of

methylcobalamine (1,000 mcg/day up to 25,000 mcg/day for those with severe neuropathy). Methyl B_{12} injections need to be obtained from a compounding pharmacy

- α-lipoic acid (300 mg–600 mg 2x per day). Lower doses should be used if hypoglycemia, and/or liver function abnormalities
- Magnesium (average dose: 500 mg/day, higher doses may be used for resistant spasm or severe constipation)
- Zinc (average dose: 15–30 mg/day)
- Omega-3 fatty acids (minimum 2 grams/day)
- Glutathione precursors such as NAC (600 mg, 1–2, PO BID), glycine, and oral liposomal glutathione (Wellness pharmacy) 500–1,000 mg/day. Higher doses can be effective for Herxheimer reactions and significant neurocognitive deficits (2000 mg, PO QD, BID)

All overlapping causes of inflammation should be addressed (infections, autoimmunity, toxins, food allergies, dysbiosis, mineral deficiencies, sleep disorders, detoxification problems, etc.) to ensure maximum efficacy.

For Multiple Chemical Sensitivity, Environmental Illness, Heavy Metals, Mold, and Neurotoxins (External and Internal Biotoxins)
HEAVY METALS:

- Oral chelation regimens (DMSA, DMPS, D-penicillamine), transdermal chelation (children), IV chelation (DMPS, EDTA), as well as using rectal suppositories (Detoxamine, EDTA) are commonly used methods of chelation after testing through an approved laboratory, like Doctor's Data (Chicago). Speak to your healthcare provider regarding side effects, dosage, and routes of administration. We generally use low-dose oral DMSA every several days at bedtime (100 mg–200 mg), or pulsed DMSA 2 days in a row on the weekends (5–10 mg/kg, PO BID, one hour before meals), as some Lyme disease patients do not tolerate standard dosages of oral chelating agents due to JH flares. You can obtain DMSA through a compounding pharmacy in various dosages: 100 mg, 250 mg, and 500 mg capsules. Local pharmacies may carry Chemet (succimer, DMSA) in lower doses of 100 mg capsules, which are usually covered by insurance. DMSA and DMPS are sulfa drugs, and should be used in caution in those with sulfa sensitivities.
- Nutritional supplements used Q 3rd night with DMSA include Chlorella (split cell, 7 tablets) with 600 mg NAC, alpha-lipoic acid (600 mg), and occasionally Med Caps DPO (Xymogen) if phase I and phase II liver detoxification pathways are not functioning efficiently. EDTA suppositories (750 mg) can also be added if there are high levels of lead. It is essential to use a good multimineral supplement on the days not chelating (with a minimum of 800–1,000 mg calcium/day, 400–600 mg magnesium/day, zinc 30 mg/day with trace minerals), as the chelation process removes essential minerals. Mineral supplements should be taken at least several hours away from the antibiotics to avoid interfering with absorption. Check a CBC, CMP and serum/RBC mineral levels (iodine, magnesium, copper, zinc) periodically during chelation.
- Higher dose DMSA 5–10 mg/kg TID, 1 hour before meals, 3 days on, 11 days off can be used when there are very high levels of heavy metals, usually once off antibiotics. EDTA suppositories can be used in conjunction with DMSA if there are significantly elevated levels of lead.

MOLD/BIOTOXINS:

- Mold Testing: Mycotoxin testing can be done through RealTime Labs (Texas). Other practitioners have used Microbiology DX in Bedford Massachusetts (for MARCoNS and fungal strains). There are controversies among medical practitioners regarding test data, but many healthcare providers have seen improvement in CFS/FMS/ Chronic Lyme patients treating mold, nasal staph, and fungi.

- Binding formulas: clay (pyrophyllite, bentonite) such as Byron White GI Detox, ⅛–¼ tsp/day, and/or charcoal (i.e., one to two capsules of GI detox/day, Bio-Botanical Research, or intestinal drawing formula, 1 tsp/day), zeolite (one to two capsules/day, Nutramedix), cholestyramine (Questran, one–two packets/day), or Welchol (co-lesevelam) 625 mg, 3 PO QD or BID. These have to be taken 2 hours away from all medication and supplements, since they will bind them and impair absorption. Binding formulas may also cause constipation and require increased fluid intake and high doses of magnesium, i.e., minimally 750 mg–1,000 mg/day.

- High-dose oral liposomal glutathione (GSH), i.e., Essential Pro, 2 PO BID, or IV GSH, 2 grams QD-BID, combined with phosphatidylcholine (PC, i.e., Phosphaline, Xymogen) 3 capsules PO BID and N-butyrate 500 mg PO BID is effective in removing mold toxins with FIR saunas and binding agents.

- Mold and MARCoNS (Multiple Antibiotic Resistant Coagulase Negative Staphylo-cocci) can colonize mucous membranes, and hide in biofilms producing inflamma-tion (e.g., chronic sinusitis, upper respiratory symptoms, resistant neurological symptoms) with toxin formation. BE or BEG (Bactroban 0.2%, EDTA 1%, and genta-micin 0.025%–3%) nasal sprays (from compounding pharmacies, like Hopkinton Drug in Massachusetts), 2 sprays up to 3x/day, may be useful for mold and nasal staph infections. Lower doses of gentamycin may be needed if there are any kidney or hearing problems (including tinnitus). To reduce "burning" sensations from a BEG spray, some practitioners use Xlear xylitol nasal spray 3–4 times a day for one week before starting the BEG spray. A deep nasal swab and culture can help determine if these sprays are necessary in resistant biotoxin illness.

- Check mold IgG antibodies, HLA-DRB, C4a, C3a, TGF-Beta 1, MMP9, ADH, MSH, Leptin levels, VIP (Vasoactive Intestinal Peptide), and a VCS (Visual Contrast Screen-ing) test for further evaluation.

- Increase nutritional supplementation to support detoxification while removing mold and environmental chemicals (magnesium, NAC, α-lipoic acid, glutathione, DIM, sulforaphane glucosinolate, methylation cofactors). Herxheimer reactions are possible. Check bloods (CBC, CMP, serum and RBC minerals) and mold levels periodically during and after treatment.

TREATING ALLERGIES

- NAET may clear resistant food allergies, but we have not had enough experience with the technique to validate its effectiveness. Immunotherapy against various allergens (food, environmental, and even certain antibiotics like penicillins) is more commonly used, after evaluation by an allergist, using PO or subcutaneous injections to build toler-ance. It can be effective in severe cases when strict avoidance of the allergen is difficult, and/or the antihistamines listed below are insufficient to control allergic reactions.

- H1 blockers include common over-the-counter antihistamines, like Zyrtec 10 mg, one PO QD-BID, Claritin 10 mg, one PO QD-BID, and Allegra, 180 mg, PO QD, as well as Benadryl 25 mg, PO QD-BID or Atarax, 25 mg, PO QD-BID. H1 blockers can be mixed together if necessary, trying to use sedating antihistamines primarily at bedtime to avoid daytime drowsiness.

- H2 blockers include over-the-counter Zantac 75–150 mg, PO BID and Pepcid, 10–20 mg, PO BID. When H1 and H2 blockers are used together, it is more difficult to break through with allergic manifestations.

- Doxepin, 10–25 mg, PO HS is an antidepressant/antianxiety drug. It is approximately 10,000 times stronger than some available antihistamines.
- Encapsulated diamine oxidase (DAO), 15–30 minutes before meals to help degrade histamine (i.e., Xymogen, HistDAO, 1–3 capsules PO 15–30 minutes before meals), along with Vitamin C (one gram up to three times a day), B6, and SAMe (S-adenosine methionine) 400 mg, up to 800 mg/day can be helpful in those with histamine intolerance.
- Gastrocrom (cromolyn sodium) is a mast cell stabilizer, helpful in those with mast cell activation disorders/mastocytosis. Dosing is QID.
- Singulair, 5–10 mg, PO QD is helpful in those with allergic rhinitis and/or asthma with elevated leukotrienes.

TREATING NUTRITIONAL AND ENZYME DEFICIENCIES

- Replace vitamins, minerals, amino acids (AAs), essential fatty acids (EFAs), enzymes (plant or pancreatic w/amylase, lipase, proteases) as per test results.
- For low Vitamin D: K2D3 once a day (10,000 units/day) may be used for several months until Vitamin D levels increase into the mid-normal range (50–60), and then can be used every other day, following levels.

TREATING MITOCHONDRIAL DYSFUNCTION:

- NT factors or ATP Fuel (glycosylated phospholipids, such as those from Researched Nutritionals) five per day, for two months, followed by 3–5/day.
- CoQ10 (200–400 mg/day) if not on Mepron or Malarone.
- Acetyl L-carnitine, 1,000 mg, PO BID.
- NADH (Enada), 5 mg per day.
- D-ribose, 5-gram scoops, two to three x per day for several months if there is an inadequate response. Avoid D-ribose for prolonged periods of time due to possible effects of increasing glycosylation, especially in patients with blood sugar problems (metabolic syndrome/diabetes).

TREATING NEUROPSYCHOLOGICAL DISORDERS:

- SSRIs: Zoloft 100–200 mg/day, Lexapro 10–20 mg/day, or Paxil 5–10 mg/day, up to a maximum dose of 60 mg/day (when there is associated severe anxiety and panic with depression, and/or OCD). SSRIs like Cymbalta are useful when there is associated fibromyalgia and neuropathy. Starting dose is 20 mg, PO QD for several weeks, followed by 30 mg, PO QD. Increase to 60 mg, PO QD after one month if lower doses are ineffective.
- Bupropion (Wellbutrin XR, 150 mg, PO BID), which can be mixed with SSRIs for greater efficacy.
- Remeron 15 mg, HS, an antidepressant with sedating effects at the lowest dose, can be used for depression with associated insomnia.
- Anxiolytics such as Xanax, Klonopin, Ativan 0.5 mg prn. We tend to avoid regular use of benzodiazepines because of the potential for addiction and withdrawal. Short-term use is preferred. For ongoing anxiety, we prefer to use Paxil, BuSpar (average dose 15 mg PO BID), or trazodone at bedtime if there is associated insomnia (see dosing below).
- Deplin (L-methyl folate) 15 mg, PO QD can help augment the efficacy of other antidepressants. It can also be used as an extra source of folic acid while on Dapsone.
- Herbal treatments include St. John's Wort and 5-HTP for depression (100–200 mg

HS, don't mix with SSRIs); valerian root capsules or tinctures, Kava Kava, and L-theanine (typically dosed 100–200 mg/day) can be helpful as an adjunctive treatment for anxiety.

- Older antidepressants (tricyclics) like Elavil or Pamelor are usually no longer first-line choices (but low doses, i.e., Elavil [amitriptyline] 10 mg can be used for insomnia, migraines, and/or neuropathy).

TREATING HORMONAL ABNORMALITIES:

Follow the guidelines in Chapter 12 regarding initial hormone testing, and follow-up studies.

- DHEA 15–25 mg in the A.M. for low DHEA levels, i.e., Biosom (Metagenics), 3–5 sprays in morning, hold under the tongue for 30 seconds and swallow.
- Mung bean extract, i.e., Testoplex (Xymogen), 4 capsules per day (in the morning) to increase free testosterone.
- Pregnenolone 30–40 mg/day in the morning for low levels, adrenal/sex hormone support.
- Adrenal adaptogenic herbs: Adrenal essence (Xymogen) or Adapten-All (Ortho Molecular), one capsule once or twice a day.
- Adrenal complex (PHP) can be used instead of Cortef (hydrocortisone) for those with milder adrenal dysfunction. See dosing below under POTS/dysautonomia.
- Clomid 50 mg, 1 half tablet two to three times a week is usually sufficient to increase luteinizing hormone and raise testosterone levels into the normal range in men with low T. Use Arimidex (anastrazole) 1 mg, PO Q each week with Clomid to help prevent aromatization of testosterone to estrogen.
- Estriol (E3) suppository (i.e., one mg, three times a week, intravaginally) for women in menopause with vaginal dryness. Vaginal DHEA can also be used (compounding pharmacies).
- Progesterone (creams, pills/capsules, from 100–200 mg HS). This can be helpful for women in menopause with sleep disorders.
- Seriphos (phosphatidylserine) can be also be helpful for sleep disorders due to elevated levels of cortisol.

TREATING SLEEP DISORDERS:

- Activating Agents in the morning, i.e., Provigil 100 mg–200 mg, PO QD, or Nuvigil 150 mg, PO QD.
- Sleep-promoting agents in the evening, especially those that encourage stage 3/stage 4 REM sleep: Lyrica 50–150 mg, PO HS; trazadone 50–150 mg, PO HS; Gabitril 4–16 mg, PO HS; Seroquel 25 mg, HS; Xyrem 3–4.5 grams (6–9 ml), taken twice per night, four hours apart.
- Ambien (zolpidem), 5–10 mg, HS, Ambien CR (6.25–12.5 mg) HS.
- Lunesta (eszopiclone) 1–3 mg, PO HS.
- Remeron (mirtazapine) 7.5–15 mg, PO HS.
- Elavil (amitriptyline), 10–20 mg, PO HS.
- Flexeril (cyclobenzaprine), 5–10 mg, PO HS.
- 5-HTP 100 mg, HS.
- GABA (100–200 mg, HS).
- SeriPhos (phosphatidylserine) may be helpful if there are elevated levels of cortisol HS.

- Valerian root (1,000–1,500 mg) HS, alone, or combined with other herbal supplements.
- L-theanine 100 mg HS.
- KaliPhos 6 X (homeopathic).
- Chinese herbal formulas (*Ziziphus jujuba*, *Schisandra Chinensis*, *Paeonia lactiflora*, and *Rehmannia glutinosa* PO HS).
- Magnesium L-threonate (Xymogen, OptiMag Neuro) 200 mg PO HS.
- Melatonin 1–6 mg. Use the lowest effective dosage, as a hangover effect can occasionally happen in the morning.

TREATING AUTONOMIC NERVOUS SYSTEM (ANS) DYSFUNCTION/POTS

- Salt (minimum 3–4 grams/day) and licorice extract (Licorice Plus, Metagenics), 1–2 QD in A.M.
- Increase fluids (3 liters+).
- Florinef: 0.1–0.2 mg/day in the morning. Higher doses may be necessary in resistant hypotension. Taper off once the blood pressure is controlled.
- Midodrine: starting dose 2.5 PO TID, maximum 5–10 mg, PO TID. This can be added to Florinef to increase efficacy. Side effects include supine blood pressure elevations, which should be monitored.
- Northera, 100 mg, PO TID, working up to a maximum dose of 600 mg, PO TID can be added to the above therapies, or used alone in resistant dysautonomia. Side effects include supine blood pressure elevations, like Midodrine, which should be monitored.
- Cortef: 5 mg, PO QD is a starting dose, but final dosing depends on the level of symptoms and the level of adrenal dysfunction/insufficiency (moderate adrenal dysfunction usually requires between 10–15 mg/day (i.e., 10 mg A.M., 5 mg at 2 P.M.); severe adrenal dysfunction usually requires 20–30 mg/day). Cortef may be necessary if natural adrenal support (like Adrenal Complex, PHP, Professional Health Products, 1–4 in A.M., 1–2 at 2:00 P.M.) is insufficient in relieving resistant symptoms.
- Beta blockers i.e., Toprol XL (metoprolol succinate ER): starting dose is 25 mg PO q A.M., working up to 100 mg/day. This is helpful in those with POTS and significant palpitations. Low doses are often adequate in controlling symptoms. Contraindications include uncontrolled asthma, certain cardiovascular conditions (heart failure, heart block, accessory conduction pathways [WPW], severe peripheral vascular disease).
- Catapres: oral 0.1 mg PO HS or BID starting dose, or Catapres TTS patches (0,1, 0,2, 0.3/24-hour patch): This is only used for hyperadrenergic POTS, where norepinephrine levels are elevated upon standing, causing significant tachycardia.
- SSRIs like Zoloft 50–100 mg/day have been found to occasionally be useful.

FOR GI DYSFUNCTION

- Rule out underlying infections, inflammation/leaky gut, SIBO/dysbiosis, malabsorption, enzyme deficiencies, gluten sensitivity/allergies, etc., and treat accordingly. Probiotic recommendations are found at the beginning of Appendix A
- Upper GI support: GlutAloeMine (Xymogen): 1 scoop/day, contains L-glutamine, arabinogalactan, Deglycyrrhizinated Licorice, aloe vera
- Lower GI support: Opticleanse GHI (Xymogen): 1–2 scoops/day, contains vitamins, minerals, amino acids, turmeric, quercetin, betain, NAC, MSM, watercress, green tea extract, pea protein, alpha-linoleic acid, L-glutamine

FOR ELEVATED LFTS

Treat symptomatically once underlying etiologies have been ruled out and addressed. Herbal support includes:

- Milk thistle (silymarin), up to 300 mg, PO BID.
- Hepa #2 (Zhang, TCM) 2 capsules PO BID.
- NAC 600mg, PO BID, up to 1200 mg, PO BID.
- Alpha-lipoic acid 300–600 mg, PO BID.
- Broccoli extracts: DIM (Xymogen) one capsule/day for phase I liver support, with Oncoplex ES (Xymogen, sulforaphane) 100 mg, PO QD-BID for phase II liver support.
- MedCaps DPO or Liver Protect (Xymogen), one PO BID.

TREATING PAIN

High-dose narcotics should be avoided if possible (or used in limited quantity unless absolutely necessary, i.e., the patient has failed other therapeutic trials for pain), due to tolerance/addiction and possible effects on sleep and hormones. Narcotics also interfere with the use of LDN, which is a very useful drug in controlling inflammation and pain in the Lyme-MSIDS patient. Treating the underlying cause of the pain using the MSIDS map often helps to decrease levels of narcotics.

- Low-dose Ultram 50 mg, PO q 6 prn may be a useful alternative in combination with non-narcotic drug regimens to control pain.

Appendix B

Glossary of Pharmaceutical Names

Brand Name	Generic Name
Actigall	ursodiol
Adderall (XR)	dextroamphetamine/amphetamine
Albenza	albendazole
Aldactone	spironolactone
Aleve	naproxen sodium
Alinia	nitazoxanide
Allegra	fexofenadine
Allegra-D	fexofenadine/pseudoephedrine
Altace	ramipril
Ambien	zolpidem
Amoxicillin	amoxicillin (generics are generally used)
Anafranil	clomipramine
Arava	leflunomide
Arimidex	anastrazole
Ativan	lorazepam
Augmentin	amoxicillin/clavulanate
Avelox	moxifloxacin
Avonex	interferon beta 1α
Baraclude	entecavir
BEG nasal spray	Bactroban 0.2%, EDTA 1%, and gentamicin 0.025%–3%
Belsomra	suvorexant
Benadryl	diphenhydramine
Benicar	olmesartan
Betaseron	interferon beta 1b
Biaxin	clarithromycin
Bicillin	penicillin G benzathine
Biest	estradiol/estriol (compounded)

Brand Name	Generic Name
Biltricide	praziquantel
BuSpar	buspirone
Catapres	clonidine
Cedax	ceftibuten
Ceftin	cefuroxime axetil
Celebrex	celecoxib
Celexa	citalopram
Chemet	DMSA
Cimzia	certolizumab pegol
Cipro	ciprofloxacin
Claforan	cefotaxime
Claritin	loratadine
Claritin-D 24 Hr.	loratadine/pseudoephedrine
Cleocin	clindamycin
Climara	estradiol transdermal
Clomid	clomiphene
Coartem	artemether/lumefantrine
Copaxone	glatiramer
Cortef	hydrocortisone
Coumadin	warfarin
Cuprimine	penicillamine
Cymbalta	duloxetine HCl
Cytomel	liothyronine
Cytotec	misoprostol
Cytovene	ganciclovir
Dapsone	diaminodiphenyl sulfone (DDS)
Daraprim	pyrimethamine
DDAVP Nasal	desmopressin nasal
Decadron	dexamethasone
Depakote	divalproex sodium
Deplin	methyltetrahydrofolate
Detrol LA	tolterodine
Diamox	acetazolamide
Dificid	fidaxomicin
Diflucan	fluconazole
Dilaudid	hydromorphone
DMSA	dimercaptosuccinic acid
DMPS	2,3-Dimercapto-1-propanesulfonic acid
Dynabac	dirithromycin
EDTA	ethylenediaminetetraacetic acid
Elavil	amitriptyline
Enbrel	etanercept
Epivir	lamivudine
Factive	gemifloxacin
Famvir	famciclovir
Fioricet	butalbital/acetaminophen/caffeine
Flagyl	metronidazole
Flexeril	cyclobenzaprine

Brand Name	Generic Name
Florinef	fludrocortisone
Fosamax	alendronate
Gabitril	tiagabine
Gammagard	immune globulin (human)
Gamunex-C	immune globulin (human)
Gastrocrom	cromolyn sodium
Glucophage	metformin
Harvoni	ledipasvir/sofosbuvir
Heltioz	tasimelteon
Hepsera	adefovir
Horizant	gabapentin enacarbil
Humira	adalimumab
Imitrex	sumatriptan
Imuran	azathioprine
Incivek	telaprevir
Ivermectin	ivermectin
Klonopin	clonazepam
Lanoxin	digoxin
Lariam	mefloquine
Lasix	furosemide
low-dose naltrexone	low-dose naltrexone
Levaquin	levofloxacin
Lexapro	escitalopram
Lunesta	eszopiclone
Lyrica	pregabalin
Malarone	atovaquone/proguanil
Medrol	methylprednisolone
Mepron	atovaquone
Mestinon	pyridostigmine
Mevacor	lovastatin
Minocin	minocycline
Mobic	meloxicam
Motrin	ibuprofen
MS Contin	morphine sulfate
Naprosyn	naproxen
Neurontin	gabapentin
Northera	droxidopa
Nuvigil	armodafinil
Oleptro	trazodone
Omnicef	cefdinir
Pamelor	nortriptyline
Parlodel	bromocriptine
Paromomycin	paromomycin
Paxil	paroxetine
Percocet	oxycodone/acetaminophen
Phenobarbital	phenobarbital
Pin-X	pyrantel pamoate
Plaquenil	hydroxychloroquine

Brand Name	Generic Name
Pred Forte (eye drops)	prednisolone acetate ophthalmic
Prilosec	omeprazole
Primaxin	imipenem/cilastatin
ProAmatine	midodrine
Procrit	epoetin alpha
Provigil	modafinil
Prozac	fluoxetine
Pyrazinamide (only generic)	pyrazinamide
Qualaquin	quinine sulfate
Questran	cholestyramine
Rebif	interferon beta 1α
Reglan	metoclopramide
Remeron	mirtazapine
Restoril	temazepam
Rheumatrex	Methotrexate
Ribasphere	ribavirin
Rifadin	rifampin
Rilutek	riluzole
Risperdal	risperidone
Ritalin	Methylphenidate
Rituxan	rituximab
Rocephin	ceftriaxone
Septra DS	trimethoprim/sulfamethoxazole
Seroquel	quetiapine
Singulair	montelukast
Solu-Medrol	methylprednisolone sodium succinate
Sonata	zaleplon
Sporanox	itraconazole
Strattera	atomoxetine
Sudafed	pseudoephedrine
Sumycin	tetracycline
Suprax	cefixime
Synthroid	levothyroxine
Tegretol	carbamazepine
Tenormin	atenolol
Tindamax	tinidazole
Topamax	topiramate
Toprol XL	metoprolol succinate
Tylenol	acetaminophen
Tyzeka	telbivudine
Ultram	tramadol
Valcyte	valganciclovir
Valium	diazepam
Valtrex	valacyclovir
Vancocin	vancomycin
Viread	tenofovir disoproxil
Victrelis	boceprevir
Viekira Pak	ombitasvir/paritaprevir/ritonavir and dasabuvir

Brand Name	Generic Name
Vivelle-Dot	estradiol transdermal
Voltaren	diclofenac sodium
Vyvanse	lisdexamfetamine dimesylate
WelChol	colesevelam
Wellbutrin	bupropion HCl
Xanax	alprazolam
Xifaxan	rifaximin
Xyrem	sodium oxybate
Zanaflex	tizanidine
Zantac	ranitidine
Zipsor	diclofenac sodium
Zithromax	azithromycin
Zocor	simvastatin
Zofran	ondansetron
Zoloft	sertraline
Zovirax	acyclovir
Zyrtec	cetirizine
Zyrtec-D	cetirizine/pseudoephedrine

Appendix C

Journal Names and Abbreviations

AAOHN Journal (American Association of Occupational Health Nurses)

Acta Neurol Scand: Acta Neurologica Scandinavica

Acta Paediatr: Acta Paediatrica

Adv Exp Med Biol: Advances in Experimental Medicine and Biology

Adv Neuroimmunol: Advances in Neuroimmunology

Alternative Medicine Review

Am Fam Physician: American Family Physician

Am J Clin Nutr: American Journal of Clinical Nutrition, The

Am J Clin Pathol: American Journal of Clinical Pathology

Am J Dig Dis: American Journal of Digestive Diseases, The

Am J Gastro: American Journal of Gastroenterology, The

Am J Gastroenterol: American Journal of Gastroenterology, The

Am J Med: American Journal of Medicine, The

Am J Ophthalmol: American Journal of Ophthalmology

Am J Physiol Cell Physiol: American Journal of Physiology—Cellular and Molecular Physiology

Am J Physiol Lung Cell Mol Physiol: American Journal of Physiology—Lung Cellular and Molecular Physiology

Am J Psychiatry: American Journal of Psychiatry, The

Am J Respir Crit Care Med: American Journal of Respiratory and Critical Care Medicine

Am J Trop Med Hyg: American Journal of Tropical Medicine and Hygiene, The

Amer Jnl Gastroenterology: American Journal of Gastroenterology, The

American Journal of Dermatopathology

American Journal of Epidemiology

American Journal of Physiology

American Journal of Public Health

Ann Allergy: Annals of Allergy, Asthma & Immunology

Ann Behav Med: Annals of Behavioral Medicine

Ann Clin Lab Sci: Annals of Clinical & Laboratory Science

Ann Intern Med: Annals of Internal Medicine

Ann Neurol: Annals of Neurology

Ann NY Acad Sci: Annals of the New York Academy of Sciences

Ann Rheum Dis: Annals of the Rheumatic Diseases

Annals of Agricultural and Environmental Medicine

Annals of Pharmacotherapy

Annals of Tropical Medicine and Parasitology

Annu Rev Med: Annual Review of Medicine

Annu Rev Genet: Annual Review of Genetics

Annual Review of Immunology

Antibiotics and Chemotherapy

Antimicrobial Agents and Chemotherapy

APMIS (Acta Pathologica Microbiologica et Immunilogica Scandinavica)

Arch Dermatol: Archives of Dermatological Research

Arch Dis Child: Archives of Disease in Childhood

Arch Intern Med: Archives of Internal Medicine

Arch Neurol: Archives of Neurology

Arch Pediatr Adolesc Med: Archives of Pediatrics & Adolescent Medicine

Arch Phys Med Rehabil: Archives of Physical Medicine and Rehabilitation

Arch Surg: Archives of Surgery

Arthritis Res Ther: Arthritis Research & Therapy

Arthritis Rhem: Arthritis & Rheumatism

Asthma

Autoimmun Rev: Autoimmunity Reviews

Autoimmunity

Auton Neurosci: Autonomic Neuroscience

Behav Brain Res: Behavioural Brain Research

Behavioural Pharmacology

Biochem Int: Biochemistry International

Biochemical Journal

Biol Psychiatry: Biological Psychiatry

BioMedCentral Neurology

Bioorg Med Chem Lett: Bioorganic & Medicinal Chemistry Letters

BJMP: British Journal of Medical Practitioners

Blood

BMC Neurol: BMC Neuroscience

BMJ: British Medical Journal

Br J Dermatol: British Journal of Dermatology

Brain Behav Immun: Brain, Behavior, and Immunity

Brit Jnl Derm: British Journal of Dermatology

Brit J Med Practit: British Journal of Medical Practitioners

British Journal of Nutrition

Can Med Assoc: Canadian Medical Association Journal

Cardiology

Case Reports in Immunology

Cell

Cell Immunology: Cellular Immunology

Cell Physiology: American Journal of Physiology

Chest

Circulation

Cleve Clin J Med: Cleveland Clinic Journal of Medicine

Clin Biochem: Clinical Biochemistry

Clin Exp Allergy: Clinical & Experimental Allergy

Clin Exp Immunol: Clinical & Experimental Immunology

Clin Exp Rheum: Clinical and Experimental Rheumatology

Clin Gastroenterol Hepatol: Clinical Gastroenterology and Hepatology

Clin Inf Dis: Clinical Infectious Diseases

Clin Infect Dis: Clinical Infectious Diseases

Clin Microbiol Infect: Clinical Microbiology and Infection

Clin Microbiol Rev: Clinical Microbiology Reviews

Clin Orthop: Clinical Orthopaedics and Related Research

Clin Ped: Clinical Pediatrics

Clin Pediatr: Clinical Pediatrics

Clin Prac of Alt Med: Clinical Practice of Alternative Medicine

Clin Rheumatol: Clinical Rheumatology

Clin Sci (Lond): Clinical Science (London)

Clin Vaccine Immunol: Clinical and Vaccine Immunology

Clinical and Developmental Immunology

Clinical Diabetes

Clinical Rheum: Clinical Rheumatology

Cochrane Database of Systematic Reviews

Contemporary Clinical Trials

CRC Crit Rev Food Sci Nutr: Critical Reviews in Food Science and Nutrition

Critical Reviews in Toxicology

Curr Allergy Asthma Rep: Current Allergy and Asthma Reports

Curr Biol: Current Biology

Current Directions in Psychological Science

Current Medical Diagnosis & Treatment

Current Medicinal Chem: Current Medicinal Chemistry

Curr Mol Med: Current Molecular Medicine

Curr Opin Biotechnol: Current Opinion in Biotechnology

Curr Opin Investig Drugs: Current Opinion in Investigational Drugs

Curr Opin Pulm Med: Current Opinion in Pulmonary Medicine

Curr Opin Rheum: Current Opinion in Rheumatology

Curr Opin Struct Biol: Current Opinion in Structural Biology

Curr Pharm Des: Current Pharmaceutical Design

Curr Rheumatol Rep: Current Rheumatology Reports

Current Opinion in Genetics & Development

Current Opinion in Neurology

Cytokine

Diabetologia

Diagn Microbiol and Infect Dis: Diagnostic Microbiology and Infectious Disease

Dig Dis Sci: Digestive Diseases and Sciences

Directions in Psychiatry

EASD—European Association for the Study of Diabetes

EID: Emerging Infectious Diseases

Emerg Infect Dis: Emerging Infectious Diseases

Endocr Rev: Endocrine Reviews

Environment International

Epigenetics

Eur Infect Dis: European Journal of Clinical Microbiology & Infectious Diseases

Eur J Cancer: European Journal of Cancer

Eur J Clin Microbiol Infect Dis: European Journal of Clinical Microbiology & Infectious Diseases

Eur J Endocrinol: European Journal of Endocrinology

Eur J Gastroenterol Hepatol: European Journal of Gastroenterology & Hepatology

Eur J Heart Fail: European Journal of Heart Failure

Eur J Pediatr: European Journal of Pediatrics

Eur J Pharmacol: European Journal of Pharmacology

Eur Soc of Clin Microbiol and Inf Dis: European Society of Clinical Microbiology and Infectious Diseases

Eurosurveillance

Evidence-Based Complementary and Alternative Medicine

Expert Rev Anti Infect Ther: Expert Review of Anti-Infective Therapy

FEBS J: FEBS Journal (Federation of European Biochemical Societies)

Fortschritte der Medizin

Free Radic Biol Med: Free Radical Biology & Medicine

Future Microbiol: Future Microbiology

Ghana Med Jnl: Ghana Medical Journal

Health Services Research

Hepatology

Homeostasis

Hormone and Metabolic Research

Hypertension

IAMM: Indian Association of Microbiologists

IMAJ: Israel Medical Association Journal, The

Immunol Today: Immunology Today

Immunology

Indian Journal of Experimental Biology

Indian Journal of Pharmacology

Indian Pacing Electrophysiol J: Indian Pacing and Electrophysiology Journal

Infect Immun: Infection and Immunity

Infection

Infectious Agents and Disease

Infectious Disease: Infectious Disease Clinics of North America

Int J Immunopharmacol: International Journal of Immunopharmacology

Int J Infect Dis: International Journal of Infectious Diseases

Int J Neurosci: International Journal of Neuroscience

Int J Pharmalcol: International Journal of Pharmacology

Int Jnl Med: International Journal of Medicine

Int Microbiol: International Microbiology

Intern Med: Internal Medicine News

Internal Medicine (Japanese Society of Internal Medicine)

International Journal of Clinical Medicine

International Journal of Medical Sciences

International Journal of Pharmacy Practice

J Agric Food Chem: Journal of Agricultural and Food Chemistry

J Allergy Clin Immunol: Journal of Allergy and Clinical Immunology

J Alzheimers Dis: Journal of Alzheimer's Disease

J Am Acad Psychiatry Law: Journal of the American Academy of Psychiatry and the Law, The

J Am Coll Cardiol: Journal of the American College of Cardiology

J Am Diet Assoc: Journal of the American Dietetic Association

J Am Vet Med Assoc: Journal of the American Veterinary Medical Association

J Androl: Journal of Andrology

J App Physiol: Journal of Applied Physiology

J Appl Microbiol: Journal of Applied Microbiology

J Assoc Physicians India: Journal of the Association of Physicians of India

J Biol Chem: Journal of Biological Chemistry, The

J Clin Endocrinol Metab: Journal of Clinical Endocrinology & Metabolism, The

J Clin Gastroenterol: Journal of Clinical Gastroenterology

J Clin Invest: Journal of Clinical Investigation

J Clin Microbiol: Journal of Clinical Microbiology

J Clin Psychiatry: Journal of Clinical Psychiatry

J Clin Sleep Med: Journal of Clinical Sleep Medicine

J Degenerative Dis: Journal of Degenerative Diseases, The

J Endocrinol Invest: Journal of Endocrinological Investigation

J Ethnophamacol: Journal of Ethnopharmacology

J Helminthol: Journal of Helminthology

J Immunol: Journal of Immunology, The

J Immunol Methods: Journal of Immunological Methods

J Inf Dis: Journal of Infectious Diseases, The

J Infect Dis: Journal of Infectious Diseases, The

J La State Med Soc: Journal of the Louisiana State Medical Society, The

J Med Microbiol: Journal of Medical Microbiology

J Med Toxicol: Journal of Medical Toxicology

J Musculoskel Pain: Journal of Musculoskeletal Pain

J Musculoskeletal Pain: Journal of Musculoskeletal Pain

J Neuroimmunol: Journal of Neuroimmunology

J Neuroinflammation: Journal of Neuroinflammation

J Neurol Sci: Journal of Neuroscience Research

J Neuropathol Exp Neurol: Journal of Neuropathology & Experimental Neurology

J Nutr: Journal of Nutrition

J Pain: Journal of Pain, The

J Parasitol: International Journal for Parasitology

J Pharm Pharmacol: Journal of Pharmacy and Pharmacology

J Pharmacol Exp Ther: Journal of Pharmacology and Experimental Therapeutics

J Psychosom Res: Journal of Psychosomatic Research

J R Soc Med: Journal of the Royal Society of Medicine

J Rheumatol: Journal of Rheumatology, The

J Steroid Biochem Mol Biol: Journal of Steroid Biochemistry and Molecular Biology, The

J Urol: Journal of Urology

J Vet Med Sci: Journal of Veterinary Medical Science, The

J Appl Bacteriol: Journal of Applied Bacteriology

J Chronic Fatigue Syndr: Journal of Chronic Fatigue Syndrome

J Clin Microbiology: Journal of Clinical Microbiology

J Clin. Neurosci: Journal of Clinical Neuroscience

J Mol. Microbiol. Biotechnol: Journal of Molecular Microbiology and Biotechnology

J Neurol and Psychopathol: Journal of Neurology and Psychopathology, The

J Neuropath. and Exp Neur: Journal of Neuropathology & Experimental Neurology

J Physiol: Journal of Physiology, The

JAMA: Journal of the American Medical Association, The (JAMA)

JANA: Journal of the American Nutraceutical Association (JANA)

JEM: Journal of Experimental Medicine, The (JEM)

Jnl of Applied Bacteriology: Journal of Applied Bacteriology

Jnl of Chr Fatigue Syndrome: Journal of Chronic Fatigue Syndrome

Jnl of Neurosci: Journal of Neuroscience, The

Journal of Advanced Nursing

Journal of Aging and Phys Activ: Journal of Aging and Physical Activity

Journal of Alternative and Complementary Medicine, The

Journal of Antimicrobial Chemotherapy

Journal of Bacteriology

Journal of Cardiopulmonary Rehabilitation & Prevention

Journal of Cellular Biochemistry

Journal of Clin Microbiol: Journal of Clinical Microbiology

Journal of Clinical Oncology

Journal of Clinical Psychology

Journal of Consulting and Clinical Psychology

Journal of Diabetes

Journal of Internal Medicine

Journal of Nephrology

Journal of Neurochem: Journal of Neurochemistry

Journal of Nutritional and Environmental Medicine

Journal of Occupational Medicine

Journal of Perinatology

Journal of Personality and Social Psychology

Journal of Pharmacy Practice

Journal of Psychiatric Practice

Journal of Sports Medicine and Physical Fitness, The

Journal of the National Cancer Institute

Journal of the Neurological Sciences

Lancet Neurology, The

Lancet, The

Lupus

Mayo Clin Proc: Mayo Clinic Proceedings

Med Clin (Barc): Medicina Clínica (Barcelona)

Med GenMed: Medscape General Medicine

Med Hypotheses: Medical Hypotheses

Med Mal Infect: Médecine et Maladies Infectieuses

Med Sci Monitor: Medical Science Monitor

Metabolism

Microbiol Rev: Microbiological Reviews

Microbiology

MMWR: Morbidity and Mortality Weekly Report (MMWR)

Mol Microbiol: Molecular Microbiology

Mol Biol Rev: Microbiology and Molecular Biology Reviews

Mol Nutr Food Res: Molecular Nutrition & Food Research

Mol Psychiatry: Molecular Psychiatry

Morb Mortal Wkly Rep: Morbidity and Mortality Weekly Report (MMWR)

Mucosal Immunity: Mucosal Immunology

Multiple Sclerosis

Multiple Sclerosis Journal

Muscle & Nerve

N Engl J Med: New England Journal of Medicine, The

Nat Clin Pract Gastroenerol Hepatol: Nature Clinical Practice Gastroenterology & Hepatology

Nat Prod Rep: Natural Product Reports

Nature

Nature Neuroscience

Nature Reviews Neuroscience

NEJM: New England Journal of Medicine, The

Neoplasia

Nervenarzt: Nervenarzt, Der

Neurobiology of Disease

NeuroImmunoModulation

Neurology

Neurology Research International

Neuroscience & Biobehavioral Reviews

Neuroscience Letters

NeuroToxicology

New York Times, The

Novartis Found Symp: Novartis Foundation Symposia

Nutr Cancer: Nutrition and Cancer

Nutr Hosp: Nutricion Hospitalaria

Obstet Gynecol Surv: Obstetrical & Gynecological Survey

Occup Environ Med: Journal of Occupational and Environmental Medicine

Oncology Nursing Forum

Open Access

Ophthalmology

Otolaryngology—Head and Neck Surgery

PACE

Pain Med: Pain Medicine

Parasitology Today

Pediatr Infect Dis J: Pediatric Infectious Disease Journal, The

Pediatrics

Phys Ther: Physical Therapy

Phytother Res: Phytotherapy Research

Planta Med: Planta Medica

PLOS ONE

PLOS Pathogens

Polish Journal of Pharmacology

Postgrad Med: Postgraduate Medicine

Preventive Medicine

Prog Neuropsychopharmacol Biol Psychiatry: Progress in Neuro-Psychopharmacology & Biological Psychiatry

Psych Bulletin: Psychological Bulletin

Psychiatr Clin North Am: Psychiatric Clinics of North America

Psychiatric Quarterly

Psychiatric Times

Psycho-Oncology

Psychosomatic Medicine

Psychosomatics

Ren Fail: Renal Failure

Respirology

Rev Neurol (Paris): Revue Neurologique

Rheum Dis Clin North Am: Rheumatic Disease Clinics of North America

Rheumatol Int: Rheumatology International

Rocz Akad Med Bialymst: Roczniki Akademii Medycznej w Bialymstoku

Scand J Rheumatol Supp: Scandinavian Journal of Rheumatology

Scanning Electron Microscopy

Schizophr Bull: Schizophrenia Bulletin

Sci Transl Med: Science Translational Medicine

Science

Scientific American

Semin Neurol: Seminars in Neurology

Sleep

South Med J: Southern Medical Journal

Stress

Ticks and Tick-Borne Diseases

Trends Endocrinol Metab: Trends in Endocrinology & Metabolism

Trends Neurosci: Trends in Neurosciences

Trop Doct: Tropical Doctor

Turkish Journal of Pediatrics, The

Urology

Veterinary Parasitology

Wilderness & Environmental Medicine

Wilderness Medicine

World J Gastroenterol: World Journal of Gastroenterology

Yale J Biol Med: Yale Journal of Biology and Medicine, The

Zentralbl Bakteriol Mikrobiol Hyg A: Zentralblatt für Bakteriologie, Mikrobiologie und Hygiene: Serie A

Zh Mikrobiol Epidemiol Immunobiol: Zhurnal Mikrobiologii Epidemiologii I Immunobiologii

Notes

Introduction

Hook S, Nelson C, Mead P. (2013) Self-reported Lyme disease diagnosis, treatment, and recovery: results from 2009, 2011, & 2012 HealthStyles nationwide surveys. Presented at the 13th International Conference on Lyme Borreliosis and other Tick-Borne Diseases, Boston, MA, August 19, 2013.

One: Identifying Lyme Disease and Other Tick-Borne Illnesses

Allen HB, Morales D, Jones K, Joshi S. Alzheimer's disease: a novel hypothesis integrating spirochetes, biofilm, and the immune system. *J Neuroinfect Dis.* 2016;7:200. doi:10.4172/2314-7326.1000200.

Bu X-L, et al. A study on the association between infectious burden and Alzheimer's disease. *Eur J Neurol.* 2015 Dec;22(12):1519–25. doi:10.1111/ene.12477. Epub 2014 Jun 9.

Clark K, et al. Lyme borreliosis in human patients in Florida and Georgia, USA. *Int. J Med Sci.* 2013;10(7):915–931.

Girard YA, Fedorova N, Lane RS. Genetic diversity of Borrelia burgdorferi and detection of B. bissettii-like DNA in serum of north-coastal California residents. *J Clin Microbiol.* 2011;49:945–954.

Johnson L, Wilcox S, Mankoff J, Stricker RB. Severity of chronic Lyme disease compared to other chronic conditions: a quality of life survey. Wilke C, ed. *PeerJ.* 2014;2:e322. doi:10.7717/peerj.322.

Jung C-R, Lin Y-T, Hwang B-F. Ozone, particulate matter, and newly diagnosed Alzheimer's disease: a population-based cohort study in Taiwan. *J Alzheimer's Dis.* 2015;44:573–584. doi: 10.3233/JAD-140855.

Miklossy, J. Chronic inflammation and amyloidogenesis in Alzheimer's disease: role of spirochetes. *J Alzheimer's Dis.* Dec 2004;6(6):639–49; discussion 673–81; *J Alzheimer's Dis.* (review). May 13, 2008;13(4):381–391.

Pritt BS, et al. Identification of a novel pathogenic borrelia species causing Lyme borreliosis with unusually high spirochetemia: a descriptive study. *Lancet Infect Dis.* 2016 Feb 5. pii: S1473-3099(15)00464-8. doi:10.1016/S1473-3099(15)00464-8. [Epub ahead of print].

Richardson J, et al. Elevated serum pesticide levels and risk for Alzheimer disease. *JAMA Neurol.* Published online January 27, 2014. doi:10.1001/jamaneurol.2013.6030.

Soloski MJ, Crowder LA, Lahey LJ, Wagner CA, Robinson WH, et al. Serum inflammatory mediators as markers of human Lyme disease activity. (2014) *PLOS ONE.* 9(4):e93243.

Two: A Comprehensive Diagnosis: The Horowitz Sixteen-Point Differential Diagnostic Map

Aberer E, Kersten A, Klade H, Poitschek C, Jurecka W. Heterogeneity of Borrelia burgdorferi in the skin. *Am J Dermatopathology.* 1996;18(6):571–579.

Aguero-Rosenfeld ME, Wang G, Schwartz I, Wormser GP. Diagnosis of Lyme borreliosis. *Clin Microbiol Rev.* 2005;18:484–509.

Ang CW, Notermans DW, Hommes M, Simoons-Smit AM, Herremans T. Large differences between test strategies for the detection of anti-borrelia antibodies are revealed by comparing eight ELISAs and five immunoblots. *Eur J Clin Microbiol Infect Dis.* 2011;30(8):1027–1032.

Bakken LL, Callister SM, Wand PJ, Schell RF. Intralaboratory comparison of test results for detection of Lyme disease by 516 participants in the Wisconsin State Laboratory of Hygiene/ College of American Pathologists Proficiency Testing Program. *J Clin Microbiol.* Mar 1997; 35(3):537–543.

Barbour AG. Isolation and cultivation of Lyme disease spirochetes. *Yale J Biol Med.* 1984;57:521–525.

Barnett W, Sigmund D, Roelcke U, Mundt C. Endogenous paranoid-hallucinatory syndrome caused by Borrelia encephalitis. *Nervenarzt.* 1991 July;62(7):445–7.

Benke T, Gasse T, Hittmair-Delazer M, Schmutzhard E. Lyme encephalopathy: long-term neuropsychological deficits years after acute neuroborreliosis. *Acta Neurol Scand.* May 1995; 91(5):353–357.

Berman DS, Wenglin BD. Complaints attributed to chronic Lyme disease: depression or fibromyalgia? *Am J Med.* Oct 1995;99(4):440.

Bloom BJ, Wyckoff PM, Meissner HC, Steere AC. Neurocognitive abnormalities in children after classic manifestations of Lyme disease. *J Pediatric Infect Dis.* Mar 1998;17(3):189–96.

Borgermans L, Goderis G, Vandevoorde J, Devroey D. Relevance of chronic Lyme disease to family medicine as a complex multidimensional chronic disease construct: a systematic review. *International Journal of Family Medicine*, vol. 2014, Article ID 138016, 10 pages, 2014. doi:10.1155/2014/138016.

Bransfield MD, Robert C. Lyme disease, comorbid tick-borne diseases, and neuropsychiatric disorders. *Psychiatric Times.* Web. 10 Sept 2016.

Breier F, Khanakah G, Stanek G, Kunz G, Aberer E, Schmidt B, et al. Isolation and polymerase chain reaction typing of Borrelia afzelii from a skin lesion in a seronegative patient with generalized ulcerating bullous lichen sclerosus et atrophicus. *Br J Dermatol.* Feb 2001;144(2): 387–392.

Breitschwerdt EB, et al. Koch's postulates and the pathogenesis of comparative infectious disease causation associated with Bartonella species. *Comp. Path.* 2013;148:115e125.

Brown JS, Jr. Geographic correlation of schizophrenia to ticks and tick-borne encephalitis. *Schizophr Bull.* 1994;20(4):755–75.

Brunner M. New method for detection of Borrelia burgdorferi antigen complexed to antibody in seronegative Lyme disease. *J Immunol Methods.* Mar 1, 2001;249(1–2):185–190.

Buechner SA, et al. Lymphoproliferative responses to Borrelia burgdorferi in patients with erythema migrans, acrodermatitis chronica atrophicans, lymphadenosis benigna cutis, and morphea. *Arch Dermatol.* 1995;131:673–67.

Centers for Disease Control and Prevention. http://www.cdc.gov/osels/ph_surveillance/nndss

/casedef/lyme_disease_current.htm; Centers for Disease Control and Prevention. MMWR 56(23);573–576, June 15, 2007. http://www.cdc.gov/ncphi/disss/nndss/casedef/lyme_disease _2008.htm.

Cerar T, Rusic-Sabljic E, Glinsek U, Zore A, Strle F. Comparison of PCR methods and culture for the detection of borrelia spp. in patients with erythema migrans. *Clin Microbiol Infect.* 2008;14:653–658.

Chmielewska-Badora J, Cisak E, Wójcik-Fatla A, Zwoliński J, Buczek A, Dutkiewicz J. Correlation of tests for detection of Borrelia burgdorferi sensu lato infection in patients with diagnosed borreliosis. *Ann Agric Environ Med* 2006;13(2):307–11.

Coulter P, Lema C, et al. Two-year evaluation of Borrelia burgdorferi culture and supplemental tests for definitive diagnosis of Lyme disease. *J. Clin. Microbiol.* 43:5080–5084.

Coyle PK, Schutzer SE, Deng Z, Krupp LB, Belman AL, Benach JL, et al. Detection of Borrelia burgdorferi-specific antigen in antibody-negative cerebrospinal fluid in neurologic Lyme disease. *Neurology.* Nov 1995;45(11):2010–2015.

Dattwyler RJ, et al. Seronegative Lyme disease: dissociation of specific T- and B-lymphocyte responses to Borrelia burgdorferi. *N Engl J Med.* 1988;319:1441–1446.

de Martino SJ. Role of biological assays in the diagnosis of Lyme borreliosis presentations: what are the techniques and which are currently available? *Med Maladies Infect.* 2007; 37(7–8):496–506.

Dejmkova H, Hulinska D, Tegzova D, Pavelka K, Gatterova J, Vavrik P. Seronegative Lyme arthritis caused by Borrelia garinii. *Clin Rheumatol.* Aug 2002;21(4):330–334.

Dorward DW, Fischer ER, Brooks DM. Invasion and cytopathic killing of human lymphocytes by spirochetes causing Lyme disease. *Clin Infect Dis.* Jul 1997;25 Suppl 1:S2–8.

Dressler F, et al. The T-cell proliferative assay in the diagnosis of Lyme disease. *Ann Intern Med.* 1991;115:533–539.

Eshoo MW, Crowder CC, Rebman AW, Rounds MA, Matthews HE, Picuri JM, et al. (2012) Direct molecular detection and genotyping of Borrelia burgdorferi from whole blood of patients with early Lyme disease. *PLOS ONE.* 7(5):e36825. doi:10.1371/journal.pone.0036825.

Fallon BA, Kochevar JM, Gaito A, Nields JA. The underdiagnosis of neuropsychiatric Lyme disease in children and adults. *Psychiatric Clin North Am.* 1998;21:693–703.

Fallon BA, Nields JA. Lyme disease: a neuropsychiatric illness. *Am J Psychiatry.* Nov 1994; 151(11):1571–1583.

Girschick HJ, Huppertz HI, Russmann H, Krenn V, Karch H. Intracellular persistence of Borrelia burgdorferi in human synovial cells. *Rheumatol Int.* 1996;16(3):125–132.

Hajek T, Paskova B, Janovska D, et al. Higher prevalence of antibodies to Borrelia burgdorferi in psychiatric patients than in healthy subjects. *Am J Psychiatry.* Feb 2002;159:297–301.

Hess A, Buchmann J, Zettl UK, Henschel S, Schlaefke D, Grau G, Benecke R. Borrelia burgdorferi central nervous system infection presenting as an organic schizophrenia-like disorder. *Biol Psychiatry.* Mar 15, 1999;45(6):795.

Horowitz RI. Clinical roundup: selected treatment options for Lyme disease: multiple causative factors in chronic disease. *Alt and Compl Therapies (Mary Ann Libert).* Aug 2012;18:4. doi:10.1089/act.2012.18407.

Huppertz et al. Lymphoproliferative responses to Borrelia burgdorferi in the diagnosis of Lyme arthritis in children and adolescents. *Eur J Pediatr.* 1996;155:297–302.

Kaiser R. False-negative serology in patients with neuroborreliosis and the value of employing different borrelial strains in serological assays. *J Med Microbiol.* 2000 Oct;49(10):911–5.

Kaplan A. Neuropsychiatric masquerades. *Psychiatric Times.* Feb 26, 2009;(2)1–8.

Krause et al. T cell proliferation induced by Borrelia burgdorferi in patients with Lyme borreliosis. Autologous serum required for optimum stimulation. *Arthritis Rheum.* 1991;34:393–402.

Liveris D, Schwartz I, McKenna D, Nowakowski J, Wormser GP, et al. Comparison of five diagnostic modalities for direct detection of Borrelia burgdorferi in patients with early Lyme disease. *Diagn Microbiol and Infect Dis*. 2012;73:243–245.

Liveris D, Wang G, Girao G, Byrne DW, Nowakowski J, et al. Quantitative detection of Borrelia burgdorferi in 2-millimeter skin samples of erythema migrans lesions: correlation of results with clinical and laboratory findings. *J Clin Microbiol*. 2002;40:1249–1253.

Ma Y, Sturrock A, Weis JJ. Intracellular localization of Borrelia burgdorferi within human endothelial cells. *Infect Immun*. Feb 1991;59(2):671–678.

MacDonald AB. Concurrent neocortical borreliosis and Alzheimer's disease: demonstration of a spirochetal cyst form (review). *Ann NY Acad Sci*. 1988;(539):468–470.

Marangoni A, Sparacino M, Cavrini F, Storni E, Mondardini V, Sambri V, Cevenini R. Comparative evaluation of three different ELISA methods for the diagnosis of early culture-confirmed Lyme disease in Italy. *J Med Microbiol*. Apr 2005;54(Pt 4):361–7.

Miklossy J, Kasas S, Zurn, AD, McCall S, Sheng Y, McGeer PL. Persisting atypical and cystic forms of Borrelia burgdorferi and local inflammation in Lyme neuroborreliosis. *Journal of Neuroinflammation* September 25, 2008. 5:40 DOI: 10.1186/1742-2094-5-40.

Montgomery RR, Nathanson MH, Malawista SE. The fate of Borrelia burgdorferi, the agent for Lyme disease, in mouse macrophages: destruction, survival, recovery. *J Immunol*. Feb 1, 1993;150(3):909–915.

Nowakowski J, Schwartz I, Liveris D, Wang G, Aguero-Rosenfeld ME, et al. Laboratory diagnostic techniques for patients with early Lyme disease associated with erythema migrans: a composition of different techniques. *Clin Infect Dis*. 2001;33:2023–2027.

Pachner AR. Neurological manifestations of Lyme disease, the new "great imitator." *Infect Dis*. 1989;11 (Suppl 6):S1482–1486.

Pfister HW, Preac-Mursic V, Wilske B, Rieder G, Forderreuther S, Schmidt S, Kapfhammer HP. Catatonic syndrome in acute severe encephalitis due to Borrelia burgdorferi infection. *Neurology*. Feb 1993;43(2):433–435.

Pikelj F, Strle F, Mozina M. Seronegative Lyme disease and transitory atrioventricular block. *Ann Intern Med*. Jul 1, 1989;111(1):90; Oct;49(10):911–9115.

Pollack RJ, Telford SR III, Spielman A. Standardization of medium for culturing Lyme disease spirochetes. *J Clin Microbiol*. 1993;31:1251–1255.

Riedel M, Straube A, Schwarz MJ, Wilske B, Muller N. Lyme disease presenting as Tourette's syndrome. *Lancet*. Feb 7, 1998;351(9100):418–419.

Schutzer SE, Coyle PK, Belman AL, Golightly MG, Drulle J. Sequestration of antibody to Borrelia burgdorferi in immune complexes in seronegative Lyme disease. *Lancet*. Feb 10, 1990;335(8685):312–315.

Sherr VT. Panic attacks may reveal previously unsuspected chronic disseminated Lyme disease. *J Psychiatric Prac*. Nov 2000;6:352–356.

Sigal LH, et al. Cellular immune findings Lyme disease. *Yale J Biol Med*. 1984;57:595–598.

Skogman BH, Hellberg S, Ekerfelt C, Jenmalm MC. Adaptive and innate immune responsiveness to Borrelia burgdorferi sensu lato in exposed asymptomatic children and children with previous clinical Lyme borreliosis. *Clin Devel Immunol*. 2012:Article ID 294587. https://www.scienceopen.com/document?id=178452fb-c22f-4ef9-a3cb-31caffb0c940.

Stanek G, Reiter M. The expanding Lyme borrelia complex—clinical significance of genomic species? *Clin Microbiol Infect*. Apr 2011;17(4):487–493.

Steere AC. Seronegative Lyme disease. *JAMA*. Sep 15,1993 Sep 15;270(11):1369.

Stricker RB, Johnson L. Lyme wars: let's tackle the testing. *BMJ*. Nov 17, 2007; 335(7628):1008.

Valentine-Thon E, et al. A novel lymphocyte transformation test for Lyme borreliosis. *Diagn Microbiol Infect Dis*. 2007;57:27–34.

Zhang X, Meltzer MI, Pena CA, Hopkins AB, Wroth L, Fix AD. Economic impact of Lyme disease. *Emerg Infect Dis*. 2006;12(4):653–660.

Three: Lyme Disease Specifics and Treatment Options

Alban PS, et al. Serum-starvation induced changes in protein synthesis and morphology of Borrelia burgdorferi. *Microbiology*. 2000;146:119–127.

Allen HB, Morales D, Jones K, Joshi S. Alzheimer's disease: a novel hypothesis integrating spirochetes, biofilm, and the immune system. *J Neuroinfect Dis*. 2016;7:200. doi:10.4172/2314-7326.1000200.

Allison KR, Brynildsen MP, Collins JJ. Metabolite-enabled eradication of bacterial persisters by aminoglycosides. *Nature*. May 12, 2011;473(7346):216–20. doi:10.1038/nature10069.

Bakkiyaraj D, Nandhini JR, Malathy B, Pandian SK. The anti-biofilm potential of pomegranate (Punica granatum L.) extract against human bacterial and fungal pathogens. *Biofouling*. 2013 Sep;29(8):929–37. doi:10.1080/08927014.2013.820825.

Beck G, Benach JL, Habicht GS. Isolation of interleukin-1 from joint fluids of patients with Lyme disease. *J Rheumatol*. 1989;16:802–806.

Brorson O, Brorson SH. A rapid method for generating cystic forms of Borrelia burgdorferi, and their reversal to mobile spirochetes. *APMIS*. 1998;106:1131–1141.

Brorson O, et al. Transformation of cystic forms of Borrelia burgdorferi to normal, mobile spirochetes. *Infection*. 1997;25;(4):240–245.

Cerhan JR, et al. Antioxidant micronutrients and risk of rheumatoid arthritis in a cohort of older women. *Am J Epidemiol*. 2003;157(4):345–354.

Dashper S, Ang C-S, Liu SW, Paolini R, Veith P, Reynolds E. Inhibition of porphyromonas gingivalis biofilm by Oxantel. *Antimicrob Agents Chemother*. Mar 2010:1311–1314.

Delong A, Blossom B, Maloney E, Phillips SE. Antibiotic retreatment of Lyme disease in patients with persistent symptoms: a biostatistical review of randomized, placebo-controlled, clinical trials. *Contemp Clin Trials*. Nov 2012;33(6):1132–1142. ISSN 1551-7144, 10.1016/j.cct.2012.08.009.

Feng J, Wang T, Shi W, Zhang S, Sullivan D, Auwaerter PG, et al. Identification of novel activity against Borrelia burgdorferi persisters using an FDA approved drug library. *Emerg Microbes Infect*. 2014;3:1–8.

Feng J, Weitner M, Shi W, Zhang S, Zhang Y. Eradication of biofilm-like microcolony structures of Borrelia burgdorferi by daunomycin and daptomycin but not Mitomycin C in combination with doxycycline and cefuroxime. *Front. Microbiol*. 2016:62. doi:10.3389/fmicb.2016.00062.

Ferrante A, et al. Tetrandrine, a plant alkaloid, inhibits production of tumor necrosis factor-alpha by human monocytes, *Clin Exp Immunol*. 1990;80(2):232–235.

Goc A, Niedzwiecki A, Rath M. In vitro evaluation of antibacterial activity of phytochemicals and micronutrients against Borrelia burgdorferi and Borrelia garinii. *J Appl Microbiol*. Dec 2015;119(6):1561–1572.

Hall-Stoodley L, Hu FZ, Gieseke A, Nistico L, Nguyen D, et al. Direct detection of bacterial biofilms on the middle-ear mucosa of children with chronic otitis media. *JAMA*. 2006;296:202–211.

Jacovides CL, Kreft R, Adeli B, Hozack B, Ehrlich GD, et al. Successful identification of pathogens by polymerase chain reaction (PCR)-based electron spray ionization time-of-flight mass spectrometry (ESI-TOF-MS) in culture-negative periprosthetic joint infection. *J Bone Joint Surg Am*. 2012;94:2247–2254.

Kung F, et al. Borrelia burgdorferi and tick proteins supporting pathogen persistence in the vector. *Future Microbiol*. 2013;8(1):41–56.

Lahesmaa R, Shanafelt MC, Steinman L, Peltz G. Immunopathogenesis of human inflammatory arthritis: lessons from Lyme and reactive arthritis. *J. Infect. Dis*. 1994;170:978–985.

Lewis K. Persister cells, dormancy and infectious disease. *Nature Rev Microbiol.* 2007;5(1):48–56. doi:10.1038/nrmicro1557. PMID 17143318.

MacDonald AB. Spirochetal cyst forms in neurodegenerative disorders, hiding in plain sight. *Med Hypotheses.* 2006; 67:819–832.

Mah TF. Regulating antibiotic tolerance within biofilm microcolonies. *J Bacteriol.* 2012;194:4791–4792.

Maisuria VB, et al. Polyphenolic extract from maple syrup potentiates antibiotic susceptibility and reduces biofilm formation of pathogenic bacteria. *Appl Environ Microbiol.* March 2015, doi:10.1128/AEM.00239-15.

Maurin et al. Phagolysosomal alkalinization and the bactericidal effect of antibiotics: the coxiella burnetii paradigm. *J Inf Dis.* 1992;166:1097–1102.

Miklossy J. Historic evidence to support a causal relationship between spirochetal infections and Alzheimer's disease. *Front Aging Neurosci.* 2015;7:46.

Nicolson G, et al. Role of chronic bacterial and viral infections in neurodegenerative, neurobehavioral, psychiatric, autoimmune and fatiguing illnesses (part I). *BJMP.* 2009;2(4):20–28.

Nistico L, et al. Pathogenic biofilms in adenoids: a reservoir for persistent bacteria. *J Clin Microbiol.* 2011;49(4):1411–1120.

Preac-Mursic V, et al. Formation and cultivation of Borrelia burgdorferi spheroplast-L-form variants. *Infection.* 1996;24(3):218–226.

Sapi E, Bastian SL, Mpoy CM, Scott S, Rattelle A, et al. Characterization of biofilm formation by Borrelia burgdorferi in vitro. *PLOS ONE.* 2012; 7(10):e48277. doi:10.1371/journal.pone.0048277.

Sapi E, MacDonald A. Biofilms of Borrelia burgdorferi in chronic cutaneous borreliosis. *Am J Clin Pathol.* 2008;129:988–989.

Sapi E, et al. Effectiveness of Stevia rebaudiana whole leaf extract against the various morphological forms of Borrelia burgdorferi in vitro. *Eur J Microbio Immunol.* 2015. doi: 10.1556/1886.2015.00031.

Stewart PS. Mechanisms of antibiotic resistance in bacterial biofilms. *Int J Med Microbiol.* 2012:107–113.

Todd S, Dahlgren F, Traeger M, et al. No evidence of tooth staining following doxycycline administration in children for treatment of Rocky Mountain spotted fever (abstract). *J Pediatr.* 2015;166:1246–1251.

Zientek J, Dahlgren FS, McQuiston JH, Regan J. Self-reported treatment practices by healthcare providers could lead to death from Rocky Mountain spotted fever. *J Pediatr.* 2014 Feb;164(2):416–8. doi:10.1016/j.jpeds.2013.10.008. Epub 2013 Nov 16.

Four: "Persisters" and Pulsing for Treating Resistant Lyme Disease

Berende A, ter Hofstede HJM, Vos FJ, et al. Randomized trial of longer-term therapy for symptoms attributed to Lyme disease. *New Engl J Med.* 2016;374(13):1209–1220.

Bonnet S, Michelet L, Moutailler S, Cheval J, Hébert C, Vayssier-Taussat M, et al. (2014) Identification of parasitic communities within European ticks using next-generation sequencing. *PLOS Negl. Trop Dis.* 8(3):e2753. doi:10.1371/journal.pntd.0002753.

Braun J, Laitko S, Treharne J, Eggens U, Wu P, Distler A, Sieper J. Chlamydia pneumoniae—a new causative agent of reactive arthritis and undifferentiated oligoarthritis. *Ann Rheum Dis.* 1994;Feb;53:100–105.

Breitschwerdt EB, Linder KL, Day MJ, Magg RG, Chomel BB, Kempf VA. Koch's postulates and the pathogenesis of comparative infectious disease causation associated with Bartonella species. *J Compar Path.* 2013;148(115):e125.

Cai H, Caswell JL, Prescott JF. Nonculture molecular techniques for diagnosis of bacterial disease in animals: a diagnostic laboratory perspective. *Veterinary Pathol.* Mar 2014;51(2):341–350.

Cameron DJ, Johnson LB, Maloney EL. Evidence assessments and guideline recommendations in Lyme disease: the clinical management of known tick bites, erythema migrans rashes and persistent disease. *Expert Rev Anti-Infective Ther.* Sep 2014;12(9):1103–1135.

Cappellini MD, Fiorelli G. Glucose-6-phosphate dehydrogenase deficiency. *Lancet.* Jan 2008;371(9606):64–74.

Caskey JR, Embers ME. Persister development by B. burgdorferi populations in vitro. *Antimicrob Agents Chemother.* 2015 Oct;59(10):6288–95. doi:10.1128/AAC.00883-15. Epub 2015 Jul 27.

Donta ST. Tetracycline therapy in chronic Lyme disease. *Chronic Infect Dis.* 1997;25(Suppl 1):552–556.

Elsner RA, Hastey CJ, Olsen KJ, Baumgarth N. Suppression of long-lived humoral immunity following Borrelia burgdorferi infection. *PLOS Pathol.* 2015;11(7):e1004976.

Fallon BA, Keilp JG, Corbera KM, Petkova E, Britton CB, Dwyer E, et al. A randomized, placebo-controlled trial of repeated IV antibiotic therapy for Lyme encephalopathy. *Neurology.* Mar 2008;25:992–1003.

Feng F, Shi W, Zhang S, Zhang Y. Identification of novel activity against Borrelia burgdorferi persisters using an FDA approved drug library. *Emerging Microbes Infect.* 2014;3:e49.

Feng J, Shi W, Zhang S, Zhang Y, Identification of new compounds with high activity against stationary phase Borrelia burgdorferi from the NCI compound collection. *Emerging Microbes Infect.* 2015;4:e31.

Fried MD, et al. Borrelia burgdorferi persists in the gastrointestinal tract of children and adolescents with Lyme disease. *J Spirochetal Tick-borne Dis.* Spring/Summer 2002;9:11–15.

Haupl T, et al. Persistence of Borrelia burgdorferi in ligamentous tissue from a patient with chronic Lyme borreliosis. *Arthritis Rheum.* 1993;36:1621–1626.

Hodzic E, Imai D, Feng S, Barthold SW. Resurgence of persisting non-cultivable Borrelia burgdorferi following antibiotic treatment in mice. (2014) *PLOS ONE.* 9(1):e86907. doi:10.1371/journal.pone.008690.

Hong Kong Chest Service, Medical Research Council (1981). Controlled trial of four thrice weekly regimens and a daily regimen given for 6 months for pulmonary tuberculosis. *Lancet.* 1981;1(8213):171–174.

Horowitz RI, Freeman PR. The use of dapsone as a novel "persister" drug in the treatment of chronic Lyme disease/post treatment Lyme disease syndrome. *J Clin Exp Dermatol Res.* 2016;7:345.

Horowitz RI. Chronic persistent Lyme borreliosis: PCR evidence of chronic infection despite extended antibiotic therapy: a retrospective review. International Science Conference on Lyme Disease. Mar 24–26, 2000: Abstract XIII.

Johnson BJB, Pilgard MA, Russell TM. 2014. Assessment of new culture method to detect borrelia species in serum of Lyme disease patients. *J. Clin. Microbiol.* 52:721–724. 10.1128/JCM.01674-13.

Keszler K, Tilton RC. Persistent PCR positivity in a patient being treated for Lyme disease. *J Spirochetal Tick-Borne Dis.* 1995;2(3):57–58.

Klempner M, Hu L, Evans J, Schmid C, Johnson G, Trevino R, et al. Two controlled trials of antibiotic treatment in patients with persistent symptoms and a history of Lyme disease. *New Engl J Med.* Jul 2001; Jul 12:85–92.

Krause PJ, Telford SR 3rd, Spielman A, et al. Concurrent Lyme disease and babesiosis: Evidence for increased severity and duration of illness. *JAMA.* 1996; 275(21):1657–1660.

Krupp LB, Hyman LG, Grimson R, Coyle PK, Melville P, Ahnn S, et al. Study and treatment of post Lyme disease (STOP-LD): a randomized double masked clinical trial. *Neurology.* Jun 24, 2003;60(12):1923–1930.

Lawrence C, Lipton RB, Lowy RD, Coyle PK. Seronegative chronic relapsing neuroborreliosis. *Eur Neurol*. 1995;35:113–117.

Livengood JA, Gilmore RD Jr. Invasion of human neuronal and glial cells by an infectious strain of Borrelia burgdorferi. *Microbes Infect*. Nov–Dec 2006;8(14–15):2832–2840.

Ma Y, et al. Intracellular localization of Borrelia burgdorferi within human endothelial cell. *Infect Immun*. Feb 1991;59(2):671–678.

Marques A, et al. Xenodiagnosis to detect Borrelia burgdorferi infection: a first-in-human study. *Clin Infect Dis*. 2014 Apr;58(7):937–45. doi:10.1093/cid/cit939. Epub 2014 Feb 11.

Masters EJ, et al. Spirochetemia after continuous high-dose oral amoxicillin therapy. *Infect Dis Clin Practice*. 1994;3:207–208.

Montgomery RR, Nathanson MH, Malawista SE. The fate of Borrelia burgdorferi, the agent for Lyme disease, in mouse macrophages. Destruction, survival, recovery. *J Immunol*. Feb 1, 1993;150(3):909–915.

Moutailler S, Valiente Moro C, Vaumourin E, et al. Coinfection of ticks: the rule rather than the exception. *PLOS Negl Trop Dis*. 2016;10(3):e0004539. doi:10.1371/journal.pntd.0004539.

Namrata P, Miller JM, Shilpa M, Reddy PR, Bandoski C, Rossi MJ, Sapi E. Filarial nematode infection in Ixodes scapularis ticks collected from southern Connecticut. *Veterinary Sci*. 2014;1(1):5–15.

Pausa M, et al. Serum resistant strains of Bb evade complement mediated killing by expressing a CD 59–like complement inhibitory molecule. *J Immunol*. Mar 15, 2003;170(6):3214–322.

Preac-Mursic V, et al. Persistence of Borrelia burgdorferi and histopathological alterations in experimentally infected animals. A comparison with histopathological findings in human Lyme disease. *Infection*. 1990;18(6):332–341.

Preac-Mursic V, et al. Survival of Borrelia burgdorferi in antibiotically treated patients with Lyme borreliosis. *Infection*. 1989;17:355–359.

Rehman HU. Methemoglobinemia. *West J Med*. 2001;175(3):193–196.

Rogovskyy AS, Bankhead T. Variable VlsE is critical for host reinfection by the Lyme disease spirochete. (2013) *PLOS ONE*. 8(4):e61226. doi:10.1371/journal.pone.0061226.

Sapi E, Balasubramanian K, Poruri A, Maghsoudlou JS, Socarras KM, Timmaraju KR., et al. Evidence of in vivo existence of borrelia biofilm in borrelial lymphocytomas. *Eur J Microbiol Immunol*. 2016;0:1–16.

Sapi E, Pabbati N, Datar A, Davies EM, Rattelle A, Kuo BA. Improved culture conditions for the growth and detection of borrelia from human serum. *Int J Med Sci*. 2013;10(4):362–76.

Schubbert R, Renz D, Schmitz B, Doerfler W. Foreign (M13) DNA ingested by mice reaches peripheral leukocytes, spleen, and liver via the intestinal wall mucosa and can be covalently linked to mouse DNA. *Proc Natl Acad Sci U. S*. Feb 4, 1997;94(3):961–966.

Sharma B, Brown AV, Matluck NE, Hu LT, Lewis K. Borrelia burgdorferi, the causative agent of lyme disease, forms drug-tolerant persister cells. *Antimicrob. Agents Chemother*. 2015;59:4616–4624. doi:10.1128/AAC.00864-15.

Straubinger RK, et al. Persistence of Borrelia burgdorferi in experimentally infected dogs after antibiotic treatment. *J Clin Microbiol*. 1997;35(1):111–116.

Tunev SS, Hastey CJ, Hodzic E, Feng S, Barthold SW, et al. Lymphoadenopathy during Lyme borreliosis is caused by spirochete migration-induced specific B cell activation. *PLOS Pathol*. 2011;7(5):e1002066.

Zhang Y, Yew WW, Barer MR. Targeting persisters for tuberculosis control. *Antimicrob Agents Chemother*. 2012;56(5):2223–2230.

Zhang Y. Persisters, persistent infections and the Yin–Yang model. *Emerging Microbes and Infect*. 2014;3:e3. doi:10.1038/emi.2014.3.

Zhang Y. Drug combinations against Borrelia burgdorferi persisters in vitro: eradication achieved by using daptomycin, cefoperazone and doxycycline. *PLOS ONE*. 2015;10(3):e0117207.

Zosel A, Rychter K, Leikin JB. Dapsone-induced methemoglobinemia: case report and literature review. *Am J Ther.* 2007;14(6):585–587.

Five: Ticks Can Carry More Than Lyme: Associated Bacterial Infections

Annen K, et al. Two cases of transfusion-transmitted Anaplasma phagocytophilum. *Am J Clinl Path.* Apr 2012;137(4):562–565.

Aranda EA. Treatment of tularemia with levofloxacin. *Clin.Microbiol Infect.* 2001;7:167–168.

Bacon RM, Kugeler KJ, Griffith KS, Mead PS, Centers for Disease Control and Prevention. http://www.cdc.gov/osels/psurveillance/nndss/casedef/lymediseasecurrent.htm; Centers for Disease Control and Prevention. MMWR56(23);573–576, June 15, 2007. http://www.cdc.gov/ncphi/disss/nndss/casedef/lyme disease_2008.htm.

Berghoff W. Chronic Lyme disease and co-infections: differential diagnosis. *Open Neurol J.* 2012;6:158–178.

Bergmans AMC, Peeters MF, Schellekens JFP, Vos MC, Saabe LJM, Ossewaarde JM, Verbakel H, et al. Pitfalls and fallacies of cat scratch disease serology: evaluation of Bartonella henselae-based indirect fluorescence assay and enzyme-linked immunoassay. *J Clin Microbiol.* 1997;35:1931–1937.

Bernit E, et al. Neurological involvement in acute Q fever, a report of 29 cases and review of the literature. *Arch Intern Med.* 2002;162(6):693–700.

Breitschwerdt EB, Maggi RG, Cadenas MB, de Paiva Diniz PP. A groundhog, a novel Bartonella sequence, and my father's death. *Emerging Infectious Diseases.* 2009;15(12):2080–2086. doi:10.3201/eid1512.090206.

Breitschwerdt EB, Maggi RG, Farmer P, Mascarelli PE. Molecular evidence of perinatal transmission of Bartonella vinsonii subsp. berkhoffii and B. henselae to a child. *J Clin Microbiol.* 2010;48:2289–2293. doi:10.1128/JCM.00326-10.

Breitschwerdt E. Did Bartonella henselae contribute to the deaths of two veterinarians? *Parasites Vectors.* 2015;8:317.

Breitschwerdt E, et al. Bartonella sp. bacteremia in patients with neurological and neurocognitive dysfunction. *J Clin Microbiol.* Sept 2008:2856–2861.

Centers for Disease Control and Prevention. Three sudden cardiac deaths associated with Lyme carditis—United States, November 2012–July 2013. MMWR. 201(62):993–996.

Chagnon S. Child neurology: tick paralysis, a diagnosis not to miss. *Neurology.* Mar 18, 2014; 82:(11):e91-e93.

Chmielewski T. Bacterial tick-borne diseases caused by Bartonella spp., Borrelia burgdorferi sensu lato, Coxiella burnetii, and Rickettsia spp. among patients with cataract surgery. *Med Sci Monit.* 2014;20:927–931.

Chowdri HR, et al., Borrelia miyamotoi Infection presenting as human granulocytic anaplasmosis: a case report. *Ann Intern Med.* 2013;159(1):21–27. doi:10.7326/0003-4819-159-1-201307020-00005.

Clark KL, Leydet B, Hartman S. Lyme borreliosis in human patients in Florida and Georgia, USA. *Int J Med Sci.* 2013;10(7):915–931. doi:10.7150/ijms.6273.

Cook MJ. Lyme borreliosis: a review of data on transmission time after tick attachment. *International Journal of General Medicine.* 2015;8:1–8. doi:10.2147/IJGM.S73791.

Dworkin MS, Schwan TG, Anderson DE Jr, Borchardt SM. Tick-borne relapsing fever. *Infect Dis Clin North Am.* 2008;22:449–68, viii.

Fernandes EC, et al. Exposure to air pollutants and disease activity in juvenile-onset systemic lupus Erythematosus patients. *Arthr Care Res.* Nov 2015;67,(11):1609–1614.

Fernandez SV, et al. Bartonella henselae infection detected in patients with inflammatory breast cancer. Thirty-Fifth Annual CTRC-AACR San Antonio Breast Cancer Symposium, San Antonio, Tx, Dec 4–8, 2012 (abstracts).

Flexman JP, Chen SC, Dickeson DJ, Pearman JW, Gilbert GL. Detection of antibodies to Bartonella henselae in clinically diagnosed cat scratch disease. *Med J Aust.* May 19, 1997;166(10):532–535.

Forrester JD, Kjemtrup AM, Fritz CL, et al. Tickborne relapsing fever—United States, 1990–2011. *Morb Mortal Wkly Report.* 2015;64:58–60.

Girard YA, Fedorova N, Lane RS. Genetic diversity of Borrelia burgdorferi and detection of B. bissettii–like DNA in serum of north-coastal California residents. *J Clin Microbiol.* 2011; 49:945–54.

Hartzell J, et al. Q fever: epidemiology, diagnosis, and treatment. *Mayo Clin Proc.* May 2008; 83(5):574–579.

Herman-Giddens ME. Erythema migrans-like lesions in the South require treatment given the current state of knowledge. *Vector-Borne Zoonotic Dis.* 2014;14(X): 2014. doi:10.1089/vbz .2013.1545.

Horowitz RI, et al. Bartonella henselae: limitations of serological testing. Evaluation of ELISA and polymerase chain reaction testing in a cohort of Lyme disease patients and implications for treatment (abstract). Sixteenth International Scientific Conference on Lyme Disease and Other Tick-Borne Disorders. Hartford, CT, June 2003.

Horowitz RI, et al. Borrelia burgdorferi and Bartonella henselae: a study comparing tetracyclines in combination with quinolones in co-infected patients. Abstract, 16th International Scientific Conference on Lyme Disease & Other Tick-Borne Disorders. Hartford, Connecticut, June 2003.

Horowitz RI, et al. Mycoplasma infections in chronic Lyme disease: a retrospective analysis of co-infection and persistence demonstrated by PCR analysis despite long term antibiotic treatment (abstract). 16th International Scientific Conference on Lyme Disease & Other Tick-Borne Disorders. Hartford, Connecticut, June 2003.

Inman et al. Heavy metal exposure reverses genetic resistance to Chlamydia-induced arthritis. *Arthritis Research & Therapy.* 2009;11:R19. doi:10.1186/ar2610.

Jensen WA, Fall MZ, Rooney J, Kordick DL, Breitschwerdt EB. Rapid identification and differentiation of Bartonella species using a single-step PCR assay. *J Clin Microbiol.* 2000;38(5):1717–1722.

Jones JM. Notes from the field: tickborne relapsing fever outbreak at an outdoor education camp—Arizona, 2014. *Morb Mortal Wkly Report.* June 19, 2015;64(23);651–652.

Kaya A, et al. tularemia in children: evaluation of clinical, laboratory and therapeutic features of 27 tularemia cases. *Turkish J Pediat.* 2012;54:105–112.

Kempf VA, Volkmann B, Schaller M, et al. Evidence of a leading role for VEGF in Bartonella henselae-induced endothelial cell proliferations. *Cell Microbiol.* 2001;3(9):623–632.

Kosoy OI, Lambert AJ, Hawkinson DJ, Pastula DM, Goldsmith CS, Hunt DC, et al. Novel thogotovirus species associated with febrile illness and death, United States, 2014. *Emerg Infect Dis.* May 2015. https://wwwnc.cdc.gov/eid/article/21/5/pdfs/15-0150.pdf.

La Scola B, Raoult D. Culture of Bartonella quintana and Bartonella henselae from human samples: a 5-year experience (1993 to 1998). *J. Clin. Microbiol.* 1999;37:1899–1905.

Lantos PM, Brinkerhoff RJ, Wormser GP, Clemen R. Empiric antibiotic treatment of erythema migrans-like skin lesions as a function of geography: a clinical and cost-effectiveness modeling study. *Vector-Borne Zoonotic Dis* 2013;13:877–883.

Lee SH, Vigliotti J, Vigliotti V, Jones W, Shearer DM. Detection of borreliae in archived sera from patients with clinically suspect lyme disease. *Int. J. Mol. Sci.* 2014, 15(3), 4284–4298; doi:10.3390/ijms15034284.

Li H, Zheng YC, Ma L, Jia N, Jiang BG, Jiang RR, Huo QB, Wang YW, Liu HB, Chu YL, Song YD, Yao NN, Sun T, Zeng FY, Dumler JS, Jiang JF, Cao WC. Human infection with a novel tickborne anaplasma species in China: a surveillance study. *Lancet Infect Dis.* 2015 Jun;15(6): 663–70. doi:10.1016/S1473-3099(15)70051-4. Epub 2015 Mar 29.

Maggi RG, et al. Bartonella spp. bacteremia and rheumatic symptoms in patients from Lyme disease–endemic region. *Emerg Infect Dis.* May 2012; 18(5) 783–791.

Margos G, Piesman J, Lane RS, Ogden NH, Sing A, Straubinger RK, Fingerle V. Borrelia kurtenbachii sp. nov., a widely distributed member of the Borrelia burgdorferi sensu lato species complex in North America. *Int J Syst Evol Microbiol.* 2014 Jan;64(Pt 1):128–30. doi:10.1099/ijs.0.054593-0. Epub 2013 Sept 18.

Masters EJ, Donnell HD. Lyme and/or Lyme-like disease in Missouri. *Mo Med.* 1995;92:346–353.

Na Jia N, Zheng YC, Jiang JF, Ma L, Cao WC. Human infection with candidatus rickettsia tarasevichiae. *N Engl J Med.* Sept 19, 2013; 369:1178–1180.

Nicolson G, et al. Role of chronic bacterial and viral infections in neurodegenerative, neurobehavioral, psychiatric, autoimmune and fatiguing illnesses (part 1). *BJMP.* 2009;2(4) 20–28.

Nicolson GL. Chronic infections as a common etiology for many patients with chronic fatigue syndrome, fibromyalgia syndrome and Gulf War illnesses. *Intern J Med.* 1998;1:42–46.

Paul J. Colorado health officials: tularemia cases on record-breaking pace. *Denver Post* [Denver] 24 June 2015: http://www.denverpost.com/news/ci_28374467/colorado-health-officials-tularemia-cases-record-breaking-pace.

Pritt BS, et al. Identification of a novel pathogenic borrelia species causing Lyme borreliosis with unusually high spirochaetaemia: a descriptive study. *Lancet.* Online Feb 5, 2016. http://thelancet.com/journals/laninf/article/PIIS1473-3099(15)00464-8/abstract.

Raoult D, et al. Treatment of Q fever endocarditis. *Arch Intern Med.* Jan 25, 1999:159.

Rolain JM, Brouqui P, Koehler JE, Maguina C, Dolan MJ, Raoult D. Recommendations for treatment of human infections caused by Bartonella species. *Antimicrob Agents Chemother.* 2004;48(6):1921–1933.

Rudenko N, et al. Isolation of live Borrelia burgdorferi sensu lato spirochetes from patients with undefined disorders and symptoms not typical for Lyme borreliosis. *Clin Microbiol Infect.* Dec 2015 7. pii: S1198-743X(15)00991-X. doi:10.1016/j.cmi.2015.11.009.

Shah J, Horowitz R. Human babesiosis and ehrlichiosis—current status. *Eur Infect Dis.* Spring 2012;6(1).

Sriram S, Stratton CW, Yao S, et al. (1999). Chlamydia pneumoniae infection of the central nervous system in multiple sclerosis. *Ann Neurol.* 46(1):6–14.

Stanek G, Strle F. Lyme disease: European perspective. *Infect. Dis. Clin. North Am.* June 2008; 22(2):327–39, vii.

Todd S, Dahlgren F, Traeger M, et al. No evidence of tooth staining following doxycycline administration in children for treatment of Rocky Mountain spotted fever. *J Pediatr.* 2015;166:1246–1251.

Vineyard Gazette. May 21, 2015. http://vineyardgazette.com/news/2015/05/21/education-key-stop-tick-borne-illnesses-white-clothes-help-too?k=vg556221f10aedc&r=1.

Yeşilyurt M, Kılıç S, Bekir ÇB, Mesure Ç, Serdar G, Fikret E, et al. Antimicrobial susceptibilities of Francisella tularensis subsp. holarctica strains isolated from humans in the Central Anatolia region of Turkey. *J. Antimicrob. Chemother.* 2011.

Zemtsova GE, Killmaster LF, Montgomery M, Schumacher L, Burrows M, Levin Michael L. First report of rickettsia identical to R. slovaca in colony-originated D. variabilis in the United States: detection, laboratory animal model, and vector competence of ticks. *Vector Borne Zoonotic Dis* 2016 Feb 25;16(2):77–84. Epub 2016 Jan 25.

Six: Lyme and Other Co-infections: Parasitic, Viral, and Fungal Infections

Allred, DR. Babesiosis: persistence in the face of adversity. *Parasitol Today.* 2003;19:51–55.

Bonnet S, Michelet L, Moutailler S, Cheval J, Hébert C, Vayssier-Taussat M, et al. (2014) Identification of parasitic communities within European ticks using next-generation sequencing. *PLOS Negl Trop Dis.* 8(3):e2753. doi:10.1371/journal.pntd.0002753.

Bugyei KA, et al. Clinical efficacy of a tea-bag formulation of Cryptolepis sanguinolenta root in the treatment of acute uncomplicated falciparum malaria. *Ghana Med J.* Mar 2010;44(1).

Cursino-Santos JR, Singh M, Pham P, Rodriguez M, Lobo CA. Babesia divergens builds a complex population structure composed of specific ratios of infected cells to ensure a prompt response to changing environmental conditions. *Cell Microbiol.* 2016 Jun;18(6):859–74. doi: 10.1111/cmi.12555. Epub 2016 Jan 20.

Dupuis AP II, et al. Isolation of deer tick virus (Powassan virus, lineage II) from Ixodes scapularis and detection of antibody in vertebrate hosts sampled in the Hudson Valley, New York State. *Parasites Vectors.* 2013;6:185. doi:10.1186/1756-3305-6-185.

Hamer SA, Hickling GJ, Walker ED, Tsao JI. Increased diversity of Zoonotic pathogens and Borrelia burgdorferi strains in established versus incipient Ixodes scapularis populations across the midwestern United States. *Infect. Genetics Evol.* 2014;27:531–542.

Hersh M, et al. Reservoir competence of wildlife host species for Babesia microti. *Emerg Infect Dis.* Dec 2012;18(12). http://wwwnc.cdc.gov/eid/article/18/12/11-1392_article.

Hersh MH, Ostfeld RS, McHenry DJ, Tibbetts M, Brunner JL, Killilea ME, et al. (2014) Coinfection of blacklegged ticks with Babesia microti and Borrelia burgdorferi is higher than expected and acquired from small mammal hosts. *PLOS ONE.* 9(6):e99348. doi:10.1371/journal.pone.0099348.

Hojgaard A, Lukacik G, Piesman J. Detection of Borrelia burgdorferi, Anaplasma phagocytophilum and Babesia microti, with two different multiplex PCR assays. *Ticks Tick-Borne Dis.* 2014 Apr;5(3):349–51. doi:10.1016/j.ttbdis.2013.12.001. Epub 2014 Jan 18.

Horowitz, R. Chronic persistent babesiosis after C+Q/ M+Z (abstract). Twelfth Int Conference on Lyme Borreliosis, New York City. April 1999.

Horowitz RI, Freeman PR. Are mycobacterium drugs effective for treatment resistant Lyme disease, tick-borne co-infections, and autoimmune disease? *JSM Arthritis* (2016) 1(2):1008.

Horowitz RI, Freeman PR. The use of Dapsone as a novel "persister" drug in the treatment of chronic Lyme disease/post treatment Lyme disease syndrome. *J Clin Exp Dermatol Res.* 2016;7:(3).

Joseph JT, Purtill K, Wong SJ, Munoz J, Teal A, Madison-Antenucci S, et al. Vertical transmission of Babesia microti, United States. *Emerg Infect Dis.* Aug 18, 2012;18(8):1318–1321.

Juven B, et al. Studies on the mechanism of antimicrobial action of oleuropein. *J of App Bacteriol.* 1970;35: 559–567.

Krause PJ, et al. Persistent parasitemia after acute babesiosis. *NEJM.* 1998 Jul 16;339(3):160–5.

Kumar P, Marshall BC, Deblois G, Koch WC. A cluster of transfusion-associated babesiosis in extremely low birthweight premature infants. *J Perinatol.* 2012;32:731–733.

Lempereur L, et al. A retrospective serological survey on human babesiosis in Belgium. *Clin Microbiol Infect.* Jan 2015;21(1):96.e1–7.

Lieberman, S, Enig MG, Preuss HG. A review of monolaurin and lauric acid: natural virucidal and bactericidal agents. *Alt Complement Thera.* 2006;12(6):310–314.

Martinsen ES, McInerney N, Brightman H, Ferebee K, Walsh T, McShea WJ, et al. Hidden in plain sight: cryptic and endemic malaria parasites in North American white-tailed deer (Odocoileus virginianus). *Sci Adv.* Feb 2016; 5;2(2):e1501486.

Mechelli R, et al. Epstein-Barr virus genetic variants are associated with multiple sclerosis. *Neurology.* Mar 31, 2015;84(13):1362–1368.

Middelveen MJ, Burugu D, Porur A, et al. Association of spirochetal infection with Morgellons disease. *F1000 Res.* 2013;2:25 v1.

Middelveen MJ, et al. Exploring the association between Morgellons disease and Lyme disease: identification of Borrelia burgdorferi in Morgellons disease patients. *BMC Dermatol.* Feb 12, 2015;15(1):1.

Miotto O, et al. Multiple populations of artemisinin-resistant Plasmodium falciparum in Cambodia. *Nat Genet.* Jun 2013;45(6):648–55.

Moutailler S, Valiente Moro C, Vaumourin E, Michelet L, Tran FH, Devillers E, et al. Coinfection of ticks: the rule rather than the exception. *PLOS Negl Trop Dis.* 2016;10(3).

Murray PK, Jennings FW, Murray M, Urquhart GM. The nature of immunosuppression in Trypanosoma brucei infections in mice: II. The role of the T and B lymphocytes. *Immunology.* 1974;27(5):825–840.

Plerer M, et al. Association of anti-cytomegalovirus seropositivity with more severe joint destruction and more frequent joint surgery in rheumatoid arthritis. *Arthritis Rheum.* 2012;64: 1740–1749.

Sayler KA, Barbet AF, Chamberlain C, Clapp WL, Alleman R, et al. Isolation of tacaribe virus, a Caribbean arenavirus, from host-seeking Amblyomma americanum ticks in Florida. *PLOS ONE.* 2014;9(12):e115769.

Tanyel E, et al. A case of severe babesiosis treated successfully with exchange transfusion. *International Journal of Infectious Diseases* 38 (2015) 83–85.

Wormser GP, Prasad A, Neuhaus E, Joshi S, Nowakowski J, Nelson J, Mittleman A, Aguero-Rosenfeld M, Topal J, Krause PJ. Emergence of resistance to azithromycin-atovaquone in immunocompromised patients with Babesia microti infections. *Clin Infect Dis.* 2010 Feb 1; 50(3):381–6. doi:10.1086/649859.

Yang Y-S, Murciano B, Moubri K, Cibrelus P, Schetters T, Gorenflot A, et al. Structural and functional characterization of Bc28.1, major erythrocyte-binding protein from *Babesia canis* merozoite surface. *J Biol Chem.* 2012;287(12):9495–9508.

Zanet S, Trisciuoglio A, Bottero E, Garcia de Mera I, Gortazar C, Grazia Carpignano MG, et al. Piroplasmosis in wildlife: Babesia and Theileria affecting free-ranging ungulates and carnivores in the Italian Alps. *Parasites Vectors.* 2014;7:70.

Zhang X, Norris DE, Rasgon JL. Distribution and molecular characterization of Wolbachia endosymbionts and filarial nematodes in Maryland populations of the lone star tick (Amblyomma americanum). *FEMS Microbiol. Ecol.* 2011, 77, 50–56.

Seven: Lyme and Immune Dysfunction

Alaedini A, Latov N. Antibodies against OspA epitopes of Borrelia burgdorferi cross-react with neural tissue. *J Neuroimmunol.* 2005;(159):192–195.

Braun J, Laitko S, Treharne J, et al. Chlamydia pneumoniae—a new causative agent of reactive arthritis and undifferentiated oligoarthritis. *Annals of the Rheumatic Diseases.* 1994;53(2):100–105.

Buzzard EF. The treatment of disseminated sclerosis. *Lancet,* January 1911, vol. 177, No 4559(11):98.

Campfield BT, Nolder CL, Marinov A, Bushnell D, Davis A, Spychala C, et al. Follistatin-like protein 1 is a critical mediator of experimental Lyme arthritis and the humoral response to Borrelia burgdorferi infection. *Microb Pathog.* 2014 Aug;73:70–9. doi:10.1016/j.micpath .2014.04.005. Epub 2014 Apr 24.

Cimmino MA, Trevisan G. Lyme arthritis presenting as adult onset Still's disease. *Clin Exp Rheumatol.* May–June 1989;7(3):305–308.

Coblyn JS, Taylor P. Treatment of chronic Lyme arthritis with hydroxychloroquine. *Arthritis Rheum.* Dec 1981;24(12):1567–1569.

Cree BA, Kornyeyeva E, Goodin DS. Pilot trial of low-dose naltrexone and quality of life in MS. *Ann Neurol.* 2010 Aug;68(2):145–50. doi: 10.1002/ana.22006.

Dorward D, et al. Invasion and cytopathic killing of human lymphocytes by spirochetes causing Lyme disease. *Clin Infect Dis.* July 1997;25(Suppl 1):S2–8,209.

Fritzsche M. Chronic Lyme borreliosis at the root of MS—is a cure with antibiotics attainable? *Med Hypotheses.* 2005;64(3):438–448.

Furr PM, Taylor-Robinson D, Webster AD. Mycoplasmas and ureaplasmas in patients with hypogammaglobulinaemia and their role in arthritis: microbiological observations over twenty years. *Ann Rheum Dis.* 1994;(53):183–184.

Garcia-Monco JC, et al. Multiple sclerosis or Lyme disease? A diagnostic problem of exclusion. *Med/Clin* (Barcelona). May 12, 1990;94(18):685–688.

Halperin JJ, et al. Lyme neuroborreliosis: central nervous system manifestations. *Neurology.* Jun 1989;39(6):753–759.

Hansen K, et al. Oligoclonal B burgdorferi-specific IgG antibodies in CSF in Lyme neuroborreliosis. *J Inf Dis.* Jun 1990;161(6):1194–1202.

Inman RD, Chui B. Heavy metal exposure reverses genetic resistance to Chlamydia-induced arthritis. *Arth Res Ther.* Feb 2009;11:R19. doi:10.1186/ar2610.

Irie S, Saito T, Kanazawa N, et al. Relationships between anti-ganglioside antibodies and clinical characteristics of Guillain-Barré syndrome. *Intern Med.* 1997;36(9):607–612. doi:10.2169/internalmedicine.36.607.

"Joint Pain From the Gut." *The Atlantic.* 12 Jan. 2015. Web. http://www.theatlantic.com/health/archive/2015/01/joint-pain-from-the-gut/383772/.

Karma A, et al. Diagnosis and clinical characteristics of ocular Lyme borreliosis. *Am J Ophthalmol.* Feb 1995;119(2):127–135.

Kharrazian D. The potential roles of Bisphenol A (BPA) pathogenesis in autoimmunity. *Autoimmune Diseases.* 2014;(743616):12.

Kohler J, et al. Chronic central nervous system involvement in Lyme borreliosis. *Neurology.* Jun 1988;38(6):863–867.

Kologrivova EN, et al. Intensity of the production of rheumatoid factor in patients with different degrees of sensitization to B. garinii antigens. *Zh Mikrobiol Epidemiol Immunobiol.* Mar–Apr 2005;(2):80–83.

Kurtz SK. Relapsing fever/Lyme disease, multiple sclerosis. *Med Hypotheses.* Nov 1986;21(3): 335–343.

Linden J, Fischetti VA, Vartanian T. Isolation of Clostridium perfringens type B in an individual at first clinical presentation of multiple sclerosis provides clues for environmental triggers of the disease. *PLOS ONE.* 2013;8(10):e76359.

Maggi RG, et al. Bartonella spp. bacteremia and rheumatic symptoms in patients from Lyme disease–endemic region. *Emerg Infect Dis.* May 2012;18(5):783–791.

Marshall V. Multiple sclerosis is a chronic central nervous system infection by a spirochetal agent. *Med Hypotheses.* Feb 1988;25:2: 89–92.

Mechelli R, et al. Epstein-Barr virus genetic variants are associated with multiple sclerosis. *Neurology.* Mar 31, 2015;84(13):1362–1368.

Miner J, et al. Chikungunya viral arthritis in the United States: a mimic of seronegative rheumatoid arthritis. *Arthritis & Rheumatology,* 2015; 67:1214–1220. doi:10.1002/art.39027.

Mühlradt PF, Quentmeier H, Schmitt E. Involvement of interleukin-1 (IL-1), IL-6, IL-2 and IL-4 in generation of cytolytic T cells from thymocytes stimulated by a Mycoplasma fermentans-derived product. *Infect Immun.* 1991;59:3962–3968.

Munger K, et al. Vitamin D intake and incidence of multiple sclerosis. *Neurology.* Jan 13, 2004;62(1): 60–65.

Nicolson GL, Haier J. Role of chronic bacterial and viral Infections in neurodegenerative, neurobehavioral, psychiatric, autoimmune and fatiguing illnesses, part 2. *Br J Med. Pract.* 2010;3(1):301a–311.

Olivares JP, et al. Lyme disease presenting as isolated acute urinary retention caused by transverse myelitis; an electrophysiological and urodynamical study. *Arch Phys Med Rehabil.* Dec 1995;76(12):1171–1172.

Pfau J, et al. Autoimmunity and asbestos exposure. *Autoimmune Dis.* 2014. doi:10.1155/2014/782045.

Plerer M, et al. Association of anti-cytomegalovirus seropositivity with more severe joint destruction and more frequent joint surgery in rheumatoid arthritis. *Arthritis Rheum.* 2012;64: 1740–1749.

Rogers HJ. Short notes and clinical cases: the question of silver cells as proof of the spirochætal theory of disseminated sclerosis. *J Neurol Psychopathol.* 1932 Jul;13(49):50–1.

Roush JK, et al. Rheumatoid arthritis subsequent to Borrelia burgdorferi infection in two dogs. *J Am Vet Med Assoc.* 1989 Oct 1;195(7):951–3.

Saulsbury FT. Lyme arthritis in 20 children residing in a non-endemic area. *Clin Pediatr* (Phila). Jun 2005;44(5):419–421.

Schnarr S, et al. *Chlamydia* and *Borrelia* DNA in synovial fluid of patients with early undifferentiated oligoarthritis: results of a prospective study. *Arthritis Rheum.* 2001;44(11):2679–2685.

Simecka JW, et al. Interactions of mycoplasmas with B cells: antibody production and nonspecific effects. *Clin Infect Dis.* 1993;17(Suppl 1):S176–S182.

Smith JP, Stock H, Bingaman S, Mauger D, Rogosnitzky M, Zagon IS. Low-dose naltrexone therapy improves active Crohn's disease. *Am J Gastroenterol.* 2007 Apr;102(4):820–8. Epub 2007 Jan 11.

Steere A, et al. Antibiotic-refractory Lyme arthritis is associated with HLA-DR molecules that bind a Borrelia burgdorferi peptide. *JEM.* April 17, 2006;203(4): 961–971.

Steere AC, Dwyer E, Winchester R. Association of chronic Lyme arthritis with HLA-DR4 and HLA-DR2 alleles. *N Engl J Med.* 1990;(323):219–23.

Steiner G. Acute plaques in MS, their pathogenetic significance and the role of spirochetes as the etiological factor. *J. Neuropath & Exp Neur.* 1954;11(4):343.

Steiner G. Morphology of Spirochaeta myelophthora in multiple sclerosis. *J Neuropath Exp Neurol.* 1954 Jan;13(1):221–9.

Summerday NM, et al. Vitamin D and multiple sclerosis: review of a possible association. *J Pharm Practice.* 2012:75–84.

Walsh N. Beyond asbestos: autoimmunity, pollution, and particles. *MedPage Today.* Aug 13, 2014; http://www.medpagetoday.com/rheumatology/generalrheumatology/47186.

Weigelt W, Schneider T, Lange R. Sequence homology between spirochete flagellin and human myelin basic protein. *Immunol Today.* Jul 1992;13(7):279–280.

Weiss NL, Sadock VA, Sigal LH, et al. False-positive seroreactivity to Borrelia burgdorferi in systemic lupus erythematosus: the value of immunoblot analysis. *Lupus.* 1995;4:131–137.

Whitmire WM, Garon CF. Specific and nonspecific responses of murine B cells to membrane blebs of Borrelia burgdorferi. *Infect Immun.* 1993;(61):1460–1467.

Wilder RL, Crofford LJ. Do infectious agents cause rheumatoid arthritis? *Clin Orthop Relat Res.* 1991 Apr;(265):36–41.

Zeft A. Beyond asbestos: autoimmunity, pollution, and particles. *Ped Rheum.* Aug 13, 2014..

Eight: Lyme and Inflammation

Alaedini A, Latov N. Antibodies against OspA epitopes of Borrelia burgdorferi cross-react with neural tissue. *J Neuroimmunol.* 2005;159:192–195.

Allen HB, Morales D, Jones K, Joshi S. Alzheimer's disease: a novel hypothesis integrating spirochetes, biofilm, and the immune system. *J Neuroinfect Dis.* 2007;(7):200. doi:10.4172/2314-7326.1000200.

Braun J, et al. Chlamydia pneumoniae, a new causative agent of reactive arthritis and undifferentiated oligoarthritis. *Ann Rheum Dis.* 1994;(53):100–105.

Casjens S, et al. Borrelia genomes in the year 2000. *J. Mol. Microbiol Biotech.* 2000;2(4):401–410.

Clarkson T, Magos L. The toxicology of mercury and its chemical compounds. *Critic Rev Toxicol*. 2006;(36):609–662.

Clauw DJ, et al. Chronic pain and fatigue syndromes: overlapping clinical and neuroendocrine features and potential pathogenic mechanisms. *Neuroimmunomodulation*. 1997;(4):134–153.

Fallon BA, Levin ES, Schweitzer PJ, Hardesty D. Inflammation and central nervous system Lyme disease. *Neurobiol Dis*. 2010;(10)534–541.

Fraser CM, et al. Genomic sequence of a Lyme disease spirochaete, Borrelia burgdorferi. *Nature*. Dec 11, 1997;390(6660):580–586.

Furr PM, Taylor-Robinson D, Webster AD. Mycoplasmas and ureaplasmas in patients with hypogammaglobulinemia and their role in arthritis: microbiological observations over twenty years. *Ann Rheum Dis*. 1994;53;183–184.

Gallagher CM, Meliker JR. Mercury and thyroid autoantibodies in U.S. women, NHANES 2007–2008. *Environ Intl*. Apr 2012;(40):39–43. Published online Dec 27, 2011.

Haack M, Kraus T, Schuld A, Dalal M, Koethe D, Pollmächer T. Diurnal variations of interleukin-6 plasma levels are confounded by blood drawing procedures. *Psychoneuroendocrinology*. 2002;27:921–31.

Hawn TR, Misch EA, Dunstan SJ, et al. A common human TLR1 polymorphism regulates the innate immune response to lipopeptides. *Eur J Immunol*. 2007;37:2280–2289.

Inman RD, et al. Heavy metal exposure reverses genetic resistance to Chlamydia-induced arthritis. *Arthritis Res Ther*. Feb 2009;(11):R19.

Johnson CM, Lyle EA, Omueti KO, Stepensky VA, Yegin O, Alpsoy E, Hamann L, Schumann RR, Tapping RI. Cutting edge: a common polymorphism impairs cell surface trafficking and functional responses of TLR1 but protects against leprosy. *J Immunol*. 2007 Jun 15;178(12):7520–4.

Kharrazian D. The potential roles of Bisphenol A (BPA) pathogenesis in autoimmunity. *Autoimmune Diseases*. 2014;2014:743616. doi:10.1155/2014/743616.

Lorton D, et al. Bidirectional communication between the brain and the immune system: implications for physiological sleep and disorders with disrupted sleep. *Neuroimmunomodulation*. 2006;13(5–6):357–374. Published online Aug 2007.

Maggi RG, Mozayeni BR, Pultorak EL, Hegarty BC, Bradley JM, Correa M, Breitschwerdt EB. Bartonella spp. bacteremia and rheumatic symptoms in patients from Lyme disease–endemic region. *Emerg Infect Dis*. 2012 May;18(5):783–791.

Moldofsky H. Sleep and the immune system. *Int J Immunopharmacol*. 1995;(17):649–654.

Mühlradt PF, Quentmeier H, Schmitt E. Involvement of interleukin-1 (IL-1), IL-6, IL-2, and IL-4 in generation of cytolytic T cells from thymocytes stimulated by a Mycoplasma fermentans-derived product. *Infect Immun*. Nov 1991;59(11):3962–3968.

Nathan C, Ding A. Nonresolving inflammation. *Cell*. 2010;140:871–882.

Nicolson GL, Gan R, Haier J. Evidence for Brucella spp. and Mycoplasma spp. coinfections in the blood of chronic fatigue syndrome patients. *J. Chron Fatigue Syndr*. 2005;12(2):5–17.

Nielsen JB, Hultman P. Experimental studies on genetically determined susceptibility to mercury-induced autoimmune response. *Renal Failure*. May–Jul 1999;21(3–4):343–348.

Pachner AR, Steiner I. Lyme Neuroborreliosis: infection, immunity and inflammation. *Lancet Neurology*. 2007;(6):544–552.

Parks CG, Cooper GS. Occupational exposures and risk of systemic lupus erythematosus: a review of the evidence and exposure assessment methods in population-and clinic-based studies. *Lupus*. 2006;(15):728–736.

Pfau JC, Serve KM, Noonan CW. Autoimmunity and asbestos exposure. *Autoimmune Diseases*. 2014; 2014, Article ID 782045, doi:10.1155/2014/782045.

Prasad AS, et al. Zinc supplementation decreases incidence of infections in the elderly: effect of zinc on generation of cytokines and oxidative stress1,2,3. *Am J Clin Nutr*. 2007;(85):837–844.

Recchiuti A. Immunoresolving lipid mediators and resolution of inflammation in aging. *J Gerontol Geriat Res.* 2014;3:151.

Roe HR, Jumper JM, Fu AD, et al. Ocular Bartonella infections. *International Ophthalmology Clinics.* 2008;48:93–105.

Russell IJ. Neurochemical pathogenesis of fibromyalgia syndrome. *J Musculoskel Pain.* 1996; 4:61–92.

Schnarr S, et al. Chlamydia and Borrelia DNA in synovial fluid of patients with early undifferentiated oligoarthritis: results of a prospective study. *Arthritis Rheumatism.* 2001;44(11):2679–2685.

Simecka JW, et al. Interactions of mycoplasmas with B cells: antibody production and nonspecific effects. *Clin Infect Dis.* 1993;1(Supplement 1):S176–S182.

Soloski MJ, Crowder LA, Lahey LJ, Wagner CA, Robinson WH, et al. Serum inflammatory mediators as markers of human Lyme disease activity. *PLOS ONE.* 9(4):e93243. http://doi.org/10 .1371/journal.pone.0093243.

Sommer C, et al. Recent findings on how proinflammatory cytokines cause pain: peripheral mechanisms and inflammatory and neuropathic hyperalgesia. *Neurosci.* 2004:184–187(Letters: 361).

Steere A, et al. Antibiotic-refractory Lyme arthritis is associated with HLA-DR molecules that bind a Borrelia burgdorferi peptide. *JEM.* Apr 17, 2006;203(4):961–971.

Steere AC, et al. Association of chronic Lyme arthritis with HLA-DR4 and HLA-DR2 alleles. *N Engl J Med.* 1990;(323):219–223.

Strle K, Drouin EE, Shen S, et al. Borrelia burgdorferi stimulates macrophages to secrete higher levels of cytokines and chemokines than Borrelia afzelii or Borrelia garinii. *The Journal of Infectious Diseases.* 2009;200(12):1936–1943. doi:10.1086/648091.

Strle K, Shin JJ, Glickstein LJ, Steere AC. (2012) Association of a Toll-like receptor 1 polymorphism with heightened Th1 inflammatory responses and antibiotic-refractory Lyme arthritis. *Arthritis & Rheumatism.* 64:1497–1507. Strle et al. *Am J Pathol.* 2011;(178):2726–2739.

Szczepanski B. Lyme borreliosis: host responses to Borrelia burgdorferi. *Microbio Mol Biol Rev.* March 1991;55(1): 21–34.

Tabas I, Glass CK. Anti-inflammatory therapy in chronic disease: challenges and opportunities. *Science.* 2013;339:166–172.

Tobinick E, Gross H, Weinberger A, Cohen H. TNF-alpha modulation for treatment of Alzheimer's disease: a 6-month pilot study. *Medscape General Medicine.* 2006;8(2):25.

Walsh N. Rheumatology: beyond asbestos: autoimmunity, pollution, and particles. *MedPage Today.* Aug 13, 2014. http://www.medpagetoday.com/rheumatology/generalrheumatology /47186.

Weis JJ, et al. Biological activities of native and recombinant Borrelia burgdorferi outer surface protein A: dependence on lipid modification. *Infect Immun.* 1994;62 (10):4632.

Weiss G, et al. Lactobacilli and bifidobacteria induce differential interferon-β profiles in dendritic cells. *Cytokine.* Nov 2011;56(2):520–530.

Whalen KA, McCullough ML, Flanders WD, Hartman TJ, Judd S, Bostick RM. Paleolithic and Mediterranean diet pattern scores are inversely associated with biomarkers of inflammation and oxidative balance in adults. *J Nutr.* 2016 Jun;146(6):1217–26. doi:10.3945/jn.115.224048. Epub 2016 Apr 20.

Wolfe F, et al. The prevalence and characteristics of fibromyalgia in the general population. *Arthritis Rheum.* 1995;(38):19–28.

Nine: Lyme and Environmental Toxins

Bartczak S. Would you like to have a cup of lead? Le Point.fr. Jun 12, 2013. http://www.lepoint.fr /sante/vous-prendrez-bien-une-tasse-de-plomb-06-12-2013-1765645_40.php.

Braidy N, Grant R, Adams S, Guillemin GJ. Neuroprotective effects of naturally occurring polyphenols on quinolinic acid-induced excitotoxicity in human neurons. *Fed Euro Biochem Soc J.* Jan 2010;277(2):368–382.

Bralley Alexander and Richard S, Lord. Laboratory Evaluations in Molecular Medicine. Norcross, GA: Institute for Advancement in Molecular Medicine, 2001.

Brewer J. Detection of mycotoxins in patients with chronic fatigue syndrome. *Toxins.* 2013; 5:605–617.

Cascinu S. Neuroprotective effect of reduced glutathione on oxaliplatin-based chemotherapy in advanced colorectal cancer: a randomized, double-blind, placebo-controlled trial. *J Clin Oncol.* Aug 15, 2002;20(16):3478–34383.

Chen A, Yolton K, Rauch SA, Webster GM, Hornung R, Sjödin A, Dietrich KN, Lanphear BP. Prenatal polybrominated diphenyl ether exposures and neurodevelopment in U.S. children through 5 years of age: the HOME Study. *Environmental Health Perspectives*, 2014; doi:10 .1289/ehp.1307562.

Civileats.com. http://civileats.com/2015/12/22/atrazine-the-latest-pesticide-on-trial/.

Clarkson TW, et al. Toxicology of mercury and its chemical compounds. *Crit Rev Toxicol.* 2006;(36):609–662.

CNN. http://www.cnn.com/2015/08/10/us/animas-river-toxic-spill-colorado/index.html.

Consumer Reports. http://www.consumerreports.org/cro/consumer-reports-magazine-january -2012/arsenic-in-your-juice/index.htm. [Author's comment: And federal (safe) levels don't exist]; http://www.fda.gov/ForConsumers/ConsumerUpdates/ucm319827.htm.

Cooper GS, et al. Occupational risk factors for the development of systemic lupus erythematosus. *J Rheumatol.* 2004;31:1928–1933.

Environmental Working Group's 2014 Shopper's Guide to Pesticides in Produce. April 2014. http://www.ewg.org/release/ewgs-2014-shoppers-guide-pesticides-produce.

Exley C. Why industry propaganda and political interference cannot disguise the inevitable role played by human exposure to aluminum in neurodegenerative diseases, including Alzheimer's disease *Front. Neurol.*, 27 October 2014 | http://dx.doi.org/10.3389/fneur.2014.00212.

Exposure to common household chemicals may cause IQ drop, 11 Dec 2014 http://www.cnn.com /2014/12/11/health/chemical-link-to-lower-iq/index.html?hpt=he_c2.

Fernandes EC, et al. Exposure to air pollutants and disease activity in juvenile-onset systemic lupus erythematosus patients. *Arthritis Care Res.* Nov 2015;67(11):1609–1614.

Grandjean P, Landrigan PJ. Neurobehavioural effects of developmental toxicity. *Lancet Neurol.* 2014;13:330–338. Published online February 15, 2014. http://dx.doi.org/10.1016/S1474-4422 (13)70278-3.

Guillemin G. Quinolinic acid selectively induces apoptosis of human astrocytes: potential role in AIDS dementia complex. *J Neuroinflammation.* 2005;2(16).

Guillemin GJ, Smith DG, Smythe GA, Armati PJ, Brew BJ. Expression of the kynurenine pathway enzymes in human microglia and macrophages. *Adv Exp Med Biol.* 2003;527:105–12.

Hibberd AR, et al. Mercury from dental amalgam fillings: studies on oral chelating agents for assessing and reducing mercury burdens in humans. *J Nutr Environ Med.* Jan 1998;8(3):219–231.

Hsu CW, et al. Association of urinary cadmium with mortality in patients at a coronary care unit. *PLOS ONE.* Jan 7, 2016;11(1):e0146173. doi:10.1371/journal.pone.0146173.

Kalonia H, Kumar P, Kumar A, Nehru B. Protective effect of rofecoxib and nimesulide against intra-striatal quinolinic acid-induced behavioral, oxidative stress and mitochondrial dysfunctions in rats. *Neurotoxicology.* Mar 2010;31(2):195–203.

Koga M, et al. Glutathione is a physiologic reservoir of neuronal glutamate. *Biochem Biophys Res Commun.* Jun 17, 2011;409(4):596–602. doi:10.1016/j.bbrc.2011.04.087. Epub Apr 24, 2011.

Larsson SC, et al. Urinary cadmium concentration and risk of breast cancer: a systematic review and dose-response meta-analysis (review article). *Am. J. Epidemiol.* 2015;182(5):375–380.

Lee BK, et al. Provocative chelation with DMSA and EDTA: evidence for differential access to lead storage sites. *Occup Environ Med.* 1995;52(1):13–19.

Müller N. COX-2 inhibitors as antidepressants and antipsychotics: clinical evidence. *Curr Opin Investig Drugs.* Jan 2010;11(1):31–42. PMID 20047157.

Mutter J, et al. Comments on the article "The Toxicology of Mercury and Its Chemical Compounds" by Clarkson and Magos (2006). *Crit Rev Toxicology.* 2007;37:537–549.

Navas-Acien A. Arsenic exposure and prevalence of type 2 diabetes in U.S. adults. *JAMA.* 2008;300(7):814–822.

Pfau JC, Serve KM, Noonan CW. Autoimmunity and asbestos exposure, autoimmune diseases, 2014; 2014, Article ID 782045, doi:10.1155/2014/782045.

Prasad AS, et al. Zinc supplementation decreases incidence of infections in the elderly: effect of zinc on generation of cytokines and oxidative stress. *Am J Clin Nutr.* 2007;844; 85:837–844.

Richardson JR, Roy A, Shalat SL, von Stein RT, Muhammad M, Hossain MM, et al. Elevated serum pesticide levels and risk for Alzheimer disease. *JAMA Neurol.* Published online Jan 27, 2014. doi:10.1001/jamaneurol.2013.6030.

Sagiv SK, Thurston SW, Bellinger DC, Amarasiriwardena C, Korrick SA. Prenatal exposure to mercury and fish consumption during pregnancy and attention-deficit/hyperactivity disorder–related behavior in children. *Arch Pediatr Adolesc Med.* 2012 Dec;166(12):1123–31. doi:10.1001/archpediatrics.2012.1286.

Shanker AH, et al. Zinc and immune function: the biological basis of altered resistance to infection. *Am J Clin Nutr.* 1988;68(Suppl):447s–63s.

Shelton JF, Geraghty EM, Tancredi DJ, Delwiche LD, Schmidt RJ, Ritz B, et al.; and the CHARGE Study. Neurodevelopmental disorders and prenatal residential proximity to agricultural pesticides. *Environ Health Perspect.* doi:10.1289/ehp.1307044. http://ehp.niehs.nih.gov/1307044/.

Usberti M, et al. Effects of a vitamin E-bonded membrane and of glutathione on anemia and erythropoietin requirements in hemodialysis patients. *J Nephrology.* Sept–Oct 2002;15(5):558–564.

Ten: Lyme, Functional Medicine, and Nutritional Therapies

Calabro AR, Gazarian DI, Barile FA. Effect of metals on beta-actin and total protein synthesis in cultured human intestinal epithelial cells. *J Pharmacol Toxicol Methods.* 2011, 63:47–58.

Castagliulo I, Riegler, MF, Valenick L., LaMont JT, Pothoulakis C. Saccharomyces boulardii protease inhibits the effects of Clostridium difficile toxins A and B in human colonic mucosa. *Infect Immun.* 1999 Jan;67(1):302–7.

Environmental Working Group. http://www.ewg.org/release/landmark-federal-study-cell -phone-radiation-linked-brain-cancer.

Fasano A. Zonulin and its regulation of intestinal barrier function: the biological door to inflammation, autoimmunity, and cancer. *Physiol Rev.* 2011;91:151–175.

Groschwitz KR, Hogan SP. Intestinal barrier function: molecular regulation and disease pathogenesis. *The Journal of Allergy and Clinical Immunology.* 2009;124(1):3–22. doi:10.1016/j.jaci.2009.05.038.

Jan RL, Yeh KC, Hsieh MH, Lin YL, Kao HF, Li PH, Chang YS, Wang JY. Lactobacillus gasseri suppresses Th17 pro-inflammatory response and attenuates allergen-induced airway inflammation in a mouse model of allergic asthma. *Br J Nutr.* Oct 14, 2011:1–10.

Lewis KN, Mele J, Hayes JD, Buffenstein R. Nrf2, a guardian of healthspan and gatekeeper of species longevity. *Integrative and Comparative Biology.* 2010;50(5):829–843. doi:10.1093/icb/icq034.

Lorenz W, et al. Bacterial lipopolysaccharides form procollagen-endotoxin complexes that trigger cartilage inflammation and degeneration: implications for the development of rheumatoid arthritis. *Arthritis Res Ther.* 2013;15:R111.

Ouwehand AC, Bergsma N, Parhiala R, Lahtinen S, Gueimonde M, Finne-Soveri H, Strandberg T, Pitkälä K, Salminen S Bifidobacterium microbiota and parameters of immune function in elderly subjects. *FEMS Immunology & Medical Microbiology.* 53:18–25. doi:10.1111/j.1574-695X.2008.00392.x.

Packer L, Tritschler HJ, Wessel K; and Department of Molecular and Cell Biology, University of California, Berkeley. Neuroprotection by the metabolic antioxidant alpha-lipoic acid. *Free Radic Biol Med.* 1997;22(1–2):359–378.

Patrick L. Mercury toxicity and antioxidants (part 1): role of glutathione and alpha-lipoic acid in the treatment of mercury toxicity. *Altern Med Rev.* Dec 2002;7(6):456–471.

Patrick L. Toxic metals and antioxidants (part 2). The role of antioxidants in arsenic and cadmium toxicity. *Altern Med Rev.* May 2003;8(2):106–128.

Roony PJ, et al. A short review of the relationship between intestinal permeability and inflammatory joint disease. *Clin Exp Rheum.* 1990;8:75–83.

Rowe AH, et al. Bronchial asthma due to food allergy alone in 95 patients. *JAMA.* 1959;169:1158.

Singh K, Connors S, Macklin EA, Smith, KD, Fahey JW, Talalay P, Zimmerman A. Sulforaphane treatment of autism spectrum disorder (ASD). Oct 2014 *PNAS* vol. 111 no. 43, 15550–15555, doi:10.1073/pnas.1416940111.

Smith JP, et al. Low-dose naltrexone therapy improves active Crohn's disease. *Am J Gastroenterology.* Apr 2007;102:1–9.

Soleas GJ, Diamandis EP, Goldberg DM. Resveratrol: a molecule whose time has come? And gone? *Clin Biochem.* Mar 1997;30(2):91–113.

Suzuki T, et al. Epigenetic control using natural products and synthetic molecules. *Current Medicinal Chem.* 2006;11:935–958.

Theophilus PAS, et al. Effectiveness of Stevia rebaudiana whole leaf extract against the various morphological forms of Borrelia burgdorferi in vitro. *Euro J Microbiol Immunol.* 2015. doi:10.1556/1886.2015.00031.

Tjellström B, et al. Oral immunoglobulin treatment in Crohn's disease. *Acta Paediatrica.* Feb 1997;86(2):221–223.

U.S. Department of Agriculture. Dietary Reference Intakes for Energy, Carbohydrate, Fiber, Fat, Fatty Acids, Cholesterol, Protein, and Amino Acids (Macronutrients) (2005), Chapter 7: "Dietary, Functional and Total Fiber." National Agricultural Library and National Academy of Sciences, Institute of Medicine, Food and Nutrition Board. http:/www.nal.usda.gov/fnic /DRI//DRI_Energy/339-421.pdf.

Valenzano DR, Terzibasi E, Genade T, Cattaneo A, Domenici L, Cellerino A. Resveratrol prolongs lifespan and retards the onset of age-related markers in a short-lived vertebrate. *Curr Biol.* Feb 7, 2006;16(3):296–300.

Waller P, et al. (2011) Dose-response effect of Bifidobacterium lactis HN019 on whole gut transit time and functional gastrointestinal symptoms in adults. *Scandinavian Journal of Gastroenterology,* 46:9, 1057–1064, doi:10.3109/00365521.2011.584895.

Yadav VS, et al. Immunomodulatory effects of curcurmin. *Immunopharmacol Immunotox.* 2005;27(3):485–497.

Eleven: Lyme and Mitochondrial Dysfunction

Ash M, Nicolson G. Mechanisms of membrane repair and the novel role of oral phospholipids (lipid replacement therapy) and antioxidants to improve membrane function. *Clinical Education.* Oct

2012. http://www.clinicaleducation.org/resources/reviews/mechanisms-of-membrane-repair-and-the-novel-role-of-oral-phospholipids-lrt-and-antioxidants/.

Balaban RS, et al. Mitochondria, oxidants, and aging. *Cell*. 2005;120:483–495.

Castro-Marrero J, et al. Could mitochondrial dysfunction be a differentiating marker between chronic fatigue syndrome and fibromyalgia? *Antioxidants & Redox Signaling*. Nov 20, 2013; 19(15):1855–1860. Published online May 29, 2013 doi:10.1089/ars.2013.5346.

Cohen BH, et al. Mitochondrial cytopathy in adults: what we know so far. *Cleveland Clin J Med*. 2001;68:625–626, 629–642.

Conley KE, et al. Ageing, muscle properties and maximal O(2) uptake rate in humans. *J. Physiol*. 2000;526(Part 1):211–217.

Einat H, et al. Increased anxiety-like behaviors and mitochondrial dysfunction in mice with targeted mutation of the Bcl-2 gene: further support for the involvement of mitochondrial function in anxiety disorders. *Behav Brain Res*. 2005;165:172–180.

Fattal O, et al. Review of literature on major mental disorders in patients with mitochondrial diseases. *Psychosomatics*. 2006;47:1–7.

Fosslien E. Mitochondrial medicine—molecular pathology of defective oxidative phosphorylation. *Ann Clin Lab Sci*. 2001;31:25–67.

Frye RE, Rossignol D. Mitochondrial physiology and autism spectrum disorder. *OA Autism*. Mar 1, 2013;1(1)3.

Fukui H, et al. The mitochondrial impairment, oxidative stress and neurodegeneration connection: reality or just an attractive hypothesis? *Trends Neurosci*. 2008;31:251–256.

Gu M, et al. Mitochondrial DNA transmission of the mitochondrial defect in Parkinson's disease. *Ann Neurol*. 1998;44:177–186.

Howitz KT, Bitterman KJ, Cohen HY, Lamming DW, Lavu S, Wood JG, Zipkin RE, Chung P, Kisielewski A, Zhang LL, Scherer B, Sinclair DA. Small molecule activators of sirtuins extend Saccharomyces cerevisiae lifespan. *Nature*. 2003 Sept 11;425(6954):191–6. Epub 2003 Aug 24.

IntraCellular Diagnostics. Magnesium depletion depresses ATP production in diabetic cells .http://exatest.com/MITOCHONDRIA%20SEMINAR/Mitochondria%20Seminar%20%20P1-2.htm.

Jacobs TL, Epel ES, Lin J, Blackburn EH, Wolkowitz OM, Bridwell DA, Zanesco AP, Aichele SR, Sahdra BK, MacLean KA, King BG, Shaver PR, Rosenberg EL, Ferrer E, Wallace BA, Saron CD. Intensive meditation training, immune cell telomerase activity, and psychological mediators. *Psychoneuroendocrinology*. 2011;36:664–681.

Koike, K. Molecular basis of hepatitis C virus-associated hepatocarcinogenesis: lessons from animal model studies. *Clin Gastroenterol Hepatol*. 2005;3:S132–135.

Lamkanfi M, Dixit VM. Modulation of inflammasome pathways by bacterial and viral pathogens. *J Immunol*. 2011;187:597–602.

Lieber CS, et al. Model of nonalcoholic steatohepatitis. *Am J Clin Nutr*. 2004;79: 502–509.

Lisanti CL, et al. Antibiotics that target mitochondria effectively eradicate cancer stem cells, across multiple tumor types: treating cancer like an infectious disease. *Oncotarget*, January 2015. http://www.sciencedaily.com/releases/2015/01/150128081957.htm.

Maalouf M, Rho JM, Mattson MP. The neuroprotective properties of calorie restriction, the ketogenic diet, and ketone bodies. *Brain Res Rev*. Mar 2009;59(2):293–315.

Mattman A, et al. Diagnosis and management of patients with mitochondrial disease. *BCMJ* (articles). May 2011;53(4):177–182.

Neustat J, et al. Medication-induced mitochondrial damage and disease. *Mol. Nutr. Food Res*. 2008;52:780–788.

Nicolson G. Lipid replacement as an adjunct to therapy for chronic fatigue, anti-aging and restoration of mitochondrial function. *J Am Nutraceut Assoc.* 2003;6(3):22–28.

Nicolson G. Metabolic syndrome and mitochondrial function: molecular replacement and antioxidant supplements to prevent membrane peroxidation and restore mitochondrial function. *J Cellular Biochem.* 2007;9999:1–18.

Nicolson G, et al. Lipid replacement therapy with a glycophospholipid formulation with NADH and CoQ10 significantly reduces fatigue in intractable chronic fatiguing illnesses and chronic Lyme disease patients. *Int J Clin Med.* 2012;3:163–170.

Paoli A, Rubini A, Volek JS, Grimaldi KA. Beyond weight loss: a review of the therapeutic uses of very-low-carbohydrate (ketogenic) diets. *Eur J Clin Nutr.* 2013;67:789–796.

Peppa M, et al. Glucose, advanced glycation end products, and diabetes complications: what is new and what works. *Clinical Diabetes.* Oct 2003;21(4): 186–187.

Porcellini E, Carbone I, et al. Alzheimer's disease gene signature says: beware of brain viral infections. *Immun Ageing.* Dec 2010;7:16. doi: 10.1186/1742-4933-7-16.

Puddu P, et al. Mitochondrial dysfunction as an initiating event in atherogenesis: a plausible hypothesis. *Cardiology.* 2005;103:137–141.

Saffran HA, Pare JM, Corcoran JA, et al. Herpes simplex virus eliminates host mitochondrial DNA. *Eur Molecular Biol Org* (report). Feb 2007;8(2):188–193.

Soleas GJ, Diamandis EP, Goldberg DM. Resveratrol: a molecule whose time has come? And gone? *Clin Biochem.* Mar 1997;30(2):91–113.

Stavrovskaya IG, et al. The powerhouse takes control of the cell: is the mitochondrial permeability transition a viable therapeutic target against neuronal dysfunction and death? *Free Radic. Biol. Med.* 2005;38:687–697.

Stork C, et al. Mitochondrial dysfunction in bipolar disorder: evidence from magnetic resonance spectroscopy research. *Mol. Psychiatry.* 2005;10:900–919.

Sullivan PG, et al. Mitochondrial aging and dysfunction in Alzheimer's disease. *Prog Neuropsychopharmacol Biol Psychiatry.* 2005;29:407–410.

Valenzano DR, Terzibasi E, Genade T, Cattaneo A, Domenici L, Cellerino A. Resveratrol prolongs lifespan and retards the onset of age-related markers in a short-lived vertebrate. *Curr Biol.* Feb 7, 2006;16(3):296–300.

Wallace DC, Singh G, Lott MT, et al. Mitochondrial DNA mutation associated with Leber's hereditary optic neuropathy. *Science.* 1988;242(4884):1427–1430.

Wallace DC, Singh G, Lott MT, et al. Mitochondrial DNA mutation associated with Leber's hereditary optic neuropathy. *Science.* 1988;242(4884):1427–1430.

Wallace DC. A mitochondrial paradigm of metabolic and degenerative diseases, aging and cancer: a dawn for evolutionary medicine. *Annu. Rev. Genet.* 2005;39:359–407.

Yunus MB, et al. Primary fibromyalgia syndrome and myofascial pain syndrome: clinical features and muscle pathology. *Arch Phys Med Rehabil.* 1988;69:451–454.

Twelve: Lyme and Hormones

Anisman H, et al. Neuroimmune mechanisms in health and disease. *Can Med Assoc.* Oct 15, 1996;1:155(8).

Baumert J, et al. A pattern of unspecific somatic symptoms as long-term premonitory signs of type 2 diabetes: findings from the population-based MONICA/KORA Cohort Study. 1984–2009. *BMC Endocrin Disord.* 2014;14(87).

Berczi I, et al. Hormones in self-tolerance and autoimmunity: a role in the pathogenesis of rheumatoid arthritis? *Autoimmunity.* 1993;16:45–56.

Berczi I, et al. The Pituitary Gland, Psychoneuroimmunology and Infectious Disease *Psychoneuroimmunology, Stress and Infection*, Boca Raton, FL: CRC Press 1996:79–109.

Bourdeau I, et al. Loss of brain volume in endogenous Cushing's syndrome and its reversibility after correction of hypercortisolism. *J Clin Endocrinol Metabol.* 2000;87:1949.

Clauw DJ, et al. Chronic pain and fatigue syndromes: overlapping clinical and neuroendocrine features and potential pathogenic mechanisms. *Neuro Immunomodulation.* 1997;4:134–153.

Crofts CA, et al. Hyperinsulinemia: a unifying theory of chronic disease? *Diabesity.* 2015;1(4):34–43. doi:10.15562/diabesity.2015.19.

Cunningham RL, Singh M, O'Bryant SE, Hall JR, Barber RC. Oxidative stress, testosterone, and Cognition among caucasian and Mexican-American men with and without Alzheimer's disease. *Journal of Alzheimer's Disease*, vol. 40, no. 3, pp. 563–573, 2014.

Dandona P, et al. Hypogonadotrophic hypogonadism in type 2 diabetes, obesity and the metabolic syndrome. *Curr Mol Med.* Dec 2008;8(8):816–828.

Garber JR, et al. ATA/AACE guidelines for hypothyroidism in adults. *Endocr Pract.* 2012; 18(6)989.

Gooren I. Androgen deficiency in the aging male: benefits and risks of androgen supplementation. *J Steroid Biochem Mol Biol.* Jun 2003;85(2–5):349–355.

Goto A, Noda M, Sawada N, Kato M, Hidaka A, Mizoue T, Shimazu T, Yamaji T, Iwasaki M, Sasazuki S, Inoue M, Kadowaki T, Tsugane S, and for the JPHC Study Group (2016). High hemoglobin A1c levels within the non-diabetic range are associated with the risk of all cancers. *Int. J. Cancer*, 138:1741–1753. doi:10.1002/ijc.29917.

Haddad RM, et al. Testosterone and cardiovascular risk in men: a systematic review and meta-analysis of randomized placebo-controlled trials. *Mayo Clin Proc.* Jan 2007;82(1):29–39.

Hedner LP, et al. Endogenous iridocyclitis relieved during treatment with bromocriptine. *Am J Ophthalmol.* 1985;100:618–619.

Hess A, et al. Borrelia burgdorferi central nervous system infection presenting as an organic schizophrenia like disorder. *Biol Psychiatry.* Mar 15, 1999;45(6):795.

Hoang TD, Olsen CH, Mai VQ, Clyde PW, Shakir MK. Desiccated thyroid extract compared with levothyroxine in the treatment of hypothyroidism: a randomized, double-blind, crossover study. *J Clin Endocrinol Metab.* 2013 May;98(5):1982–90. doi:10.1210/jc.2012-4107. Epub 2013 Mar 28.

Izquierdo M, et al. Effects of strength training on muscle power and serum hormones in middle-aged and older men. *J App Physiol.* 2001;90(4):1497–1507.

Jalali GR, et al. Impact of oral zinc therapy on the level of sex hormones in male patients on hemodialysis. *Ren Fail.* May 2010;32(4):417–419.

Kandaraki E, et al. Endocrine disruptors and polycystic ovary syndrome (PCOS): elevated serum levels of bisphenol A in women with PCOS. *J Clin Endocrinol Metabol.* Dec 10, 2010.

Khaw KT et al. Endogenous testosterone and mortality due to all causes, cardiovascular disease, and cancer in men: European prospective investigation into cancer in Norfolk (EPIC-Norfolk) Prospective Population Study. *Circulation.* Dec 4, 2007;116(23):2694–2701.

Kutlucan A, Kale Koroglu B, Numan Tamer M, Aydin Y, Baltaci D, Akdogan M, et al. The investigation of effects of fluorosis on thyroid volume in school-age children. *Med Glas (Zenica).* 2013;10(1):93–98.

Laaksonen DE, et al. Sex hormones, inflammation and the metabolic syndrome: a population-based study. *Eur J Endocrinol.* Dec 2003;149(6):601–608.

Liu et al. The relationship between serum thyroid hormones and fluoride levels in endemic fluorosis. *CMJ.* 1988;7(4):216–218.

Maggio M, et al. 25(OH)D serum levels decline with age earlier in women than in men and less efficiently prevent compensatory hyperparathyroidism in older adults. *J Endocrinol Invest.* 2005;28(11, suppl proceedings):116–119.

Makhsida N, et al. Hypogonadism and metabolic syndrome: implications for testosterone therapy. *J Urol.* Sept 2005;174(3):827–834.

Mazokopakis EE, Papadakis JA, Papadomanolaki MG, et al. Effects of 12 months treatment with L-selenomethionine on serum anti-TPO levels in patients with Hashimoto's thyroiditis. *Thyroid*. 2007;17(7):609–612. doi:10.1089/thy.2007.0040. PMID 17696828.

Morley JE, Charlton E, Patrick P, Kiaser FE, Cadeau P, McCready D, Perry HM III. Validation of a screening questionnaire for androgen deficiency in aging males. *Metabolism*. 2000;49: 1239–1242.

Muller M, et al. Endogenous sex hormones and metabolic syndrome in aging men. *J Clin Endocrinol Metab*. May 2005;90(5):2618–2623.

Nagata C, et al. Inverse association of soy product intake with serum androgen and estrogen concentrations in Japanese men. *Nutr Cancer*. 2000;36(1):14–18.

Ohlsson C, et al. Low serum levels of dehydroepiandrosterone sulfate predict all-cause and cardiovascular mortality in elderly Swedish men. *J Clin Endocrinol Metab*. Sept 2010;95(9): 4406–14. Published online Jul 7, 2012.

Pastan I, Macchia V, Katzen R. Effect of fluoride on metabolic activity of thyroid slices. *Endocrinology*. 1968;83(1):157–160.

Pilz S, Frisch S, Koertke H, Kuhn J, Dreier J, Obermayer-Pietsch B, et al. Effect of vitamin D supplementation on testosterone levels in men. *Hormone Metabolic Res*. Dec 10, 2010.

Russell IJ. Neurochemical pathogenesis of fibromyalgia syndrome. *J Musculoskel Pain*. 1996;4: 61–92.

Sapolsky R. Why stress is bad for your brain. *Science*. 1996;273:749–750.

Sciencecodex.com. Study suggests testosterone therapy does not raise risk of aggressive prostate cancer. May 7, 2016. http://www.sciencecodex.com/study_suggests_testosterone_therapy_does _not_raise_risk_of_aggressive_prostate_cancer-181925?utm_source=twitterfeed&utm _medium=twitter.

Shores MM, et al. Low serum testosterone and mortality in male veterans. *Arch Intern Med*. Aug 14, 2006;166(15):1660–1665.

Takihara H, et al. Zinc sulfate therapy for infertile males with or without varicocelectomy. *Urology*. Jun 1987;29(6):638–641.

Tang YJ, et al. Serum testosterone level and related metabolic factors in men over 70 years old. *J Endocrinol Invest*. Jun 2007;30(6):451–458.

Traish AM, et al. The dark side of testosterone deficiency: II. Type 2 diabetes and insulin resistance. *J Androl*. Jan–Feb 2009;30(1):23–32.

Wick G, et al. Immunoendocrine communication via the hypothalamo-pituitary adrenal axis in autoimmune diseases. *Endocr Rev*. 1993;14:539–563.

Wolfe F, et al. The prevalence and characteristics of fibromyalgia in the general population. *Arthritis Rheum*. 1995; 38:19–28.

Thirteen: Lyme and the Brain

Allen H, et al. Autoimmune diseases of the innate and adaptive immune system including atopic dermatitis, psoriasis, chronic arthritis, Lyme disease, and Alzheimer's disease. *Immunochem Immunopathol*. 2015;1:2. http://dx.doi.org/10.4172/2469-9756.1000112.

Allen HB, et al. Alzheimer's disease: a novel hypothesis integrating spirochetes, biofilm, and the immune system. *J Neuroinfect Dis*. 2016: 7:1. http://dx.doi.org/10.4172/2314-7326.1000200.

Amminger GP, Schäfer MR, Schlögelhofer M, Klier CM, McGorry PD. Longer-term outcome in the prevention of psychotic disorders by the Vienna omega-3 study. *Nature Communications*. 2015 Aug 11. pii: ncomms8934. doi:10.1038/ncomms8934.

Avery RA, Frank G, Eppes SC. Diagnostic utility of Borrelia burgdorferi cerebrospinal fluid polymerase chain reaction in children with Lyme meningitis. *Pediatr Infect Dis J*. Aug 2005;24(8):705–708.

Battistini S, et al. Severe familial ALS with a novel exon 4 mutation (L106F) in the SOD1 gene. *J Neurol Sci.* June 2010;293(1):112–115.

Blanc F, et al. Lyme neuroborreliosis and dementia. *J Alzheimer's Dis.* 2014;41(4):1087–1093. doi: 10.3233/JAD-30446. http://www.ncbi.nlm.nih.gov/pubmed/24762944.

Bransfied R. The psychoimmunology of Lyme/tick-borne diseases and its association with neuropsychiatric symptoms. *J Open Neurol.* 2012;6(Suppl 1-M3): 88–93.

Breitschwerdt EB, et al. Bartonella sp. bacteremia in patients with neurological and neurocognitive dysfunction. *J Clin Microbiol.* 46(9):2856–2861.

Breitschwerdt EB, Maggi RG, Nicholson WL, Cherry NA, Woods CW. Bartonella sp. bacteremia in patients with neurological and neurocognitive dysfunction. *J Clin Microbiol.* 46(9):2856–2861.

Breitschwerdt EB, et al. Molecular evidence of perinatal transmission of Bartonella vinsonii subsp. Berkhoffii and B. henselae to a child. *J Clin Microbiol.* April 14, 2010.

Briançon-Marjollet A, et al. The impact of sleep disorders on glucose metabolism: endocrine and molecular mechanisms. *Diabetology & Metabolic Syndrome.* 2015;7:25. doi:10.1186/s13098-015-0018-3.

Brouwer EJ, Evelo CT, Verplanke AJ, van Welie RT, de Wolff FA. Biological effect monitoring of occupational exposure to 1,3-dichloropropene: effects on liver and renal function and on glutathione conjugation. *Br J Ind Med.* 1991;48:167–172.

Burakgazi AZ. Lyme disease–induced polyradiculopathy mimicking amyotrophic lateral sclerosis. *Int J Neurosci.* 2014 Nov;124(11):859–62. doi:10.3109/00207454.2013.879582. Epub 2014 Feb 7.

Cerar T, et al. Differences in genotype, clinical features, and inflammatory potential of Borrelia burgdorferi sensu stricto strains from Europe and the United States. *Emerging Infect Dis.* May 2016;22:5.

Chez MG, et al. Elevation of tumor necrosis factor-alpha in cerebrospinal fluid of autistic children. *Pediatric Neurol.* 2007;36(6):361–365.

Cicciù M, Matacena G, Signorino F, Brugaletta A, Cicciù A, Bramanti E. Relationship between oral health and its impact on the quality life of Alzheimer's disease patients: a supportive care trial. *Int J Clin Experimental Med.* 2013;6(9):766–772.

Clayton EW. Beyond myalgic encephalomyelitis/chronic fatigue syndrome: an IOM report on redefining an Illness. *JAMA.* 2015;313(11):1101–1102. doi:10.1001/jama.2015.1346.

CNN.com. Salivary test to detect early Alzheimer's. July 21, 2015. http://www.cnn.com/2015/07 /20/health/saliva-test-may-catch-alzheimers-disease/.

Coyle PK, et al. Detection of Borrelia burgdorferi-specific antigen in antibody-negative cerebrospinal fluid in neurologic Lyme disease. *Neurology.* 1995;45:2012–2015.

Coyle PK, Neurologic Lyme disease. *Seminars in Neurol.* 1992;12:200–208.

Dattwyler RJ, et al. Failure of tetracycline therapy in early Lyme disease. *Arthritis Rheum.* Apr 1987 Apr;30(4):448–450.

Diamond B, et al. Brain-reactive antibodies and disease. *Annu Rev Immunol.* 2013;31:345–385.

Drexel University Team Duplicates Dr. Alan MacDonald's Findings of Bacterial Biofilms in Alzheimer's Plaques https://spirodementia.wordpress.com/drexel-university-team-duplicate -dr-alan-macdonalds'-findings-of-bacterial-biofilms-in-alzheimers-plaques. Alzheimer's/ 17767391/.

Erickson KI, et al. Exercise training increases size of hippocampus and improves memory. *PNAS.* Feb 15, 2011;108(7):3017–3022.

Erickson KI, Raji CA, Lopez OL, et al. Physical activity predicts gray matter volume in late adulthood: the Cardiovascular Health Study (e–Pub ahead of print). *Neurology.* 2010;75(16): 1415–1422. doi:10.1212/WNL.0b013e3181f88359.

Factor-Litvak P, Insel B, Calafat AM, Liu X, Perera F, Rauh VA, et al. (2014) Persistent associations between maternal prenatal exposure to phthalates on child IQ at age 7 years. *PLOS ONE.* 9(12):e114003. doi:10.1371/journal.pone.0114003.

Fallon B, et al. The neuropsychiatric manifestations of Lyme borreliosis. *Neurobiol Dis.* 2010;37:534–541.

Fallon BA, et al. Functional brain imaging and neuropsychological testing in Lyme disease. *Clin Infect Dis.* 1997;25(Suppl 1):857–863.

Fallon BA, et al. A randomized, placebo controlled trial of repeated IV antibiotic therapy for Lyme encephalopathy. *Neurology.* Mar 25, 2008;70(13):992–1003.

Fallon BA, et al. The under diagnosis of neuropsychiatric Lyme disease in children and adults. *Psychiatr Clin North Am.* Sept 1998;21(3):693–703, viii.

Fallon BA, et al. The neuropsychiatric manifestations of Lyme borreliosis. *Psychiatric Quarterly.* 1992;63:95–115.

Fattal O, et al. Review of literature on major mental disorders in patients with mitochondrial diseases. *Psychosomatics.* 2006;47: 1–7.

Feng-Chiao S, et al. Association of environmental toxins with amyotrophic lateral sclerosis. *JAMA Neurol.* Published online May 9, 2016. doi:10.1001/jamaneurol.2016.0594http://archneur .jamanetwork.com/article.aspx?articleid=2519875.

Frankola KA, Greig NH, Luo W, Tweedie D. Targeting TNF-alpha to elucidate and ameliorate neuroinflammation in neurodegenerative diseases. *CNS Neurol Disord Drug Targets.* Feb 2, 2011.

Gelber RP, Redline S, Ross GW, Petrovitch H, Sonnen JA, Zarow C, Uyehara-Lock JH, Masaki KH, Launer LJ, White LR. Associations of brain lesions at autopsy with polysomnography features before death. *Neurology.* 2015 Jan 20;84(3):296–303. doi:10.1212/WNL.0000000000001163. Epub 2014 Dec 10.

Gomm W, et al. Association of proton pump inhibitors with risk of dementia: a pharmaco-epidemiological claims data analysis. *JAMA Neurol.* 2016;73(4):410–416. doi:10.1001/jamaneurol .2015.4791.

Gozalo AS,et al. Visceral and neural larva migrans in rhesus macaques. *J. Amer. Assoc. Lab Animal Sci.* 2008;47(4):64–67.

Haack M, et al. Chronic sleep restriction leads to elevations in IL-6 and pain symptoms in healthy volunteers. *J Pain.* April 2004, Suppl 1;5(3).

Halpern JJ, et al. Nervous system abnormalities in Lyme disease. *Ann NY Acad Sci.* 1988;539:24–34.

Hornig M, et al. Distinct plasma immune signatures in ME/CFS are present early in the course of illness. *Sci Advances.* 27 Feb 2015: E1400121.

Horowitz RI, Freeman PR. The use of Dapsone as a novel "persister" drug in the treatment of chronic Lyme disease/post treatment Lyme disease syndrome. *J Clin Exp Dermatol Res.* 2016;7:3. http://dx.doi.org/10.4172/2155-9554.1000345.

Hreljac I, Filipic M. Organophosphorus pesticides enhance the genotoxicity of benzo(a)pyrene by modulating its metabolism. *Mutat Res.* 2009;671:84–92. doi:10.1016/j.mrfmmm.2009.09.011.

Innes J, et al. Cerebrospinal nematodiasis. *AMA Archives of Neurol Psychiatry.* 1953;70(3):325–349.

Itzhakia R, et al. Microbes and Alzheimer's disease. *J Alzheimer's Dis.* 2016;51(4):979–84. doi: 10.3233/JAD-160152.

Janickova H, et al. Lipid-based diets improve muscarinic neurotransmission in the hippocampus of transgenic APPswe/PS1dE9 mice. *Current Alzheimer Res.* 2015;12(10):923. doi:10.2174/156 7205012666151027130350.

Jung C-R, et al. Ozone, particulate matter, and newly diagnosed Alzheimer's disease: a population-based cohort study in Taiwan. *J Alzheimer's Dis.* 2015; 44:573–584. doi:10.3233/ JAD-140855 IOS Press.

Kirvan CA, Swedo SE, Snider LA, Cunningham MW. Antibody-mediated neuronal cell signaling in behavior and movement disorders. *J Neuroimmunol*. 2006 Oct;179(1–2):173–9. Epub 2006 Jul 27.

Kisand et al. Propensity to excessive proinflammatory response in Lyme borreliosis. *Acta Pathologica Microbiologica Immun Scandinavia*. Feb 2007;115(2):134–141.

Kocaman AY, Topaktaş M. Genotoxic effects of a particular mixture of acetamiprid and α-cypermethrin on chromosome aberration, sister chromatid exchange, and micronucleus formation in human peripheral blood lymphocytes. *Environ Toxicol*. 2010;25:157–168. doi:10.1002/tox.20485.

Koranyi EK. Somatic illness in psychiatric patients. *Psychosomatics*. 1980;21:887–891.

Kozuli M, et al. Research Report. Atorvastatin and pitavastatin protect cerebellar Purkinje cells in AD model mice and preserve the cytokines MCP-1 and TNF-α (research report). *Brain Res*. May 4, 2011;1388,(4):32–38. http://www.sciencedirect.com/science/article/pii/S000689931100521X.

Krause PJ, et al. Concurrent Lyme disease and babesiosis, evidence for increased severity and duration of illness. *JAMA*. June 5, 1996;275:21.

Krupp LB, et al. Cognitive functioning in late Lyme borreliosis. *Arch Neurol*. 1991; 48:1125–1129.

Leonard HL, Swedo SE, Garvey M, et al. Postinfectious and other forms of obsessive-compulsive disorder. *Child Adolescent Psych Clin North Am*. Jul 1999;8(3):497–511.

Levin EC, et al. Brain-reactive autoantibodies are nearly ubiquitous in human sera and may be linked to pathology in the context of blood-brain barrier breakdown. *Brain Res*. July 23, 2010;1345:221–1332.

Lipid-based diets effectively combat Alzheimer's disease in mouse model. Science News, February 10, 2016. https://www.sciencedaily.com/releases/2016/02/160210142701.htm#.Vr54_nXgjaA.

Liu F, et al. Minocycline supplementation for treatment of negative symptoms in early-phase schizophrenia: a double blind, randomized, controlled trial. *Schizophr Res*. Feb 3, 2014. pii: S0920–9964(14)00014–0. doi:10.1016/j.schres.2014.01.011. [Epub ahead of print]. http://www.ncbi.nlm.nih.gov/pubmed/24503176.

Logigian EL, et al. Chronic neurologic manifestations of Lyme disease. *NEJM*. 1990;323:1438–1444.

Lyme.net.(Europe). http://www.lymeneteurope.org/forum/viewtopic.php?t=6122.

Manzardo M, et al. Plasma cytokine levels in children with autistic disorder and unrelated siblings. *Int J Developmental Neurosci*. 2012;30(2):121–127.

Meek ME, et al, eds. Risk assessment of combined exposure to multiple chemicals, a WHO/IPCS framework WHO supplement. *Regulatory Toxicol and Pharmacol*. Jul 1, 2011;60(2, Suppl): S1–S14.

Miklossy J. Alzheimer's disease—a neurospirochetosis: analysis of the evidence following Koch's and Hill's criteria. *J Neuroinflammation*. 2011;8:90. doi:10.1186/1742-2094-8-90.

Miklossy J. Historic evidence to support a causal relationship between spirochetal infections and Alzheimer's disease. *Front. Aging Neurosci*. Apr 16, 2015;7:46.

Moldofsky H. Sleep, neuroimmune and neuroendocrine functions in fibromyalgia and chronic fatigue syndrome. *Advances Neuroimmuno*. 1995;5:39–56.

Monti JM, et al. Identifying and characterizing the effects of nutrition on hippocampal memory. *Adv Nutr*. 2014;5:337S–343S.

Morris MC, et al. Association of seafood consumption, brain mercury level, and APOE ε4 status with brain neuropathology in older adults. *JAMA*. 016;315(5):489–497. doi:10.1001/jama.2015.19451.

Nicolson GL, Gan R, Nicolson NL, Haier J. Evidence for Mycoplasma ssp., Chlamydia pneumo-miae, and human herpes virus-6 coinfections in the blood of patients with autistic spectrum disorders. *J Neurosci Res.* 2007 Apr;85(5):1143–8.

Nicolson GL, Nasralla M, Haier, J, Pomfret J. High frequency of systemic mycoplasmal infec-tions in Gulf War veterans and civilians with amyotrophic lateral sclerosis (ALS). *J Clin. Neurosci.* 2002;9:525–529.

Nields JA, Fallon BA. Differential diagnosis and treatment of Lyme disease, with special refer-ence to psychiatric practice. *Directions in Psychiatry.* 1998;18:209–228.

Okonkwo OC, et al. Physical activity attenuates age-related biomarker alterations in preclinical AD. *Neurology.* Nov 4, 2014;83(19):1753–1760. http://www.neurology.org/content/83/19/1753 .abstract.

Olmos-Alonso A, et al. Pharmacological targeting of CSF1R inhibits microglial proliferation and prevents the progression of Alzheimer's-like pathology. *Brain.* Jan 3, 2016. doi:http://dx.doi .org/10.1093/brain/awv379 awv379. First published online January 8, 2016. http://brain .oxfordjournals.org/content/early/2016/01/07/brain.awv379.

Pachner AR. Borrelia burgdorferi in the nervous system: the new "great imitator." In Jorge L. Benach, *Lyme Disease and Related Disease and Related Disorders.* NY: New York Acadamy of Science, 1988. *Annals NY Academy Sci.* 1988;539:56–64.

Pachner AR. Early disseminated Lyme disease: Lyme meningitis. *Am J Med.* 1995;98(4A): 30S–37S.

Pachner et al. Interleukin-6 is expressed at high levels in the CNS in Lyme neuroborreliosis. *Neurology.* Jul 1997;49(1)c147–52.

Patterson-Fortin J, Kohli A, Suarez MJ, Elliott Miller P. Case report: ocular Lyme borreliosis as a rare presentation of unilateral vision loss. *Brit Med J Case Reports.* 2016. doi:10.1136/bcr-2016-215307.

Pavone P, Bianchini R, Parano E, et al. Anti-brain antibodies in PANDAS versus uncomplicated streptococcal infection. *Pediatric neurol.* Feb 2004;30(2):107–110.

Phillips C, et al. The link between physical activity and cognitive dysfunction in Alzheimer dis-ease. *Physical Ther.* July 2015. doi:10.2522/ptj.20140212. http://ptjournal.apta.org/content/95 /7/1046.

Picha D, Moravcova L, Zdarsky E, Maresova V, Hulinsky V. PCR in Lyme neuroborreliosis: a prospective study. *Acta Neurol Scand.* 2005 Nov;112(5):287–292.

Ramesh G, Didier PJ, England JD, et al. Inflammation in the pathogenesis of Lyme neurobor-reliosis. *The American Journal of Pathology.* 2015;185(5):1344–1360. doi:10.1016/j.ajpath. 2015.01.024.

Ratnasamy N, et al. Central nervous system manifestations of human ehrlichiosis. *Clin Infect Dis.* Aug 1996;23(2);314–319.

Rawlings AW, et al. Diabetes in midlife and cognitive change over 20 years. *Ann Intern Med.* 2014; doi:10.7326/M14–0737.

Richardson J et al. Elevated serum pesticide levels and risk for Alzheimer's disease. *JAMA Neurol.* Published online January 27, 2014. doi:10.1001/jamaneurol.2013.6030.

Schaller JL, Burkland GA, Langhoff PJ. Do bartonella infections cause agitation, panic disorder, and treatment-resistant depression? *Medscape General Med.* Sept 13, 2007;9(3):54.

Schutzer SE, et al. Distinct cerebrospinal fluid proteomes differentiate post-treatment Lyme disease from chronic fatigue syndrome. *PLOS ONE.* 6(2):e17287.

Shi JQ, et al. Anti-TNF-alpha reduces amyloid plaques and tau phosphorylation and induces CD11c-positive dendritic-like cell in the APP/PS1 transgenic mouse brains. *J. Brain Res.* Jan 12, 2011;(1368):239–247.

Shroff G, et al. Safety of human embryonic stem cells in patients with terminal/incurable conditions—a retrospective analysis. *Ann Neurosci.* Jul 2015;22(3).

Singh K, et al. Sulforaphane treatment of autism spectrum disorder (ASD). *Proc Natl Acad Sci USA.* 2014 Oct 28;111(43):15550–5. doi:10.1073/pnas.1416940111. Epub 2014 Oct 13.

Steere AC, Berardi VP, Weeks KE, Logigian EL, Ackermann R. Evaluation of the intrathecal antibody response to Borrelia burgdorferi as a diagnostic test for Lyme neuroborreliosis. *J Infect Dis.* Jun 1990;161(6):1203–1209.

Stuart SA, Robertson JD, Marrion NV, Robinson ES. Chronic pravastatin but not atorvastatin treatment impairs cognitive function in two rodent models of learning and memory. *PLOS ONE.* 2013;8:e75467.

Tobinick E. Inflammatory markers and the risk of Alzheimer disease: the Framingham Study. *Neurology.* Apr 1, 2008;70(14):1222–1223.

Tobnick E. Tumour necrosis factor modulation for treatment of Alzheimer's disease: rationale and current evidence. *CNS Drugs.* Sept 1, 2009;23(9):713–725.

Tselis A, et al. Behavioral consequences of infections of the central nervous system: with emphasis on viral infections. *J Am Acad Psychiatry Law.* 2003;31:289–298.

Wei H, et al. Brain IL-6 elevation causes neuronal circuitry imbalances and mediates autism-like behaviors. *Biochim Biophys Acta.* 2012 Jun;1822(6):831–42. doi:10.1016/j.bbadis.2012.01.011. Epub 2012 Feb 2.

Wells R, et al. Meditation's impact on default mode network and hippocampus in mild cognitive impairment: a pilot study. *Neuroscience* (letters). Nov 27, 2013;556:15–19.

What's in a name? Systemic exertion intolerance disease. (Editorial) *Lancet.* Feb 21, 2015; 385(9969):663.

Witte AV, et al. Effects of resveratrol on memory performance, hippocampal functional connectivity, and glucose metabolism in healthy older adults. *J Neurosci.* June 4, 2014;34(23):7862–7870; doi:10.1523/JNEUROSCI.0385-14.2014.

Xu N, et al. Inflammatory cytokines: potential biomarkers of immunologic dysfunction in autism spectrum disorders. *Mediators of Inflammation,* vol. 2015, Article ID 531518, 2015. doi:10.1155/2015/531518.

Yang L, et al. Brain amyloid imaging—FDA approval of Florbetapir F18 injection. *N Engl J Med.* Sept 6, 2012;367:885–887.

Zhang Y, et al. Identification of novel activity against Borrelia burgdorferi persisters using an FDA approved drug library. *Emerg Microbes Infect.* 2014;3:e49.

Fourteen: Lyme and Sleep Disorders

Ancoli-Israel S, et al. The effect of nocturia on sleep. *Sleep Medicine Reviews.* 2011;15(2):91–97.

Ayas NT, et al. A prospective study of sleep duration and coronary heart disease in women. *Arch Int Med.* 163:205–209.

Cirignotta F, et al. Insomnia: an epidemiological survey. *Clin Neuropharmacol.* 1985;8 (Suppl 1):S49.

Dagan Y, et al. Circadian rhythm sleep disorders: toward a more precise definition and diagnosis. *Chronobiol Int.* Mar 1999;16(2):213–222.

Ensrud KE, et al. Effect of escitalopram on insomnia symptoms and subjective sleep quality in healthy perimenopausal and postmenopausal women with hot flashes: a randomized controlled trial. *Menopause.* Aug 2012;19:848.

Ford ES, et al. Trends in outpatient visits for insomnia, sleep apnea, and prescriptions for sleep medications among U.S. adults: findings from the National Ambulatory Medical Care Survey 1999-2010. *Sleep.* 2014;37(8):1283–1293.

Greenberg HE, et al. Sleep quality in Lyme disease. *Sleep*. Dec 1995;18(10):912–6.

Hardeland R. Antioxidative protection by melatonin: multiplicity of mechanisms from radical detoxification to radical avoidance. *Endocrine*. July 2005;27(2):119–130.

Hatta J. The impact of sleep deprivation caused by nocturia. *BJU Int*. 1999;81(Suppl 1):27–28.

Hoque R, et al. Pharmacologically induced/exacerbated restless legs syndrome, periodic limb movements of sleep, and REM behavior disorder/REM sleep without atonia: literature review, qualitative scoring, and comparative analysis. *J Clin Sleep Med*. Jan 2010;6:79.

Hublin C, et al. 2007. Sleep and mortality: a population-based 22 year follow-up study. *Sleep*. 2007;30:1245–1253.

Huffington Post Healthy Living. Eight ways working the night shift hurts your health. http://www.huffingtonpost/2014/08/14/shift-work-health-risks_n_5672965.

Jensen J, et al. Falls among frail older people in residential care. *Scandinavian J Public Health*. 2002;30(1):54–61.

Joffe H, et al. Evaluation and management of sleep disturbance during the menopause transition. *Semin Reprod Med*. Sept 2010;28:404.

Joffe H, et al. A gonadotropin-releasing hormone agonist model demonstrates that nocturnal hot flashes interrupt objective sleep. *Sleep*. Dec 2013;36:1977.

Kao C-H, Sun L-M, Liang J-A, Chang S-N, Sung F-C, Muo C-H. Relationship of Zolpidem and cancer risk: a Taiwanese population-based cohort study. *Mayo Clinic Proceedings*. 2012;87(5):430–436.

Kobelt G, et al. Productivity, vitality and utility in a group of healthy professionally active individuals with nocturia. *BJU Int*. 2003;1(3):190–195.

Manber R, Armitage R. Sex, steroids, and sleep: a review. *Sleep*. May 1999; 22:540.

Meier-Ewert HK, et al. Effect of sleep loss on C-reactive protein, an inflammatory marker of cardiovascular risk. *J Am Coll Cardiol*. Feb 18, 2004;43(4):678–83.

Moldofsky H. Sleep and the immune system. *Int J Immunopharmacol*. 1995;17:649–654.

Moldofsky H. Sleep, neuroimmune and neuroendocrine functions in fibromyalgia and chronic fatigue syndrome. *Adv Neuroimmunol* 1995;5:39–56.

Moldofsky. Management of sleep disorders in fibromyalgia. *Rheum Dis Clin North Am*. 2002;28:53–65.

Mullington JM, et al. Mediators of inflammation and their interaction with sleep: relevance for chronic fatigue syndrome and related conditions. *Ann NY Acad Sci*. 2001;933:201–210.

Pall ML. Microwave frequency electromagnetic fields (EMFs) produce widespread neuropsychiatric effects including depression. *J. Chem. Neuroanatomy*. Volume 75, Part B, September 2016, Pages 43–51.

Parish JM. Sleep-related problems in common medical conditions. *Chest*. Feb 2009; 135(2):563–572.

Reiter RJ, et al. Free radical-mediated molecular damage. Mechanisms for the protective actions of melatonin in the central nervous system. *Ann NY Acad Sci*. Jun 2001;939:200–215.

Rossini SR, et al. Chronic insomnia in workers poisoned by inorganic mercury: psychological and adaptive aspects. *Arq Neuro-Psiquiatr*, Mar 2000; 58(1):32–38. http://dx.doi.org/10.1590/S0004-282X2000000100005.

Rottach K, et al. Restless legs syndrome as side effect of second generation antidepressant. *J Psychiatric Res*. 2008;43(1):70–75.

Schatzl G, et al. Cross-sectional study of nocturia in both sexes: analysis of a voluntary health screening project. *Urology*. 56(1):71–75.

Spath-Schwalbe E, et al. Sleep disruption alters nocturnal ACTH and cortisol secretory patterns. *Biol Psychiatry*. 1991;29:575–584.

Stamatakis E, Rogers K, Ding D, et al. All-cause mortality effects of replacing sedentary time with physical activity and sleeping using an isotemporal substitution model: a prospective study of 201,129 mid-aged and older adults. *Intl J Behav Nutr Physical Activity.* 2015 Sept 30;12:121. doi:10.1186/s12966-015-0280-7.

Walsh JK, et al. Effects of triazolam on sleep, daytime sleepiness, and morning stiffness in patients with rheumatoid arthritis. *J Rheumatol.* 23:245–252.

Winston AP, Hardwick E, Jaberi N. Neuropsychiatric effects of caffeine. *Adv Psychiatric Treatment.* Oct 11, 2005;11(6):432–439.

Xie L, Kang H, Xu Q, et al. Sleep drives metabolite clearance from the adult brain. *Science.* 2013;342(6156):10.1126/science.1241224. doi:10.1126/science.1241224.

Zee PC, Turek FW. Sleep and health: everywhere and in both directions. *Arch Intern Med.* 2006;166:1686–1688.

Fifteen: Lyme and Autonomic Nervous System Dysfunction/POTS

Garcia-Monoco JC, et al. Experimental immunization with Borrelia burgdorferi induces development of antibodies to gangliosides. *Infection and Immunity.* 1995;63(10):4130–4137.

Jacob G, et al. Hypovolemia in syncope and orthostatic intolerance: role of the renin-angiotensin system. *Am J Med.* 1997;103:1008–1014.

Jordan J, et al. Increased sympathetic activation in idiopathic orthostatic intolerance: role of systemic adrenoreceptor sensitivity. *Hypertension.* 2002;39:173–178.

Karas B, et al. The postural orthostatic tachycardia syndrome: a potentially treatable cause of chronic fatigue, exercise intolerance, and cognitive impairment in adolescents. *PACE.* 2000; 3:344–351.

Raj S. The postural tachycardia syndrome (POTS): pathophysiology, diagnosis and management. *Indian Pacing Electrophysiol J.* Apr–Jun 2006;6(2):84–99.

Rupprecht TA, et al. Autoimmune-mediated polyneuropathy triggered by borrelial infection? *Muscle and Nerve.* 2008;37(6):781–785.

Staud R. Autonomic dysfunction in fibromyalgia syndrome: postural orthostatic tachycardia. *Curr Rheumatol Rep.* Dec 2008;10(6):463–466.

Stewart JM. Microvascular filtration is increased in postural tachycardia syndrome. *Circulation.* Jun 2003;10(107):2816–2822. Epub May 2003.

Streeten DH, et al. Excessive gravitational blood pooling caused by impaired venous tone is the predominant non-cardiac mechanism of orthostatic intolerance. *Clin Sci* (London). 1996;90:277–285.

Tanaka M, et al. Noradrenaline systems in the hypothalamus, amygdala and locus coeruleus are involved in the provocation of anxiety: basic studies. *Euro J Pharmacol.* 2000; 405(1–3):397–406.

Tani H, et al. Splanchnic-mesenteric capacitance bed in the postural tachycardia syndrome (POTS). *Autonomic Neurosci.* 2000;86:107–113.

Thieben M, et al. postural orthostatic tachycardia syndrome: the Mayo Clinic experience. *Mayo Clin Proc.* Mar 2007;82(3):308–313.

U.S. Food and Drug Administration FDA Safety Information and Adverse Event Reporting Program. Safety Labeling Changes: Epogen/Procrit (epoetin alfa) and Aranesp (darbepoetin alfa). *MedWatch.* Aug 8, 2011. http://www.fda.gov/Safety/MedWatch/SafetyInformation /ucm267698.htm.

Vernino S, et al. Autoantibodies to ganglionic AchR's in autoimmune autonomic neuropathies. *N Engl J Med.* 2000;343:847–855.

Younger D, et al. Lyme neuroborreliosis: preliminary results from an urban referral center employing strict CDC criteria for case selection. *Neurology Res Int.* 2010:525206.

Sixteen: Lyme and Allergies

Akin C. Mast cell activation syndromes presenting as anaphylaxis. *Immunol and Allergy Clin North Am.* 2015;35(2):277–285. doi:10.1016/j.iac.2015.01.010.

Andresen AFR. Ulcerative colitis—an allergic phenomenon. *Am J Digestive Dis.* 1942;9:91.

Atherton DJ, et al. A double-blind controlled crossover trial of an antigen-avoidance diet in atopic eczema. *Lancet.* 1978;1:401–403; cited by *Textbook of Natural Medicine,* 3rd ed., vol. 1.

Berg S, Tackling the peanut allergy. *Asthma Magazine.* 2004;9(4):13–15.

Carter CM, et al. Effects of a few food diet in attention deficit disorder. *Arch Dis Child.* 1993;69:564–568.

Chang, K. "Organic Meat and Milk Higher in Healthful Fatty Acids." *New York Times.* 15 Feb 2016.

Crous-Bou M, et al. Mediterranean diet and telomere length in Nurses' Health Study: population-based cohort study. *BMJ.* 2014;349:g6674.

Edwards AM. Food allergic disease. *Clin Exp Allergy.* 1995;25:16–19.

Egger J, et al. Controlled trial of oligoantigenic treatment in the hyperkinetic syndrome. *Lancet.* 1985;1:540–545.

Egger J, et al. Is migraine food allergy? A double-blind controlled trial of oligoantigenic diet treatment. *Lancet.* 1983;2:865–869.

Fagan DL, et al. Monoclonal antibodies to immunoglobulin G4 induce histamine release from human basophils in vitro. *J Allergy Clin Immunol.* 1982;70:399–404.

Fasano A. Zonulin and its regulation of intestinal barrier function: the biological door to inflammation, autoimmunity, and cancer. *Physiol Rev.* Jan 2011;91(1):151–175. doi:10.1152/physrev.00003.2008. PMID 21248165.

Finn DF, Walsh JJ. Twenty-first century mast cell stabilizers. *Br. J. Pharmacol.* 2013;170(1):23–37. doi:10.1111/bph.12138. PMC 3764846. PMID 23441583.

Fleischer DM, et al. Peanut allergy: recurrence and its management. *J Allergy Clin Immunol.* 2004;114(5):1195–1201.

Gibson PR, et al. Evidence-based dietary management of functional gastrointestinal symptoms: the FODMAP approach. *J Gastroenterol Hepatol.* 2010;25(2):252–258. doi:10.1111/j.1440-1746.2009.06149.x. PMID 20136989.

Gunter MJ, Xianhong X, Xiaonan X, Geoffrey C, Kabat GC, Rohan TE, et al. Breast cancer risk in metabolically healthy but overweight postmenopausal women. *Am Assoc Cancer Res.* http://cancerres.aacrjournals.org/content/75/2/270.abstract.

Hipkiss AR. Energy metabolism, altered proteins, sirtuins and ageing: converging mechanisms? *Biogerontology.* Feb 2008;9(1):49–55.

Jang AS, et al. Obesity in aspirin-tolerant and aspirin-intolerant asthmatics. *Respirology.* Nov 2008;13(7):1034–1038.

Ji J, Sundquist J, Sundquist K. Lactose intolerance and risk of lung, breast and ovarian cancers: aetiological clues from a population-based study in Sweden. *British J Cancer.* 2015 Jan 6;112(1):149–52. doi:10.1038/bjc.2014.544. Epub 2014 Oct 14.

Jiang Y, Pan Y, Rhea PR, Tan L, Gagea M, Cohen L, Fischer SM, Yang P. A sucrose-enriched diet promotes tumorigenesis in mammary gland in part through the 12-Lipoxygenase Pathway. *Cancer Research.* 2016 Jan 1;76(1):24–9. doi:10.1158/0008-5472.CAN-14-3432.

Kivity S, et al. Adult-onset food allergy. *Israel Med Assn J.* Jan 2012;14(1):70–72.

Klimberg VS, et al. Oral glutamine accelerates healing of the small intestine and improves outcome after whole abdominal radiation. *Arch Surg.* 1990;125:1040–1045.

Lernera A, et al. Changes in intestinal tight junction permeability associated with industrial food additives explain the rising incidence of autoimmune disease. *Autoimmunity Reviews.* June 2015;14(6):479–489. http://www.sciencedirect.com/science/article/pii/S1568997215000245.

Maintz L, Novak N. Histamine and histamine intolerance. *Am J Clin Nutr.* 2007;85:1185–1196.

Manzel A, et al. Role of "Western diet" in inflammatory autoimmune diseases. *Curr Allergy Asthma Rep.* 2014;14:404.

Milner J, and Dysautonomia International Conference and CME (Washington, DC). Dysautonomia International Research Update: POTS, EDS, MCAS genetics. 2015. http://www .dysautonomiainternational.org/page.php?ID=151.

Morris MC, et al. Association of seafood consumption, brain mercury level, and APOEε4 status with brain neuropathology in older adults. *JAMA.* 2016;315(5):489–497. doi:10.1001/ jama.2015.19451.

Munro J, et al. Food allergy in migraine: study of dietary exclusion and RAST. *Lancet.* 1980;2:1–4.

Paoli A, et al. Beyond weight loss: a review of the therapeutic uses of very-low-carbohydrate (ketogenic) diets. *Eur J Clin Nutr.* 2013;67:789–796.

Pizzorno, Joseph E., and Michael Murray. *Textbook of Natural Medicine,* 3rd ed., vol 1. Melbourne, Australia: Elsevier Ltd., 2006.

Rowe AH, et al. Bronchial asthma due to food allergy alone in 95 patients. *JAMA.* 1959;169:1158.

Ruskin DN, Masino SA. The nervous system and metabolic dysregulation: emerging evidence converges on ketogenic diet therapy. *Frontiers Neurosci.* 2012;6:33.

Russell GW, et al. Biological activities of IgA In Mucosal Immunity, Ogra PL, Mestecky J, Lamm ME, et al., eds. San Diego, CA: Academic Press. 2004:225–240.

Savage J, et al. The natural history of peanut allergy: extending our knowledge beyond childhood. *J Allergy and Clin Immuno.* Sept 2007;120(3):717–719.

Science Daily. Red meat allergies likely result of lone star tick. (Source: Vanderbilt University Medical Center). Feb 20, 2014. http://www.sciencedaily.com/releases/2014/02/140220102727 .htm.

Szczawinska-Poplonyk A. An overlapping syndrome of allergy and immune deficiency in children. *J Allergy.* 2012. http://www.hindawi.com/journals/ja/2012/658279/.

Talkington J, Nickell SP. Borrelia burgdorferi spirochetes induce mast cell activation and cytokine release. McGhee JR, ed. *Infection and Immunity.* 1999;67(3):1107–1115.

Terfel T. Skin manifestations in food allergy. *Allergy.* 2001;56 (Suppl)(67):98–101.

Toledo E, Salas-Salvadó J, Donat-Vargas C, et al. Mediterranean diet and invasive breast cancer risk among women at high cardiovascular risk in the PREDIMED trial: a randomized clinical trial. *JAMA Intern Med.* 2015;175(11):1752–1760.

Walen KA, et al. Paleolithic and Mediterranean diet pattern scores are inversely associated with biomarkers of inflammation and oxidative balance in adults. *J Nutr.* June 1, 2016 vol. 146 no. 6 1217–1226.

Weng Z, et al. Quercetin is more effective than cromolyn in blocking human mast cell cytokine release and inhibits contact dermatitis and photosensitivity in humans. *PLOS ONE.* 2012;7(3):e33805. doi:10.1371/journal.pone.0033805.

Witte A, et al. Long-chain omega-3 fatty acids improve brain function and structure in older adults. *Cereb. Cortex* (2014) 24 (11): 3059–3068. doi:10.1093/cercor/bht163 http://cercor .oxfordjournals.org/content/24/11/3059.long.

Yang Q, Zhang Z, Gregg EW, Flanders W, Merritt R, Hu FB. Added sugar intake and cardiovascular diseases mortality among U.S. adults. *JAMA Intern Med.* 2014;174(4):516–524.

Zhao L-G, et al. Fish consumption and all-cause mortality: a meta-analysis of cohort studies. *Eur Journal Clin Nutr.* 2015;70:155–161. (Feb 2016) | doi:10.1038/ejcn.2015.72.

Seventeen: Lyme and Gastrointestinal Health

Albrecht, J. Roles of neuroactive amino acids in ammonia neurotoxicity. *J Neurosci.* Jan 1998;15:5(2):133–138.

Aschner M, Syversen T, Souza DO, Rocha JBT, Farina M. Involvement of glutamate and reactive oxygen species in methylmercury neurotoxicity. *Brazil J Med Biol Res.* 2007;40:285–291.

Bittner A, et al. Prescript-assist probiotic-prebiotic treatment for irritable bowel syndrome: a methodologically oriented, 2 week, randomized, placebo-controlled, double blind clinical study. *Clin Therapeutics.* 2005 Jun;27(6):755–61.

Brooks M; Movement Disorder Society (MDS). H pylori eradication important in Parkinson's disease. Seventeenth International Congress of Parkinson's Disease and Movement Disorders. June 18, 2013: Abstract LBA-32. Presented June 18, 2013, reported by M Brooks, June 27, 2013. http://emedicine.medscape.com/article/176938-overview.

Brown JP. Role of gut bacterial flora in nutrition and health: a review of recent advances in bacteriological techniques, metabolism, and factors affecting flora composition. *CRC Crit Rev Food Sci Nutr.* 1977;8(3):229–336.

Burton Goldberg Group. *Alternative Medicine: The Definitive Guide.* London: Future Medicine. 1993, p. 589.

Calabro AR, Gazarian DI, Barile FA. Effect of metals on beta-actin and total protein synthesis in cultured human intestinal epithelial cells. *J Pharmacol Toxicol Methods.* 2011;63:47–58.

Castro-Nallar E, et al. Composition, taxonomy and functional diversity of the oropharynx microbiome in individuals with schizophrenia and controls. *Peer J.* 2015;3:e1140. doi:10.7717/peerj.1140.

Chen W, Li D, Paulus B, Wilson I, Chadwick VS. High prevalence of Mycoplasma pneumoniae in intestinal mucosal biopsies from patients with inflammatory bowel disease and controls. *Dig Dis Sci.* 2001;46(11):2529–2535.

Chiang BL, Sheih YH, Wang LH, Liao CK, Gill HS. Enhancing immunity by dietary consumption of a probiotic lactic acid bacterium (Bifidobacterium lactis HN019): optimization and definition of cellular immune responses. *Eur J Clin Nutr.* 2000;54:849–855.

Conway P. "Microbial Ecology of the Human Large Intestine," in *Human Colonic Bacteria: Role in Nutrition, Physiology, and Pathology,* G. Gibson and G. Macfarlane, eds. Boca Raton, FL: CRC Press. 1995, p. 292.

Deguchi R, Nakaminami H, Rimbara E, Noguchi N, Sasatsu M, Suzuki T, et al. Effect of pretreatment with Lactobacillus gasseri OLL2716 on first-line Helicobacter pylori eradication therapy. *J Gastroenterol Hepatol.* May 2012;27(5):888–892. doi:10.1111/j.1440–1746.2011. 06985.x.

Dienst FT Jr. tularemia: a perusal of three hundred thirty nine cases. 1963. *J LA State Med Soc.* 1963;115:114–124.

Dinan TG, et al. Psychobiotics: a novel class of psychotropic. *Biol Psychiatry.* 2013;74:708–709, 720–726.

Domingue GJ Sr, Woody HB. Bacterial persistence and expression of disease. *Clin Microbiol Rev.* 1997;10(2):320–344.

Dunbar K, et al. Association of acute gastroesophageal reflux disease with esophageal histologic changes. *JAMA.* 2016;315(19):2104–2112. doi:10.1001/jama.2016.5657.

Engelhaupt E. *Science News.* 4:38 P.M., June 2014. www.sciencenews.org/blog/gory-details-/here%E2%80%99s-poop-getting-your-gut-microbiome-analyzed.

JE Everhart, ed. The Burden of Digestive Diseases in the United States, Bethesda, MD: National Institute of Diabetes and Digestive and Kidney Diseases, U.S. Dept of Health and Human Services. 2008, NIH publication 09-6433. https://www.niddk.nih.gov/about-niddk/strategic-plans-reports/Pages/burden-digestive-diseases-united-states.aspx.

Federal Food and Drug Administration. Low magnesium levels can be associated with long-term use of proton pump inhibitor drugs (PPIs). Mar 2, 2011. http://www.fda.gov/Drugs/DrugSafety/ucm245011.htm.

Ferran C, et al. Anti-tumor necrosis factor modulates anti-CD3 triggered T cell cytokine gene expression in vivo. *J Clin Invest.* 1994;93:2189–2196.

FODMAP food list: IBS diets. http://www.ibsdiets.org/fodmap-diet/fodmap-food-list/.

Foligne B, Nutten S, Grangette C, Dennin V, Goudercourt D, Poiret S, et al. Correlation between in vitro and in vivo immunomodulatory properties of lactic acid bacteria. *World J Gastroenterol.* Jan 14, 2007;13(2):236–243.

Fried M, et al. Borrelia burgdorferi persists in the gastrointestinal tract of children and adults with Lyme disease. *J Spirochetal and Tick-Borne Dis.* Spring/Summer 2002;9:11–15.

Fried MD, et. al,. Bartonella henselae is associated with heartburn, abdominal pain, skin rash, mesenteric adenitis, gastritis and duodenitis in children and adolescents. http:// www.healthydays .info/bartonella-henselae-is-associated-with-heartburn-abdominal-pain-skin-rash-mesenteric -adenitis-gastritis-and-duodenitis-in-children-and-adolescents.html#sthash.56rh8iyD.dpuf.

Gomm W, et al. Association of proton pump inhibitors with risk of dementia: a pharmacoepidemiological claims data analysis. *JAMA Neurol.* 2016;73(4):410–416. doi:10.1001/jamaneurol.2015.4791.

Gopal PK, Prasad J, Gill HS. Effects of the consumption of Bifidobacterium lactis HN019 (DR10) and galacto-oligosaccharides on the microflora of the gastrointestinal tract in human subjects. *Nutr Res.* 2003;23:1313–1328.

Goto Y, Kurashima Y, Kiyono H. The gut microbiota and inflammatory bowel disease. *Curr Opin Rheumatol.* 2015;27(4):388–396.

Harsharnjit S, Gill HS, Rutherfurd J, Cross ML, Pramod K, Gopal PK. Enhancement of immunity in the elderly by dietary supplementation with the probiotic Bifidobacterium lactis HN0191,2,3. *Am J Clin Nutr.* 2001;74(6):833–839.

Itoh H, Uchida M, Sashihara T, Ji ZS, Li J, Tang Q, et al. S Lactobacillus gasseri OLL2809 is effective especially on the menstrual pain and dysmenorrhea in endometriosis patients: randomized, double-blind, placebo-controlled study. *Cytotechnology.* Mar 2011;63(2):153–1 61. Epub Dec 10, 2010.

Jan RL, Yeh KC, Hsieh MH, Lin YL, Kao HF, Li PH, Chang YS, Wang JY. Lactobacillus gasseri suppresses Th17 pro-inflammatory response and attenuates allergen-induced airway inflammation in a mouse model of allergic asthma. *Br J Nutr.* 2012 Jul 14;108(1):130–9. doi:10.1017/ S0007114511005265.

Ji J, Sundquist J, Sundquist K. Lactose intolerance and risk of lung, breast and ovarian cancers: aetiological clues from a population-based study in Sweden. *British J Cancer.* 2015 Jan 6;112(1):149–52. doi:10.1038/bjc.2014.544. Epub 2014 Oct 14.

Johnson DH, Cunha BA. Atypical pneumonias. Clinical and extrapulmonary features of Chlamydia, Mycoplasma, and Legionella infections. *Postgrad Med.* 1993;93(7):69–72, 75–76, 79–82.

Jumppanen, Sarah Jane, DuPont probiotics reduce risk of respiratory symptoms. http://www .danisco.com/about-dupont/news/news-archive/2013/clinical-study-results-show-dupont -probiotics-reduce-risk-of-respiratory-symptoms-in-healthy-adults/.

Kadooka Y, Sato M, Imaizumi K, Ogawa A, Ikuyama K, Akai Y, et al. Regulation of abdominal adiposity by probiotics (Lactobacillus gasseri SBT2055) in adults with obese tendencies in a randomized controlled trial. *Eur J Clin Nutr.* June 2010;64(6):636–643. Epub Mar 10, 2010.

Kawase M, He F, Kubota A, Harata G, Hiramatsu M. Oral administration of lactobacilli from human intestinal tract protects mice against influenza virus infection (letter). *Appl Microbiol.* Jul 2010;51(1):6–10. Epub Apr 5, 2010.

Kerlin P, Wong L. (1988) Breath hydrogen testing in bacterial overgrowth of the small intestine. *Gastroenterology.* 1988;95(4):982–988.

Kumar H, et al. Gut microbiota as an epigenetic regulator: pilot study based on whole-genome methylation analysis. *mBio.* 2014;5(6):e02113–14. doi:10.1128/mBio.02113-14.

Lawley TD, Clare S, Walker AW, Stares MD, Connor TR, Raisen C, et al. Targeted restoration of the intestinal microbiota with a simple, defined bacteriotherapy resolves relapsing Clostridium difficile disease in mice. *PLOS Pathog.* (2012) 8(10): e1002995. doi:10.1371/journal.ppat.1002995.

Lembo A, Pimentel M, Rao SS, et al. Efficacy and safety of repeat treatment with rifaximin for diarrhea-predominant irritable bowel syndrome (IBS-D): results of the TARGET 3 study. Presented at: American College of Gastroenterology (ACG) 2014 Annual Scientific Meeting; October 17–22 2014; Philadelphia, PA.

Lerner A, et al. Changes in intestinal tight junction permeability associated with industrial food additives explain the rising incidence of autoimmune disease. *Autoimmunity Rev.* Jun 2015;14(6):479–489. http://dx.doi.org/10.1016/j.autrev.2015.01.009.

Lo WK, Chan WW. Proton pump inhibitor use and the risk of small intestinal bacterial overgrowth: a meta-analysis. *Clin Gastroenterol Hepatol.* May 2013;11(5):483–90. doi:10.1016/j.cgh.2012.12.011.

Louie TJ, et al. Fidaxomicin versus vancomycin for Clostridium difficile infection. *NEJM.* Feb 3, 2011;364:5.

Malhotra SL. Faecal urobilinogen levels and pH of stools in population groups with different incidence of cancer of the colon, and their possible role in its aetiology. *J R Soc Med.* 1982;75(9):709–714.

McFarland LV. Meta-analysis of probiotics for the prevention of antibiotic associated diarrhea and the treatment of Clostridium difficile disease. *Am J Gastroenterol.* Apr 2006;101(4):812–822.

Million M, Angelakis E, Paul M, Armougom F, Leibovici L, Raoult D. Comparative meta-analysis of the effect of Lactobacillus species on weight gain in humans and animals. *Microb Pathology.* May 24, 2012; (Epub ahead of print).

Muir JG, Gibson PR. The low FODMAP diet for treatment of irritable bowel syndrome and other gastrointestinal disorders. *Gastroenterology & Hepatology.* 2013;9(7):450–452.

Musso G, et al. Interactions between gut microbiota and host metabolism predisposing to obesity and diabetes. *Annu Rev Med.* 2011;62:361–380.

Na X, et al. Probiotics in Clostridium difficile infection. *J Clin Gastroenterol.* Nov 2011;45(Suppl):S154–S158.

National Institutes of Health, U.S. Dept. of Health and Human Services. Opportunities and Challenges in Digestive Diseases Research: Recommendations of the National Commission on Digestive Diseases. Bethesda, MD: National Institutes of Health. 2009, NIH publication 08–6514. https://www.niddk.nih.gov/about-niddk/strategic-plans-reports/Documents/NCDD%20Research%20Plan/NCDD_04272009_ResearchPlan_CompleteResearchPlan.pdf.

Oprins JC, et al. TNF-alpha potentiates the ion secretion induced by muscarinic receptor activation in HT29cl. 19A cells. *Am J Physiol Cell Physiol.* 2000;278:C463–C472.

Ouwehand AC, Salminen S. In vitro adhesion assays for probiotics and their in vivo relevance: a review. *Microbial Ecol Health and Dis.* 2003;15:175–184.

Pimentel M, et al. Eradication of small intestinal bacterial overgrowth reduces symptoms of irritable bowel syndrome. *Am J Gastroenterol.* 2000;95:3503–3506.

Reisinger E, et al. Diarrhea caused by primarily non-gastrointestinal infections. *Nat Clin Pract Gastroenerol Hepatol.* 2005;2(5): 216–222.

Ringel Y, Ringel-Kulka T, Maier D, et al. Clinical trial: probiotic bacteria Lactobacillus acidophilus NCFM and Bifidobacterium lactis Bi-07 versus placebo for the symptoms of bloating in patients with functional bowel disorders—a double-blind study. *J Clin Gastroenterol.* 2011; 45(6): 518–525.

Roediger WE. Intestinal mycoplasma in Crohn's disease. *Novartis Found Symp.* 2004;263: 85–98.

Roediger WE, Macfarlane GT. A role for intestinal mycoplasmas in the aetiology of Crohn's disease? *J Appl Microbiol*. 2002;92(3):377–381.

Rumah KR, Linden J, Fischetti VA, Vartanian T (2013) Isolation of clostridium perfringens Type B in an individual at first clinical presentation of multiple sclerosis provides clues for environmental triggers of the disease. *PLOS ONE*. 2013;8(10):e76359.

Saavedra JM, et al. Human studies with probiotics and prebiotics: clinical indications. *Br J Nutri*. 2002;87(Suppl 2):S241–S246.

Sampo Lahtinn, et al. *Lactic Acid Bacteria, Microbiological and Functional Aspects,* 4th ed. Boca Raton, FL: CRC Press, 2011.

Saulnier DMA, et al. Mechanisms of probiosis and prebiosis: considerations for enhanced functional foods. *Curr Opin Biotechnol*. Apr 2009;20(2):135–141.

Shah NH, LePendu P, Bauer-Mehren A, Ghebremariam YT, Iyer SV, Marcus J, et al. Proton pump inhibitor usage and the risk of myocardial infarction in the general population. *PLOS ONE*. 2015;10(6):e0124653. doi:10.1371/journal.pone.0124653.

Smith JP, et al. Low-dose naltrexone therapy improves active Crohn's disease. *Am J Gastroenterol*. 2007 Apr;102(4):820–8. Epub 2007 Jan 11.

Staudacher HM, et al. Mechanisms and efficacy of dietary FODMAP restriction in IBS (review). *Nat Rev Gastroenterol Hepatol*. Apr 2014;11(4): 256–266. doi:10.1038/nrgastro.2013.259. PMID 24445613.

Tang M, Ponsonby A, Orsini F, Tey D, Robinson M, Su E. Administration of a probiotic with peanut oral immunotherapy: a randomized trial. *J Allergy and Clin Immunol*. 2015.

Tillisch K, et al. Consumption of fermented milk product with probiotic modulates brain activity. *Gastroenterology*. Jun 2013;144(7):1394–1401.e.

Tillisch K, Rex DK, et al. Probiotics may alter brain activity involving emotional regulation. *Gastroenterology*. Jun 2013:61.

Van de Wetering MD, et al. Severity of enterocolitis is predicted by IL-8 in pediatric oncology patients. 2004. *Eur J Cancer*. 2004;40:571–578.

Vojdani A., Perlmutter D. Differentiation between celiac disease, nonceliac gluten sensitivity, and their overlapping with Crohn's disease: a case series. *Case Reports Immunol*. 2013:248482.

Vrieze A, et al. Transfer of intestinal microbiota from lean donors increases insulin sensitivity in individuals with metabolic syndrome. *Gastroenterology* 143, 913–916(2012).

Waller PA, Gopal PK, Leyer GJ, Ouwehand AC, Reifer C, Stewart ME, Miller LE. Dose-response effect of Bifidobacterium lactis HN019 on whole gut transit time and functional gastrointestinal symptoms in adults. *Scand J Gastroenterol*. 2011;46:1057–1064.

Weiss G, Christensen HR, Zeuthen LH, Vogensen FK, Jakobsen M, Frøkiær H. Lactobacilli and bifidobacteria induce differential interferon-β profiles in dendritic cells. *Cytokine*. Nov 2011;56(2):520–530.

West NP, Horn PL, Pyne DB, Gebski VJ, Lahtinen SJ, Fricker PA, et al. Supplementation for respiratory and gastrointestinal illness symptoms in healthy physically active individuals. *Clin Nutr*. 2014;33(4):581–587.

Zaidi SA, et al. Gastrointestinal and hepatic manifestations of tick-borne diseases in the United States. *Clin Infect Dis*. 34:1206–1212.

Zamakhchari M, et al. Gluten degradation by Rothia bacteria. *PLOS ONE*. 2011;6(9):e24455.

Zaura E, et al. Same exposure but two radically different responses to antibiotics: resilience of the salivary microbiome versus long-term microbial shifts in feces. *mBio*. 2015;6(6):e01693-15. doi:10.1128/mBio.01693-15.

Zeneng W., et al. Non-lethal inhibition of gut microbial trimethylamine production for the treatment of atherosclerosis. *Cell*. 2015;163(7):1585. doi:10.1016/j.cell.2015.11.055.

Zimmer C. Tending the body's microbial garden. *New York Times,* Jun 18, 2012.

Eighteen: Lyme and Liver Dysfunction

Cecil Textbook of Medicine, 17th ed. Wyngaarden James B., Smith, Jr., Lloyd H., eds. Philadelphia: W. B. Saunders. 1985.

Chowdri HR, et al. Borrelia miyamotoi infection presenting as human granulocytic anaplasmosis: a case report. *Ann Intern Med.* July 2, 2013;159(1).

Hashizume H, et al. Primary liver cancers with nonalcoholic steatohepatitis. *Eur J Gastroenterol Hepatol.* 2007;19:827–834.

Horowitz HW, et al. Liver function in early Lyme disease. *Hepatology.* Jun 1996;23 (6):1412–1417.

Mizejewski G. Levels of alpha-fetoprotein during pregnancy and early infancy in normal and disease states. *Obstet Gynecol Surv.* Dec 2003;58(12):804–826.

Nadelman RB, et al. The clinical spectrum of early Lyme borreliosis in patients with culture confirmed erythema migrans. *Am J Med.* May 1996;100(5):502–508.

Newsweek.com. NASH is the 21st century's looming public health threat. Jan 30, 2016. http://www.newsweek.com/2016/02/12/nash-deadly-liver-disease-obesity-big-pharma-421363.html.

Papadakis M., et al. *Current Medical Diagnosis and Treatment 2013.* New York: McGraw-Hill. 2013, p. 675.

Runyon BA, et al. The spectrum of liver disease in systemic lupus erythematosus. Report of 33 histologically proven cases and review of the literature. *Am J Med.* 1980;69:187–194.

Shedlofsky S. I., et al. "Hepatic dysfunction due to cytokines" in *Cytokines and Inflammation,* Kimball E. S., ed. Boca Raton: CRC Press, 1991, pp. 235–261.

Shimizu Y. Liver in systemic disease. *World J Gastroenterol.* 2008;14(26):4111–4119.

Silverman JF, et al. Liver pathology in morbidly obese patients with and without diabetes. *Am J Gastroenterol.* 1990;85:1349–1355.

Tojo J., et al. Autoimmune hepatitis, accompanied by systemic lupus erythematosus. *Intern Med.* 2004;43:258–262.

Nineteen: Lyme and Pain

Aberer E, et al. Molecular mimicry and Lyme borreliosis: a shared antigenic determinant between Borrelia burgdorferi and human tissue. *Ann Neurol.* Dec 1989;26(6):732–737.

Berkson B, Windham D, Smith J. LDN 2013 Conference. http://www.ldnresearchtrust.org/node/245.

Block ML, Zecca L, Hong JS. Microglia-mediated neurotoxicity: uncovering the molecular mechanisms. *Nature Rev Neurosci.* Jan 2007;8(1):57–69.

Casjens J, et al. Borrelia genomes in the year 2000. *J Mol Microbiol Biotechnol.* 2000;2(4):401–410.

Crous-Bou M, Fung TT, Prescott J, Julin B, Du M, Sun Q, et al. Mediterranean diet and telomere length in Nurses' Health Study: population based cohort study. *BMJ.* 2014;349:g6674.

Das UN. Angiotensin-II behaves as an endogenous pro-inflammatory molecule. *J Assoc Physicians India.* May 2005;53:472–476.

Fraser CM, et al. Genomic sequence of a Lyme disease spirochete, Borrelia burgdorferi. *Nature.* 1997;390:580–586.

Gironi M, et al. A pilot trial of low-dose naltrexone in primary progressive multiple sclerosis. *Multiple Sclerosis.* Sept 2008;14(8):1076–1083.

Horowitz RI, Freeman PR. The use of Dapsone as a novel "persister" drug in the treatment of chronic Lyme disease/post treatment Lyme disease syndrome. *J Clin Exp Dermatol Res.* 2016;7:345. doi:10.4172/2155-9554.1000345.

Rettner R. Women feel pain more intensely than men do. *Scientific American.* Jan 23, 2012.

Lindeberg S, Jönsson T, Granfeldt Y, Borgstrand E, Soffman J, Sjöström K, et al. A palaeolithic diet improves glucose tolerance more than a Mediterranean-like diet in individuals with ischaemic heart disease. *Diabetologia.* 2007 Sept;50(9):1795–807. Epub 2007 Jun 22.

Lomaestro BM, et al. Glutathione in health and disease: pharmacotherapeutic issues. *Annals of Pharmacotherapy.* 1995;29:1263–1273.

Maintz L, Novak N. Histamine and histamine intolerance. *Am J Clin Nutr.* 2007;85:1185–1196.

Mangin M, et al. Inflammation and vitamin D: the infection connection. *Inflamm Res.* 2014;63:803–819.

Marshall RP, et al. Angiotensin II and the fibroproliferative response to acute lung injury. *Am J Physiol Lung Cell Mol Physiol.* 286(1):156–164.

Morris MC, et al. Association of seafood consumption, brain mercury level, and APOEε4 status with brain neuropathology in older adults. *JAMA.* Feb 2, 2016;315(5):489–497. doi:10.1001/jama.2015.19451.

Oh H-M, Chung ME. Botulinum toxin for neuropathic pain: a review of the literature. *Toxins.* 2015;7(8):3127–3154.

Park SH, Araki S, Nakata A, Kim YH, Park JA, Tanigawa T, Yokoyama K, Sato H. Effects of occupational metallic mercury vapour exposure on suppressor-inducer (CD4+CD45RA+) T lymphocytes and CD57+CD16+ natural killer cells. *Int Arch Occup Environ Health.* 2000 Nov;73(8):537–42.

Rodieux F, Piguet V, Berney P, Desmeules J, Besson M. Pharmacogenetics and analgesic effects of antidepressants in chronic pain management. *Personalized Medicine.* 2015;12(2):163–175.

Smith JP, et al. Low-dose naltrexone therapy improves active Crohn's disease. *Am J Gastroenterol.* Apr 2007;102:1–9.

Smith JP, et al. Therapy with the opioid antagonist naltrexone promotes mucosal healing in active Crohn's disease: a randomized placebo-controlled trial. *Digestive Dis Sci.* Mar 8, 2011.

Sommer C, et al. Recent findings on how proinflammatory cytokines cause pain: peripheral mechanisms and inflammatory and neuropathic hyperalgesia. *Neuroscience Letters.* 2004;361: 184–187.

Szczepanski A, Benach JL. Lyme borreliosis: host responses to Borrelia burgdorferi. *Microbiol Rev.* Mar 1991;55(1):21–34.

Trollmo C, et al. Molecular mimicry in Lyme arthritis demonstrated at the single cell level: LFA-1 alpha L is a partial agonist for outer surface protein A-reactive T cells. *J Immunol.* Apr 151, 2001;166(8):5286–5291.

Vojdani A, Perlmutter D. Differentiation between celiac disease, nonceliac gluten sensitivity, and their overlapping with Crohn's disease: a case series. *Case Reports Immunol.* 2013:248482.

Weis JJ, Ma Y, Erdile LF. Biological activities of native and recombinant Borrelia burgdorferi outer surface protein A: dependence on lipid modification. *Infect Immun.* 1994;62 (10):4632.

Whalen KA, McCullough ML, Flanders WD, Hartman TJ, Judd S, Bostick RM. Paleolithic and Mediterranean diet pattern scores are inversely associated with biomarkers of inflammation and oxidative balance in adults. *J Nutr.* Apr–Jun;146(6):1217–26. doi:10.3945/jn.115.224048. Epub 2016 Apr 20.

Twenty: Lyme and Exercise

Alentorn-Geli E, et al. Six weeks of whole-body vibration exercise improves pain and fatigue in women with Fibromyalgia. *J Alternative Complemen Med.* 2008;14(8):975–981.

Black SA. Diabetes, diversity, and disparity: what do we do with the evidence? *Am J Public Health.* 2002;92:543–548.

Booth F, et al. Exercise and gene expression: physiological regulation of the human genome through physical activity. *J Physiol.* 2002;543(2):399–411.

Broman G, Quintana M, Engardt M, Gullstrand L, Jansson E, Kaijser L. Older women's cardiovascular responses to deep-water running. *J Aging and Phys Activ.* 2006;14:29–40.

Cider A, Svealv BG, Tang MS, Schaufelberger M, Andersson B. Immersion in warm water induces improvement in cardiac function in patients with chronic heart failure. *Eur J Heart Fail.* 2006;8(3):308–313.

Folsom AR, Yatsuya H, Nettleton JA, et al., and ARIC Study investigators. Community prevalence of ideal cardiovascular health, by the American Heart Association definition, and relationship with cardiovascular disease incidence. *J Am Coll Cardiol.* 2011;57:1690–1696.

Hu FB, et al. Diet, lifestyle, and the risk of type 2 diabetes in women. *NEJM.* 345: 790–797.

Hu FB, et al. Physical activity and the risk of stroke in women. *JAMA.* 283: 961–967.

Hu FB, et al. Walking compared with vigorous physical activity and the risk of type 2 diabetes in women: a prospective study. *JAMA.* 282:1433–1439.

Janssen I, Carson V, Lee I-M, Katzmarzyk PT, Blair SN. Years of life gained due to leisure-time physical activity in the United States. *Am J Preventive Med.* 2013;44(1):23–29. doi:10.1016/j.amepre.2012.09.056.

Jancin B, Kearney-Strouse J. eds. Heart healthy lifestyles also cut cancer risks. *Internal Medicine News.* February 15, 2012.

Kremer JM, et al. Fish oil fatty acid supplementation in active rheumatoid arthritis. A double blinded, controlled, crossover study. *Ann Intern Med.* 1987;106 (4):497–503.

Lane AM, et al. The effects of exercise on mood changes: the moderating effect of depressed mood. *J Sports Med and Physical Fitness.* 2001;41(4):539–545.

Lotshaw AM, Thompson M, Sadowsky S, Hart MK, Millard MW. Quality of life and physical performance in land- and water-based pulmonary rehabilitation. *J Cardiopulmonary Rehab and Prev.* 2007;27:247–251.

Martinez ME, et al. Leisure time physical activity, body size, and colon cancer in women. Nurses' Health Study Research Group. *J Natl Cancer Institute.* 89:948–955.

Mock V, et al. Exercise manages fatigue during breast cancer treatment: a randomized controlled trial. *Psycho-Oncology.* 2005;14:464–477.

Moser MMC. Treatment for a 14-year-old girl with Lyme disease using therapeutic exercise and gait training. *Phys Ther.* 2011;91:1412–1423.

Naziroglu M, et al. Vitamins C and E treatment combined with exercise modulates oxidative stress markers in blood of patients with fibromyalgia: a controlled clinical pilot study. *Stress.* Nov 2010;13(6):498–505.

Oken B, et al. Randomized controlled trial of yoga and exercise in multiple sclerosis. *Neurology.* 2004; 62:2058–2064.

Ramos JS, Dalleck LC, Tjonna AE, Beetham KS, Coombes JS. The impact of high-intensity interval training versus moderate-intensity continuous training on vascular function: a systematic review and meta-analysis. *Sports Med.* May 2015;45(5):679–692. doi:10.1007/s40279-015-0321-z.

Sedel F, Papeix C, Bellanger A, Touitou V, Lebrun-Frenay C, et al. High doses of biotin in chronic progressive multiple sclerosis: a pilot study. *MS Related Disorders.* 2015;4:159–169.

Tomassini V, et al. Comparison of the effects of acetyl L-carnitine and amantadine for the treatment of fatigue in multiple sclerosis: results of a pilot, randomized, double-blind, crossover trial. *J Neurological Sci.* 204;218(1–2):103–108.

World Health Organization. Global Health Risks: Mortality and Burden of Disease Attributable to Selected Major Risks. Geneva, Switzerland: World Health Org. 2009. http://www.who.int/healthinfo/global_burden_disease/GlobalHealthRisks_report_full.pdf.

Twenty-one: Meditation and the MSIDS Model

Alexander CN, Robinson P, Orme-Johnson DW, Schneider RH, Walton KG. The effects of transcendental meditation compared to other methods of relaxation and meditation in reducing risk factors, morbidity, and mortality. *Homeostasis.* 1994:35:243–263.

Carlson LE, Speca M, Faris P, Patel KD. One year pre- post intervention follow-up of psychological, immune, endocrine and blood pressure outcomes of mindfulness-based stress reduction (MBSR) in breast and prostate cancer outpatients. *Brain, Behavior, and Immunity.* 2007;21:1038–1049.

Carlson LE, Speca M, Patel KD. Goodey. Mindfulness stress reduction in relation to quality of life, mood, symptoms of stress, and immune parameters in breast and prostate cancer outpatients. *Psychosomatic Med.* 2003;5:571–581.

Carrington P, Collins GH, Benson H, et al. The use of meditation-relaxation techniques for the management of stress in a working population. *J Occupational Med.* 1980;22:221–231.

Coe C. L. "All roads lead to psychoneuroimmunology" in *Handbook of Health Psychology and Behavioral Medicine,* M. Suls, K. W. Davidson, R. M. Kaplan, eds. NY: Guilford Press. 2010, 182–199.

Davidson RJ, Kabat-Zinn J, Schuacher J, et al. Alterations in brain and immune function produced by mindfulness meditation. *Psychosomatic Medicine.* 2003;65:564–570.

Davidson RJ, McEwen BS. Social influences on neuroplasticity: stress and interventions to promote well-being. *Nature Neurosci.* 2012;15(5): 689–695.

Foley E, Baillie A, Huxter M, Price M, Sinclair E. Mindfulness-based cognitive therapy for individuals whose lives have been affected by cancer: a randomized controlled trial. *J Consulting and Clin Psych.* 2010;78:72–79.

Fredrickson B, et al. Open hearts build lives: positive emotions, induced through loving-kindness meditation, build consequential personal resources. *J Personality and Social Psych.* 2008;95(5):1045–1062.

Gerbarg PL, Jacob VE, Stevens L, et al. The effect of breathing, movement, and meditation on psychological and physical symptoms and inflammatory biomarkers in inflammatory bowel disease: a randomized controlled trial. *Inflamm Bowel Dis.* Dec 2015;21(12):2886–2896. doi: 10.1097/MIB.0000000000000568.

Goyal M, Singh S, Sibinga EM, Gould NF, Rowland-Seymour A, Sharma R, Berger Z, Sleicher D, Maron DD, Shihab HM, Ranasinghe PD, Linn S, Saha S, Bass EB, Haythornthwaite JA. Meditation programs for psychological stress and well-being: a systematic review and meta-analysis. *JAMA Intern Med.* 2014 Mar;174(3):357–368. doi:10.1001/jamainternmed.2013.13018.

Grossman P, et al. Mindfulness-based stress reduction and health benefits, a meta-analysis. *J Psychosomatic Res.* 2004;57:35–43.

Hölzel BK, Carmody J, Vangel M, et al. Mindfulness practice leads to increases in regional brain gray matter density. *Psychiatry Res.* 2011 Jan 30;191(1):36–43. doi:10.1016/j.pscychresns.2010.08.006. Epub 2010 Nov 10.

Jacobs TL, et al. Intensive meditation training, immune cell telomerase activity, and psychological mediators. *Psychoneuroendocrinology.* 2011;36:664–681.

Karl A, et al. A meta-analysis of structural brain abnormalities in PTSD. *Neurosci Biobehavioral Rev.* 2006;30:1004–1031.

Kiecolt-Glaser G, McGuire JK, Robles TF. Psychoneuroimmunology and psychosomatic medicine: back to the future. *Psychosomatic Med.* 2002;64:15–18.

Miller GE, Chen Z. If it goes up, must it come down? Chronic stress and the hypothalamic-pituitary-adrenocortical axis in humans. *Psyc Bulletin.* 2007;133:25–45.

Robles TF, Kiecolt-Glaser G. Out of balance: a new look at chronic stress, depression, and immunity. *Cur Directions Psych Sci.* 2005;14:111–115.

Segerstrom SC, Miller GE. Psychological stress and the human immune system: a meta-analysis study of 30 years of inquiry. *Psych Bulletin.* 2004;130:601–630.

Wallace RK, Benson, H. The physiology of meditation. *Sci American.* 1972;226: 84–90.

Xiong G, et al. Longevity, regeneration, and optimal health. *Ann Academic Sci.* 2009;1172:63–69.

Index

risk, underestimation of, 3
Ritalin, 289
Robbin, Sidney, 14
Rocephin, 92–93, 111, 388
Rocky Mountain spotted fever (RMSF), 32, 132, 134, 327–328, 341
Rogers, Sherry, 211
Rosen Method Bodywork, 280, 373
rotation diet, 323
round bodies. *See* Cystic forms of *Borrelia burgdorferi*
RST-1 strain of Borrelia, 185, 354

S
Saccharomyces boulardii, 152, 161, 213, 322, 335–336
S-adenosinemethionine (SAMe), 278
salicylates, 320
salivary metabolomics, 271
salt, POTS and, 308
salt and vitamin C protocol, 224
samento, 221–222
Sapi, Eva, 96, 98, 100, 102, 129, 154, 221
sauna treatments, 258
schizophrenia, 265–266
Schutzer, Steven, 272
scleroderma, 174
Scrimenti, Rudolph, 14
secretory IgA, 320
SEID. *See* Systemic exertional intolerance disease
selective serotonin reuptake inhibitors (SSRI), 277, 309, 397
selenium, 243
sensory neuropathy, 263
Septra DS, 152, 386
Seroquel, 291, 293
serotonin, 328
serotonin syndrome, 292–293
serrapeptase, 73–74, 221
severe Impairment Battery, 272
sex hormone-binding globulin (SHBG), 255
sex hormones, 252–257
sexual dysfunction, 54
S-forms. *See* Cystic forms of *Borrelia burgdorferi*
Shadick, Nancy, 29
shift worker syndrome, 288, 289
short-chain fatty acids, 338

SIBO. *See* Small intestinal bacterial overgrowth
sickness syndrome, 168, 182
Sida Acuta, 391
signs of Lyme disease and co-infections, 36–37
silver treatments, 224
single nucleotide polymorphisms (SNP), 185–186
single-photon emission computed tomography (SPECT) scans, 270
sirtuin genes, 233
sleep
 Action Plan for Lyme disease and, 7
 Alzheimer's disease and, 283–284
 assessment of, 289–290
 case study, 297–300
 conditions associated with disorders of, 286–287
 differential diagnosis and, 64
 herbal remedies for, 295–297
 inflammation and, 187–188
 medications for MSIDS, 290–295
 medications interfering with, 288–289
 need for sleep study and, 289–290
 overview of with Lyme disease, 286–288
 testosterone and, 256
 treating disorders of, 398–399
sleep apnea, 288, 289, 290
small intestinal bacterial overgrowth (SIBO), 329–332
smilax, 85, 222
soft ticks, 135
Southern tick associated rash illness (STARI), 121, 138–140
spheroplasts. *See* Cystic forms of *Borrelia burgdorferi*
spinal cord, 262–263
spinal taps. *See* Cerebrospinal fluid analysis
Spirotest, 29
Sporanox, 160
spread of Lyme disease, 2–3, 16
STARI. *See* Southern tick associated rash illness
Steere, Alan, 13, 14–15, 172–173
stem cell therapies, 224
Stephania root, 85, 222
Steve (heavy metals and minerals patient), 189